AF779282

Hippocratic Commentaries in the Greek, Latin, Syriac and Arabic Traditions

Studies in Ancient Medicine

Managing editor

Philip J. van der Eijk (*Humboldt-Universität zu Berlin*)

Editors

Ann Ellis Hanson (*Yale University*)
Brooke Holmes (*Princeton University*)
Orly Lewis (*The Hebrew University of Jerusalem*)
John Scarborough (*University of Wisconsin-Madison*)
Joseph Ziegler (*University of Haifa*)

VOLUME 56

The titles published in this series are listed at *brill.com/sam*

Hippocratic Commentaries in the Greek, Latin, Syriac and Arabic Traditions

Selected Papers from the XVth Colloque Hippocratique, *Manchester*

Edited by

Peter E. Pormann

BRILL

LEIDEN | BOSTON

Library of Congress Cataloging-in-Publication Data

Names: International Hippocrates Colloquium (15th : 2015 : Manchester, England), author. | Pormann, Peter E., editor.
Title: Hippocratic commentaries in the Greek, Latin, Syriac and Arabic traditions : selected papers from the XVth Colloque hippocratique, Manchester / edited by Peter E. Pormann.
Description: Leiden ; Boston : Brill, [2021] | Series: Studies in ancient medicine, 0925-1421 ; volume 56 | Includes bibliographical references and index.
Identifiers: LCCN 2021033303 (print) | LCCN 2021033304 (ebook) | ISBN 9789004470194 (hardback) | ISBN 9789004470200 ebook)
Subjects: LCSH: Hippocrates–Criticism and interpretation–History–Congresses. | Medical literature–History and criticism–Congresses. | Medical literature–Criticism, Textual–Congresses. | Greek literature–Criticism, Textual–Congresses. | Latin literature, Medieval and modern–Criticism, Textual–Congresses. | Syriac literature–Criticism, Textual–Congresses. | Arabic literature–Criticism, Textual–Congresses.
Classification: LCC PA4016.Z5 I58 2015 (print) | LCC PA4016.Z5 (ebook) | DDC 610–dc23
LC record available at https://lccn.loc.gov/2021033303
LC ebook record available at https://lccn.loc.gov/2021033304

Typeface for the Latin, Greek, and Cyrillic scripts: "Brill". See and download: brill.com/brill-typeface.

ISSN 0925-1421
ISBN 978-90-04-47019-4 (hardback)
ISBN 978-90-04-47020-0 (e-book)

Copyright 2021 by Peter E. Pormann. Published by Koninklijke Brill NV, Leiden, The Netherlands.
Koninklijke Brill NV incorporates the imprints Brill, Brill Nijhoff, Brill Hotei, Brill Schöningh, Brill Fink, Brill mentis, Vandenhoeck & Ruprecht, Böhlau Verlag and V&R Unipress.
Koninklijke Brill NV reserves the right to protect this publication against unauthorized use. Requests for re-use and/or translations must be addressed to Koninklijke Brill NV via brill.com or copyright.com.

This book is printed on acid-free paper and produced in a sustainable manner.

Content

List of Figures

Notes on Contributors

Jesús Ángel y Espinós
is Professor of Ancient Greek at the Universidad Complutense de Madrid. He has published extensively on stagecraft in Greek theatre, ancient medicine, syntax, and the reception of the Hippocratic corpus, especially in Renaissance Spain. He is the author of *Comentario sintáctico-estilístico de Epidemias V y VII* (Madrid 2003).

Véronique Boudon-Millot
is Research Director at the Centre National de la Recherche Scientifique (CNRS). Apart from numerous articles and conference proceedings, she has produced two biographies (Galen, 2012; and Marcus Aurelius, 2020) and five critical editions with French translations of works by Galen for the prestigious series *Collection des Universités de France: Exhortation to the Arts* (2000); *My Own Books* and *The Order of My Own Books* (2007); *Avoiding Distress* (2010); *Theriac to Piso* (2016); and *Theriac to Pamphilianos* (2021).

Elizabeth Craik
is Honorary Professor at the University of St Andrews. She has published widely on tragedy, social history and history of medicine in ancient Greece, focussing in particular on Hippocrates and the Hippocratic Corpus. She produced critical editions and translations of four Hippocratic treatises, *Places in Man* (1998); *On Sight* and *On Anatomy* (2006); *On Glands* (2009), and recently published an influential monograph *The 'Hippocratic' Corpus* (2015).

Giulia Ecca
is a researcher at the Università di Roma Sapienza working in the fields of Hippocratic and Galenic studies. Her publications include a critical edition, translation and commentary of the Hippocratic *Precepts* (Wiesbaden 2016) and a volume entitled *Etica medica sulle orme di Ippocrate* (Milano 2018).

Sabrina L.M. Grimaudo
is Associate Professor at the Università degli Studi di Palermo. Her research focuses on Greek medicine, science and philosophy. She edited and translated Galen's *Preservation of Health* Book 1 (Palermo 2012), on which she has also published a separate study *Difendere la salute. Igiene e disciplina del soggetto nel De sanitate tuenda di Galeno* (Naples 2008).

R.J. Hankinson
is Professor of Philosophy and Classics at the University of Texas at Austin. He has published numerous articles on many aspects of ancient philosophy and science; his books include *Cause and Explanation in the Ancient Greek World* (1998); *Galen on Antecedent Causes* (1998); *Simplicius: On Aristotle On the Heavens 1* (2002–2014); and the *Cambridge Companion to Galen* (2008).

Jacques Jouanna
is Emeritus Professor at the University of Paris-Sorbonne and member of the Institut de France (Académie des inscriptions et belles-lettres). He founded the Research Group 'Greek Medicine' in Paris and instituted the *Colloque Hippocratique*. He has received numerous awards for his ground-breaking work, especially in editing Hippocrates (Officier de la Légion d'Honneur; Commandeur de l'Ordre des Palmes académiques; Chevalier des Arts et Lettres). His recent critical editions and translations for the *Collection des Universités de France* include *Prognostic* (with A. Anastassiou and C. Magdelaine; 2013); *Epidemics 1 and 3* (2016); *Hippocratic Problems* (with A. Guardasole; 2017); the *Oath* and other deontological treatises (2018); as well as a general introduction (2020). The second edition of his monumental monograph on Hippocrates (*Hippocrate*; 2017) has also appeared.

Kamran I. Karimullah
is a lecturer in Islamic thought at the University of Manchester. His research interests encompass the history of philosophy (especially logic) and medicine, combining close reading of primary sources with the analysis of multilingual electronic text corpora. He has published widely on these topics in the medieval and modern Arab world, and recent publications include articles on 'The Emergence of Verification (*taḥqīq*) in Islamic Medicine' (2019) and 'Hippocrates Transformed: Crafting a Hippocratic Discourse of Medical Semiotics in English, 1850–1930' (2020).

David Leith
is Senior Lecturer in Classics at the University of Exeter. His research focuses on Graeco-Roman medicine, and especially its interactions with philosophy. He has published on the Hellenistic and Roman medical sects and their theories, especially Herophilus, Erasistratus, Asclepiades and the Methodists, and has edited fragments of medical papyri for The Oxyrhynchus Papyri series. He is currently preparing an edition, with essays and commentary, of the testimonia on Asclepiades of Bithynia. Recent publications include *The Concept of Pneuma after Aristotle* (co-edited with Sean Coughlin and Orly Lewis; Berlin 2020).

Caroline Magdelaine
is vice-dean for the institutional affairs of the Arts and Humanities Faculty at Sorbonne University (Paris), where she teaches Greek language and literature. Her doctoral thesis in three volumes on the Hippocratic *Aphorisms* remains unsurpassed, and she has edited and translated a number of Hippocratic texts, including the *Prognostic* (with A. Anastassiou and J. Jouanna; Paris 2013).

Daniela Manetti
is Professor of Classics at the University of Florence. She has published widely on ancient Greek medicine, including the history of medical exegesis and Greek medical papyri. She is coeditor of the series *Corpus dei Papiri Filosofici*. She produced critical editions of the Hippocratic *Epidemics 6* (with Amneris Roselli; 1982) and the so-called *Anonymous of London, On Medicine* (2011), an introductory treatise on medicine.

Jean-Michel Mouton
is Research Director at the École Pratique des Hautes Études (ÉPHÉ) in Paris. His research focusses on Arabic papyrology and the history of the book, and the archaeology of the medieval Islamic world. He has published many primary sources in Arabic, but also produced a trade publication on *Saladin: Le sultan chevalier* (Paris 2001).

Peter E. Pormann
is Professor of Classics and Graeco-Arabic Studies at the University of Manchester. He focuses on the reception of Greek thought in the medieval and modern Arab world, as well as Greek-Syriac-Arabic translations. Recent publications include *Medicine and Philosophy in the Islamic World* (with Peter Adamson, 2017); *1001 Cures: Contributions in Medicine and Healthcare from Muslim Civilisation* (2017); and the *Cambridge Companion to Hippocrates* (2018).

Tommaso Raiola
is associate professor at the University of Naples L'Orientale. His research focusses on the history of medicine in ancient Greece, the medical sources of Plutarch, and the Renaissance physician and editor of Galen J. B. Rasarius. His publications include a monograph on Galen's autobiography (*Nel tempo di una vita*, Pisa 2015) and a collection of fragments by the Greek physician Sabinus (*Sabini medici eiusque discipulorum fragmenta*, Pisa 2018).

Amneris Roselli
is Professor Emerita of Classics at the University of Naples L'Orientale. She has published widely on ancient Greek medicine, especially Galen and the late antique tradition. She has edited a number of Greek texts, including the Hippocratic *Epidemics 6* (with Daniela Manetti; 1982) and *On the Sacred Disease* (1996); and Aristotle's *On Breath* (1992).

Ralph M. Rosen
is Vartan Gregorian Professor of the Humanities and Professor of Classical Studies at the University of Pennsylvania. He is co-founder of the Penn-Leiden Colloquia on Ancient Values, and has co-edited many volumes for Brill, including *Ancient Concepts of the Hippocratic* (with Lesley Dean-Jones, 2016) and *Aristophanes and Politics* (with Helene P. Foley, 2020). Other publications include *Making Mockery: The Poetics of Ancient Satire* (Oxford 2007) and *Hip Sublime: Beat Writers and the Classical Tradition* (with Sheila Murnaghan, Columbus 2018).

María Teresa Santamaría Hernández
is Professor of Latin Philology at the University of Castilla-La Mancha and director of the Toledo School of Translators. Her research focuses on medieval and early modern Latin medical texts, and especially on translations and compilations of Greek sources. She is particularly interested in the medical humanism of the Iberian Paeninsula, and has edited and translated a number of prominent texts, such as Miguel Servet's *Escritos médicos: apología contra Leonhart Fuchs. Doctrina completa de los jarabes* (Cuenca 2011) and Pedro Jaime Esteve's Latin translation of Nicander's *Theriac* (Cuenca 2018).

Peter N. Singer
is a research fellow at Birkbeck, University of London, and has published widely on topics at the interface of ancient philosophy and medicine, especially in Galen. His research focusses on psychology, the emotions, physiology, health and disease, with further interests in pharmacology and conceptions of time. He has produced a number of ground-breaking scholarly translations of Galen, both for Oxford University Press' World Classics series (*Selected Works*, 1997) and Cambridge University Press' Cambridge Galen Translations series: *Psychological Writings*, 2013; and *Works on Human Nature 1: Mixtures* (with P. van der Eijk), 2018. Other recent publications include *Mental Illness in Ancient Medicine* (co-edited with C. Thumiger), 2018.

Mathias Witt
is a plastic surgeon, jurist, classicist and historian of medicine. He is Associate Professor (Privatdozent) for History, Ethics and Theory of Medicine at the medical faculty of the Ludwig-Maximilian University of Munich. He published a collection of fragments of the lost Hippocratic *Wounds and Missiles* (2009). His edition of the fragments of the surgical manual by Antyllus, a surgeon from second-century AD Alexandria, is forthcoming as well as a critical edition of books 10 and 14 of Aëtius of Amida's *Sixteen Books on Medicine* (with Irene Calà).

Introduction

Peter E. Pormann

Scholars of ancient medicine and philosophy have come to recognise the role commentaries play in the history of ideas in areas as diverse as logic, physics, metaphysics, cosmology, anthropology, and ethics. In the field of philosophy, the last thirty years saw an increased engagement with the philosophical commentaries of late antiquity, which contain fascinating insights and debates and do not conform to the scholastic images which previous scholars have painted of them.[1] During the same period, medical historians have paid increased attention to the commentaries of late antiquity, which often reflect the teaching in the amphitheatres of Alexandria.[2] Likewise, although the importance of Galen's commentaries on the Hippocratic corpus has long been realised, recent scholarship has brought them into much clearer focus, not least because of their importance for the textual history of the various Hippocratic treatises.[3] And again, although it has long been acknowledged that the so-called 'Oriental' tradition played a crucial role in the transmission of Galenic and other commentaries on Hippocrates, it is only recently that this branch of Hippocratic scholarship has been put onto a firmer footing. Take the *Epidemics* as an example: only in the last decade has the Arabic version been studied in depth and published for the first time (although this remains an ongoing effort).[4] The influence of the Greek commentary tradition is also immense, and equally felt in the Latin and Arabic traditions, both East and West, so to speak. For instance, the Hippocratic *Aphorisms* attracted enormous exegetical attention in Latin, Arabic and Hebrew, not just during the medieval period, but also the Renaissance.

The aim of this volume (and the *colloque Hippocratique* on which it is based) is to bring the whole commentary tradition into clearer focus. Galen, to be sure,

1 See Sorabji (2005) for a synthetic overview.

2 See, for instance, the pioneering work by Duffy (1983, 1997) and Westerink (1985–1995); and also Pormann (2010b).

3 See the fundamental study by Manetti and Roselli (1994), but also more recently Flemming (2008); Jouanna (2013) provides an excellent example of what can be done for the Hippocratic text when full account is taken of the indirect tradition.

4 See Pormann (2008, 2012), and Vagelpohl (2014, 2016); Vagelpohl is currently preparing an edition of the Arabic text of Galen's commentary on book 6, but to my knowledge, no current plans exist to edit the Arabic text on book 3, which, nonetheless, is of vital importance; more on this below.

© PETER E. PORMANN, 2021 | DOI:10.1163/9789004470200_002

was a watershed, not least in our understanding of the development of the Greek exegetical tradition on the Hippocratic Corpus. Yet, his fame obscured the many contributions by earlier and contemporaneous commentators. But we also wanted to capture the richness of the subsequent exegetical tradition, and especially the importance of the Syriac and Arabic translations, as well as Renaissance developments. This variety is reflected in the first paper by Elizabeth Craik, which opens the volume with a panoramic reflection about the nature of commenting on works in the Hippocratic Corpus. Some texts in the Hippocratic Corpus attracted more exegetical attention than others, such as the *Aphorisms*, *Prognostic*, and *Epidemics*. The tradition to write commentaries goes back to early Hellenistic times, with Baccheius (c. 270–200 BC) being one of the earliest proponents. Yet we do not know much about Hippocratic commentaries prior to Galen, as he successfully superseded earlier attempts; in many cases, we only know of earlier commentaries through Galen.

Craik also explores the subject groupings that exist in the commentary tradition, where, for instance, surgery emerges as a separate theme. There is also a strong link between philological work and writing commentaries. For instance, those engaged in editing the Hippocratic Corpus in Alexandria also produced commentaries on various works within it. But this link between editorial and exegetical activity is not only present in Alexandria during the Imperial period, but also in Renaissance Italy, as she shows by surveying the commentary activity of editors of Hippocrates such as Asulanus, Cornarius, and Foesius. Another Renaissance scholar, Theodore Zwinger, comments on more theoretical works and illustrates his commentary with tables.

Hippocrates remains an important reference point in medical debates in the seventeenth century. William Harvey, for instance, quotes him repeatedly, including in his famous work on blood circulation (*De motu cordis*, 1628). The German physician active largely in the Low Countries, Anton Deusing (1612–1666), employs Hippocrates to underpin his own arguments about anatomy and physiology.[5] Many others physicians selected certain passages from the Hippocratic Corpus and reinterpreted them in light of their own conviction. In this way, the exegetical process provided renewed relevance to the works that by then are more than two millennia old.

To return to Antiquity: Craik also distinguished between 'commentary' and 'quasi-commentary', for instance in Galen's oeuvre. His *Method of Healing* 3–6 explains Hippocratic doctrine on surgery; in many cases, Galen first writes quasi-commentaries in the form of monographs on certain subjects which then

5 On Deusing, see now the groundbreaking study by Palabıyık (2019).

engage with Hippocratic material quite heavily. And such quasi-commentaries also exist, for instance, in the lecture notes which survive from the early modern period.

One of the pre-Galenic commentators about whom we know relatively little is Asclepiades of Bithynia, who lived in the second century BC and was largely active in Athens and Rome. He adopted an anti-Empiricist viewpoint and stands in contrast to the Alexandrian exegetical tradition. Only a few fragments of his commentaries on the Hippocratic treatises *Surgery*, *Aphorisms* and *Epidemics* 1 survive, and David Leith offers a critical survey of this material in his contribution. He begins with the evidence for Asclepiades' commentary on *Surgery*, for which we have the most evidence, as Galen quotes it repeatedly in his own commentary on this text. Asclepiades' commentary appears to have been a lemmatic commentary, preceded by a discussion of the Hippocratic treatise's title. Asclepiades appears to have been particularly interested in terminology as well as textual problems, and his entries consist of a good deal of analytical paraphrase.

This general picture is confirmed by the only evidence for Asclepiades' commentary on the *Aphorisms* found in Caelius Aurelianus' *On Acute and Chronic Diseases*. There, too, we see him define a technical term, *synánchē*. The newest evidence, however, comes from a recently discovered papyrus fragment. It contains an anonymous commentary on *Epidemics* 1, probably written in the late first century BC, which criticises Asclepiades' ideas. By combining this criticism with Galen's discussion, Leith reconstructs Asclepiades' exegetical approach, showing that he read his own theory of corpuscles (*ónkoi*) and passageways (*póroi*) into the Hippocratic text; and that he refuted the Hippocratic idea of critical days, whilst insisting on the necessity to observe paroxysms closely. Leith concludes by exploring two further pieces of evidence which could suggest that Asclepiades possibly wrote commentaries also on books 3 and 6 of the *Epidemics*, but his findings remain inconclusive.

The next two articles also deal with fragments of earlier commentators, in this case preserved in Galen's *Commentary on Hippocrates' 'Epidemics'*. Yet, the Greek manuscript tradition for this text is particularly poor: Galen wrote commentaries on books 1–3 and 6, but those on book 2 and the last third of book 6 are only extant in Arabic translation.[6] But even where the Greek text is extant, the manuscript tradition is often problematic. That led Ernst Wenkebach, who produced the first critical edition for the *Corpus Medicorum Graecorum*, to consult a German translation of the extant Arabic translation produced by his col-

6 Pormann (2008, 2012).

league Franz Pfaff. Where he perceived differences between the Greek and the Arabic, he often followed this German translation and translated it 'back' into what he thought was Galen's Greek.[7] There are two problems, however, with this procedure. First, Pfaff's German translation as reported in Wenkebach's apparatus is sometimes unreliable; occasionally, he simply misunderstood or misread the Arabic. Second, Wenkebach was a child of the early twentieth century when editors would often intervene in the text and rewrite the Greek in order to make it smoother; they were confident that they could reproduce authentic Greek text not attested in the manuscript tradition. The modern reader can easily be misled by Wenkebach's retroversions as printed in the CMG editions: they suggest a confidence and even certainty about the Greek text that is simply misplaced. For it is virtually impossible to translate back the Arabic target text into the Greek source text. Vagelpohl, the editor of Galen's commentary on book 1, highlights the problematic nature of Wenkebach's and Pfaff's collaboration which led, for instance, to 'additions Wenkebach made on the basis of the Pfaff's translation that could not be confirmed or need to be corrected, or some Arabic passages that may well be based on lost sections of the Greek original'.[8]

When editing Raiola's and Jouanna's contributions, I began to check the Arabic translation of Galen's commentary on *Epidemics* 3, and soon realised that Wenkebach's text was in need of correction on a number of occasions. Sometimes, the text of the Greek manuscripts could stand as a *lectio difficilior*; at other times, additions by Wenkebach were simply wrong, owing to a misunderstanding of the Arabic; at others yet, the Arabic helped fill lacunae. Therefore, I have systematically provided the Arabic translation alongside the Greek source text in these two articles (and elsewhere in this volume).

In his contribution, Raiola introduces us to Sabinus, a commentator of various Hippocratic works, including the *Epidemics*. He lived roughly two generations before Galen and was a very keen Hippocratic. After surveying the sources from which we can extract Sabinus' writings, the most prominent being Galen's extant Hippocratic commentaries, Raiola turns to Sabinus' own words and analyses how Galen portrays his writings. Galen criticises Sabinus for his 'chattiness (*periláLēsis*)', as he often employed flowery expressions that lack precision. Yet Raiola cautions against taking Galen's assessment of Sabinus as an objective opinion. By painstakingly going through quotations in Galen, Raiola reconstructs the sometimes complex arguments that Sabinus makes and that

7 Vagelpohl (2012, 125–130) describes the genesis of Wenkebach's edition and the collaboration between him and Pfaff.

8 Vagelpohl (2014), 47.

appear to have some merit, even if Galen disapproves of them. For instance, Sabinus clearly draws on a wide variety of sources, is interested in aetiology, and pays special attention to the patients' habits, age, and environment. Moreover, his language is often rich in metaphors and recherché expressions, again highlighting the great care that Sabinus took when writing his Hippocratic commentaries.

Jacques Jouanna investigates Galen's commentaries on *Epidemics* 1 and 3. These two Hippocratic books originally formed one continuous work, but in the process of copying, they were later separated by the insertion of what is now book 2. In particular, Jouanna studies Galen's attitude to other commentators as well as his own metadiscourse on his commentary activity. Jouanna's first striking observation is that Galen's attitude when commenting on books 1 and 3 is very different. He hardly ever mentions any previous commentator by name when commenting on book 1 (the exception being Quintus, quoted six times). Yet, when commenting on book 3, Galen names no fewer than fourteen commentators from the third century BC to Galen's own age.

Among the fourteen exegetes whom Galen quotes by name, Sabinus is the most prominent. Jouanna shows that Galen's attitude to his predecessors was largely critical; he inveighs against Sabinus, for instance, on a number of levels, criticising him for not paying close attention to the environment; for drawing false inferences from, and overinterpreting, the text; and for a lack of understanding of Hippocratic diction. Galen even has a whole section on 'inferior commentators' and is particularly concerned with the so-called 'characters (χαρακτῆρες)', signs at the end of the patient records, that have baffled many previous interpreters. Finally, Galen offers also some metadiscourse on his own exegetical activities, reflecting on his methods and justifying his own approach. Therefore, although the Hippocratic *Epidemics* 1 and 3 originally formed a whole, Galen's commentary on them treats them quite differently.

We have already seen the importance of the Arabic evidence for Galen's *Commentary on Hippocrates' 'Epidemics'*, where book 2 and the last third of book 6 are completely lost in Greek, but where the corrupt state of the Greek text for book 3 can also often be improved by taking the Arabic version into consideration. Caroline Magdelaine and Jean-Michel Mouton present here an example of how evidence in Arabic can fill important lacunae in our Greek text. They discovered important textual evidence for a commentary on the Hippocratic *Oath* which was originally written in Greek, and subsequently translated into Arabic and attributed to Galen. According to Galen's own testimony, he never wrote a commentary on the *Oath*, but in the Arabic tradition, Galen is credited with one. Franz Rosenthal had previously collected the quotations from this commentary in later sources, the indirect evidence, so to speak. Magdelaine and Mouton are the first to discover direct evidence for the Arabic translation and, thus, expand our knowledge about this commentary significantly.

The text is preserved in the so-called 'Damascus Papers', discarded material from the medieval period that was found in the Great Mosque of Damascus in the late nineteenth century, and then transferred to Istanbul and studied and photographed in the 1960s by two French scholars; Magdelaine and Mouton rely on these photographs for their study. They briefly argue for an early, possibly ninth-century, date for the manuscript on palaeographical grounds and establish that the text preserved in the 'Damascus Papers' is the same as previously known from the indirect tradition and studied by Rosenthal. The most important part of the extant text comprises ten continuous folios concerned with the ethical part of the *Oath*. Magdelaine and Mouton discuss in detail the topics of abortion and bladder stone surgery mentioned there, editing a number of extracts and establishing parallels with other medical texts, such as Soranus' *Gynaecology*. For instance, the commentary appears to allow therapeutic abortions, even if the *Oath* itself enjoins against 'abortive pessaries'. Magdelaine and Mouton conclude with a discussion of whether Galen was the author of this commentary, and advance arguments both for and against; in the end, this question will have to remain open, at least, for the present.

After this exciting new discovery, the focus moves to the many instances in which Galen comments on Hippocratic treatises in works by him that are not lemmatic commentaries. Singer reflects on these different modes of Hippocratic exegesis in Galen and sets up a number of theoretical dichotomies: a commentary can aim at elucidating the text or the meaning conveyed by it; it can be destined for private use or publication; it can take the form of a lemmatic commentary, going through the text line by line, or be a more systematic exploration of a Hippocratic text. Galen himself discusses these different modes or genres, notably in his 'auto-bibliographic' works, although the lines clearly get blurred in practice when he comments on Hippocrates.

One work that is not a lemmatic commentary but clearly aims at explaining Hippocratic doctrine is Galen's *Elements according to Hippocrates*.[9] In it, Galen refutes some contemporaneous philosophical positions such as monism and atomism, and attributes what Singer calls the 'element-body' theory—that the cosmos is made up of four elements, fire, air, earth, water, which each have two of the four primary qualities, dry and wet, and warm and cold—to Hippocrates. Galen argues, in particular, that this is the underlying theory of *Nature of Man*,

9 De Lacy (1996).

which famously sets out the four-humour theory—that health depends on the mixtures of blood, phlegm, yellow bile and black bile, each of which has two of the four primary qualities. Galen's trick is to blur the lines between the four-humour theory and what Singer calls the 'element-quality' theory, the idea that health depends on the mixture of the primary qualities.

Singer then explores the previous doxographical tradition, on which Galen might have drawn, and notably the famous account of medicine contained in an anonymous treatise preserved in a London papyrus, the so-called *Anonymous of London* or *Anonymus Londiniensis*, which comes from an Aristotelian milieu. Ultimately, however, Singer asks the question of whether we should take Galen's interpretation seriously that *Nature of Man* espouses the element-body theory. Singer's crude answer is no: neither the element-body nor the element-quality theories are in evidence there. And yet, Galen was highly successful in persuading scholars across the centuries of two things: a) that the element-quality theory underlies *Nature of Man*; and b) that the element-body theory, to which he adheres, is the same as the four-humour theory expressed in *Nature of Man*. In other words, Galen achieved two things: to reinterpret Hippocrates according to his own doctrine; and to be seen to be a faithful follower of Hippocrates.

In the next article, *Nature of Man* again figures prominently: Jim Hankinson looks at a concrete example of how Galen dealt with the Hippocratic question: to know which writings in the Corpus can be attributed to the historical Hippocrates; which are by other members of his entourage and reflect, at least, Hippocratic doctrine; and which works or parts of works are spurious or interpolated. In doing so, he focusses on *Nature of Man* and how Galen explained it in his lemmatic commentary on this text.

Nature of Man is a very heterogenous text; Galen usefully divided it into three parts: Part 1, consisting of chapters 1–8; Part 2, consisting of chapters 9–15; and Part 3, consisting of chapters 16–22. For Galen, Part 1 exemplified the essence of true Hippocratic doctrine, of what we nowadays label humoral pathology: health is the balance of the four humours: blood, phlegm, yellow bile, and black bile. They, in turn, each have two of the four primary (or cardinal) qualities (hot or cold, and moist or dry), and are thus linked to the four elements, fire, water, earth, and air. Yet Part 2, for instance, contains some anatomy that is patently wrong for Galen and therefore cannot go back to his hero Hippocrates; rather, he argues that it must have been authored by Polybus, a physician in Hippocrates' circle (and possibly his son-in-law).

Through painstaking analysis of key passages taken from the Corpus and Galen's oeuvre, Hankinson shows how Galen reshapes the Hippocratic text in his own image, in order to lend weight to his own medical theory. In the process,

Galen refutes many of what Hankinson calls his 'commentatorial opponents'—physicians such as Sabinus who also had penned commentaries on Hippocratic works. And, although Galen is certainly *parti pris* in his exegetical efforts, many of his arguments deserve to be taken seriously.

Next, Ralph M. Rosen gives a concrete example for a Galenic text that represents a quasi- or proto-commentary. He investigates one of the most famous Galenic treatises, *The Capacities of the Soul Depend on the Mixtures of the Body*, known through its abridged Latin title *Quod Animi Mores* (further abridged to *QAM*). Galen has often recast Hippocrates in his own image by interpreting his writings to support his own ideas. This procedure is especially apparent in his Hippocratic commentaries, which are lemmatic, that is, Galen first quotes the text to be explained and then offers his own exegesis. In *Capacities of the Soul*, Galen frequently quotes from the Hippocratic treatise *Airs, Waters, Places*, which in its second part contains a long section on how the environment influences a person's character; for instance, the Hippocratic author famously distinguishes between Asian and European character types, linked to climate and environment. At times, Galen's own discussion somewhat resembles a lemmatic commentary, as the quotations from the Hippocratic source follow in quick succession, punctured by Galen's own explanations.

Rosen investigates these quotations and notes that Galen does not really link them to his main topic, namely to explain the causative link that leads from the mixture of a place (the 'external' mixture) to the mixture of the body (the 'internal' mixture) and thence to character traits. Rosen therefore turns to Galen's *Commentary on Hippocrates' 'Airs, Waters, Places'*. Galen himself connects the *Commentary* to his earlier treatise *Capacities of the Soul*, referring the reader back to it in two places, once directly and once indirectly. It is, however, only later that Galen explains this causal link between environment and character, established through food in particular: foodstuffs specific to certain locations create particular humours and thus influence the mixture of the body, which, in turn, determines character traits.

In another book on a specific topic, we find that Galen engaged with Hippocrates as well, namely in *Difficulties in Breathing*. Manetti first considers the date of this work, arguing for 175, and its audience. Galen himself stated that he wrote it for himself, and not for publication, nor even for circulation among his own friends. He was motivated to write it, because although Hippocrates had touched upon the subject in the *Epidemics*, no one has specifically dealt with it; Galen paints himself as completing Hippocrates' work where others have neglected to do so. Although Galen composed the work for himself, he still employed the same exegetical strategies with which we are familiar from his commentaries written for publication.

At the beginning of the second book of *Difficulties in Breathing*, Galen even went so far as to suggest that the book 'is an explanation of what Hippocrates said about the difficulty of breathing'. He paid homage to previous generations of physicians who wrote on this topic, and of course, none more so than Hippocrates. Manetti then painstakingly shows how Galen interpreted various case histories from *Epidemics* 1 and 3, whilst also drawing on other writings of the Hippocratic Corpus, such as *Prognostic*. Galen contrasted Thucydides with Hippocrates in their approach to describing diseases: whereas the former wrote for laypeople, stating many obvious things but omitting technical details, the latter focussed on things that are normally missed by lay people. Therefore, although *Difficulties in Breathing* is generally considered a work on a specific topic, it often resembles a lemmatic commentary: Galen quotes Hippocratic passages, explains obscure words (and even considers conjectures), and constructs a coherent theory of breathing difficulties on the basis on these quotations, as interpreted by him.

The next two papers tackle Galen's exegesis of Hippocratic texts on surgery. Both explore in particular the close relationship between these surgical works and Galen's *Method of Healing*. Although the *Method of Healing* is not a lemmatic commentary, it still aims at explaining Hippocratic texts, with books 3 and 4 dealing with *Ulcers*; books 5 and the first half of 6 with the lost *Deadly Wounds*; and the second half of book six with *Head Wounds*. Witt offers a classification of different types of cranial injuries, ranging from line fractures with or without depressed margins to depressed fractures, so-called 'ping pong' fractures, and various forms of bottomhole fractures. In particular, he argues that Galen's arrangement of these various types of fractures can help us amend the Hippocratic text, in which the order of these fractures has been disturbed. Moreover, he also adduces cases where the juxtaposition of the Hippocratic and Galenic texts can help solve textual problems in the former.

Amneris Roselli, for her part, compares the material in the *Method of Healing* with that contained in Galen's commentaries on the Hippocratic works *Joints* and *Fractures*. She begins by considering a passage from the *Method of Healing*, in which Galen speaks about the relationship between this work and the commentaries on *Fractures*: since Galen explained the topic at length in the commentary, he can just deal with it briefly in the *Method of Healing*. Apart from the Hippocratic *Head Wounds*, *Joints* and *Fractures*, pre-Galenic works on surgery only survive in quotations, the two most prominent sources being Galen and Celsus.

Roselli therefore argues that the commentaries on *Joints* and *Fractures* are of particular importance, and that they share certain characteristics with monographs: Galen uses the Hippocratic text as a springboard to provide a full discussion of the subject. He does not quote the lemmas in full, but rather focusses on those parts that allow him to make his points. Nor is Galen overly concerned here with explaining rare Hippocratic vocabulary or other philological issues; the surgical content takes centre stage. Moreover, Galen goes to great length to show that his explanations of surgical procedures were already adopted by Hippocrates. Galen's intended audience is twofold: those who have not yet mastered anatomy, and potentially lack the experience of seeing the human skeleton themselves; and those who do have this knowledge and have seen human skeletons. He offers something to both. Roselli also shows how the commentary on the first lemma of *Fractures* serves as a preface or introduction to the topic. Galen insists on the fundamental importance of 'extension', of straightening the fractured limb and holding it in place. Finally, Roselli analyses an allusion to the Platonic idea that if you nourish bad souls, they become worse.

Galen operated in an environment of extreme competitiveness, as Jacques Jouanna already demonstrated in his contribution by highlighting his attempt to criticise earlier and contemporaneous interpreters of Hippocrates. Through painstaking philological work, Véronique Boudon-Millot reveals the author of the treatise *Theriac to Piso* to be one of these competitors. *Theriac to Piso* is generally attributed to Galen, but Boudon-Millot has shown elsewhere that Galen cannot be the author.[10] In her contribution, she looks at how Galen and the author of *Theriac to Piso*, whom she calls Pseudo-Galen, offer different interpretations of two Hippocratic passages relating to drugs. The transmission of the first passage, *Epidemics* 2.3.2, is particularly complicated, as it survives in Greek in the direct manuscript tradition and indirectly in a quotation in Pseudo-Galen; and in Arabic in the lemma quoted in Galen's *Commentary on Hippocrates' 'Epidemics'* as well as the anonymous Arabic translation of *Theriac to Piso*. Boudon-Millot shows that Galen and Pseudo-Galen understood the text differently and favoured different variant readings (some of which were known to both). Her second example, *Aphorisms* 4.5, confirms this picture and underlines the main difference in interpretation between the two: whereas Galen took the terms φάρμακα and φαρμακεῖαι narrowly to refer to purging drugs, Pseudo-Galen understood them to denotes drugs in general. In this way, Boudon-Millot reconstructed an exegetical debate that is of relevance not only in its own right, but also because it helps us reconstruct the textual history of the Hippocratic text.

10 Boudon-Millot (2016).

Next, Sabrina Grimaudo investigates a silence in Galen's exegetical activity: with one exception, he never mentions the Hippocratic treatise *Ancient Medicine* anywhere in his extant oeuvre. This is all the more surprising, as in modern Hippocratic scholarship, *Ancient Medicine* is often seen as the text within the Hippocratic Corpus that best aligns with what we know about the historical Hippocrates. Émile Littré placed this text at the beginning of his *Complete Works of Hippocrates*, and it has since gained enormous traction among historians not just of Greek medicine, but also of philosophy.[11] At first glance, it is not difficult to see why Galen would reject *Ancient Medicine*, as this treatise argues against explaining health and disease in terms of the four primary qualities—hot and cold, and dry and wet—that underly the doctrine of the four humours as articulated in the Hippocratic treatise *Nature of Man*.

Grimaudo first discusses the one mention of *Ancient Medicine* that Galen did make, namely that contained in his commentary on *Epidemics* 2, extant only in Arabic translation. She highlights the reasons why Galen doubted the authenticity of *Ancient Medicine* and painstakingly reconstructs other interpreters' arguments how the passage in *Epidemics* 2 could be construed as aligning with ideas expressed in *Ancient Medicine*. Grimaudo also shows that Galen must have been intimately familiar with this treatise, and details instances where his own opinions overlap with it. And yet, despite the shared doctrine between *Ancient Medicine* and other Hippocratic texts such as *Regimen*, on which Galen also wrote a commentary, as well as some of Galen's own views, he passes over it in silence. To be sure, there are some lost Galenic treatises in which he may have said more, but the fact remains: Galen deliberately did not mention *Ancient Medicine* in many contexts where he could easily and justifiably have done so.

With the next contribution, we move from Galen to late antiquity. Giulia Ecca studies a hitherto unedited prologue to a commentary on the Hippocratic *Aphorisms* that survives in two medieval manuscripts; the commentary itself is a mixture of commentaries by Galen and Theophilus. She edits, translates, and comments on this prologue, which can be divided into two parts: the first explains the title 'Aphorisms' and gives a two definitions of what medicine is; and the second explains a number of expressions found in the first aphorism ('Life is short, the Art long, …'). The prologue clearly comes from a Christian milieu, as the pious formulae at the beginning demonstrate. It also has strong links to the late antique Alexandrian tradition, and therefore cannot be older than the sixth century AD. Beyond this, however, it is difficult to establish its

11 1.570–636 L.

date: it may go back to the Alexandrian tradition, as there were quite a few Christian commentators active there; but it could also be a Byzantine compilation.

The material compiled here has parallels in Galen's *Commentary on Hippocrates' 'Aphorisms'*, as well as those by Stephen of Alexandria and Palladius, two late antique Alexandrian commentators. More importantly, however, Ecca shows that there is a lot of affinity with explanations found in the philosophical commentary tradition, notably by two Neoplatonic exegetes called David and Elias, who belonged to the school of Olympiodorus and probably lived in the sixth century. Moreover, there is some overlap with Christian authors such as Gregory of Nazianzus (ca. 329–390) and John of Damascus (fl. early eighth century). This confirms Ecca's suspicion that the prologue belongs to the late antique Alexandrian tradition, where medicine and philosophy were often taught in tandem. Other elements also point in this direction, such as the discussion of the title 'Aphorisms'. The title was one of the eight topics (or 'headings [*kephálaia*]') routinely discussed in introductions to medical and philosophical commentaries.

The Greek commentary tradition on the Hippocratic Corpus had a long afterlife in Syriac and Arabic, and it poses numerous scholarly problems, one of which is the textual history of source and target texts. When dealing with the Hippocratic text, one always needs to distinguish the direct and the indirect tradition, that is, the text of Hippocratic texts as transmitted in manuscripts containing these texts; and the text of lemmas and quotations in commentaries and other exegetical works.[12] In the Arabic tradition, Hippocratic texts, even when transmitted on their own, are generally extracted from the lemmas in the Arabic versions of Galenic commentaries.[13] This would suggest that they form part of the indirect tradition. Whilst this is generally true, there are, however, quite a few cases where the translator also drew on the direct tradition, as Jouanna argued for the *Prognostic*, the subject of the next article by Kamran Karimullah.[14]

We also know that Ḥunayn and his school (or 'workshop') often produced Arabic translations based on a previous Syriac translation that they or others produced. This is again the case for the *Prognostic* according to Ḥunayn's *Epistle* (*Risāla*) on his translations of Galen. Jouanna was the first to attempt to establish the place of the Syriac translation of the *Prognostic* as preserved in Paris,

12 See Jouanna (2018b).
13 Weisser (1989), Pormann (2018b).
14 Jouanna (2013), clxii–clxxvii.

Bibliothèque National de France, MS 6734 fonds arabe (henceforth P7) within the stemma.[15] He argues that this Syriac version was produced by Ḥunayn and that it displays similar characteristics to the Arabic translation in drawing both on the direct and the indirect traditions.

In his contribution, Karimullah sounds a note of caution against this first conclusion. His argument begins with a review of the different versions of the account about how the *Prognostic* was translated into Syriac and Arabic in Ḥunayn's *Epistle*, and then moves on to a number of both textual and stylistic considerations. For the *Prognostic*, he arrives at similar conclusions to those of Taro Mimura and Samuel Barry for the *Aphorisms* (also contained in P7), namely that the exemplars of the Syriac and Arabic translations are independent of each other; and that the scribe of P7 attempted to bring the Arabic version in line with the Syriac text.[16] Importantly, Karimullah (again like Mimura and Barry) argues that Ḥunayn was not the translator of the Syriac version as preserved in P7. Although these conclusions are at odds with those at which Jouanna arrived, this does not detract from the fact that the latter was the first to broach the question of how the Syriac *Prognostic* relates to the overall textual tradition.

With the last two articles we turn to the Renaissance, and, in particular, the medical humanism of the Iberian Peninsula. Both articles also deal with the *Epidemics*. María Teresa Santamaría Hernández explores the only Renaissance commentary specifically devoted to *Epidemics*, book 2, written by the Spanish humanist physician Pedro Jaime Esteve (ca. 1500–1556), who was active in Valencia. She shows that Esteve was guided by the same principles as other Renaissance humanists such as Leonard Fuchs. For instance, Esteve endeavoured to improve the Hippocratic text by offering his own conjectures. Some problems involve sentence division. In some, he relied on Galen's *Commentary on Hippocrates' 'Epidemics'*, book 6, which contains a number of parallel passages. He also criticised other Renaissance Latin translations of this text, notably that of Calvus (1525). In one case, for instance, he misread '*nótos* (south wind)' for '*nôtos* (back)'.

Esteve was not only concerned with improving the text, but also with understanding it in the correct way; he wanted to get to the 'truth of the Hippocratic text', the *Hippocratica ueritas*. According to Esteve, this truth was opposed to the medical 'barbarism' that reigned in many parts of Renaissance medical culture. The latter is characterised, for instance, by corrupt or unclassical Latin

15 Jouanna (2013), clxxxviii–cxcvii.

16 Mimura (2015), Barry (2018), *pace* Overwien (2015).

usage. Some of its exponents are arrogant physicians with little or no regard for their patients. Esteve quotes the case of one individual who would not even take critical days into consideration—although the *Epidemics* clearly shows that it is important to do so. Esteve describes his fight with vivid metaphors: his opponents dive into the dark waters of Styx, whereas he draws pure water from limpid fountains. These opponents are animated by a craving for fame and fortune; they are not just incompetent, but deliberately falsify even the doctrine of their own authorities, chief among them Avicenna. Therefore, Esteve's rhetoric and outlook chime with that of other humanist physicians such as Leonard Fuchs, who virulently inveighed against 'Arab' physicians.

Galen famously only considered books 1–3 and 6 of the *Epidemics* worthy of being commented upon, whilst dismissing books 4, 5 and 7 as spurious. Therefore, it is not difficult to see why Esteve focussed on book 2 (where the Greek text of Galen's commentary is lost and only an Arabic version survives). It was only in 1577 that the Spanish physician Francisco Vallés (1524–1592) produced a commentary on all seven books of the *Epidemics*, and this commentary is the object of the final article by Jesús Ángel y Espinós. Vallés lived under king Philip II and praised the latter's effort to stem the tide of decline in Classical learning, which was partially due to a prohibition to study abroad.

When writing his commentary on the *Epidemics*, Vallés failed to use a number of important sources that would have been available to him in the Escorial library. These include, for instance, an Arabic copy of Galen's commentary on *Epidemics*, book 2 and the last third of book 6, made by the Scottish monk David Colville (c. 1581–1629) at the Escorial; and manuscripts of Greek commentaries from late antiquity. Although Vallés missed some of these opportunities to consult relevant sources, he did draw on others, not least work by other humanists such as Esteve and Leonard Fuchs, as well as other figures from the Iberian peninsula.

This overview shows the richness of the Hippocratic commentary tradition and the importance of considering it in a holistic way. As said above, this was the main aim of the fifteenth *colloque Hippocratique* 'The Hippocratic Corpus and its Commentators: East and West', held in Manchester on 28–30 October 2015. Some papers delivered there are not, however, included here for a variety of reasons. Nathalie Rousseau gave a talk entitled 'Οὐ κυρίως, ἀλλ' ἐκ καταχρήσεως: les méthodes d'analyse du sens des mots dans les commentaires de Galien aux traités hippocratiques', in which she argued that Galen borrowed the technical terms 'κυρίως (properly)' and 'ἐκ καταχρήσεως (through misuse; i.e., improperly)' from the rhetorical tradition and applied them when discussing rare Hippocratic expressions. Stefania Fortuna addressed the delegates on the topic of 'the Medieval Commentaries on the *Hippocratic Law*' and subsequently published her revised paper elsewhere.[17] Robert Alessi broached the fascinating topic of 'Hippocrates' 'Sayings' in Ibn Abī Uṣaybiʿa', in which he analysed the roughly fifty pithy sayings attributed to Hippocrates in a highly influential thirteenth-century bio-bibliographical Arabic history, and compared them to those transmitted in other Arabic gnomologies; many of these saying were extracted from the *Aphorisms* and the *Epidemics*. Finally Rocío Martínez Prieto presented on part of her graduate work on 'Hipócrates como fuente en Libro de Theriaca (1575) de Lorenzo Pérez: interpretación de contenidos y empleo de ediciones y comentarios' and subsequently published it elsewhere.[18]

The *colloque Hippocratique* formed part of a much larger project on the 'Arabic commentaries on the Hippocratic *Aphorisms*', funded by the European Research Council. We used this venue to present our project to the delegates during a double slot. Three Ph.D. students, Samuel Barry, Rosalind Batten, and Elaine van Dalen, briefly talked about the topics of their theses, which have all now been completed.[19] Likewise, the postdocs Taro Mimura, Kamran Karimullah, and Nicola Carpentieri presented work-in-progress.[20] We have also published preliminary editions of all the extant Arabic commentaries on the *Aphorisms*, and our editions are freely available under a permissive creative commons licence; the total edited texts contain well over 1.5 m words and therefore similar in size to Kühn's edition of Galen.[21]

For me personally, one of the highlights of the conference was to discover the new evidence for the Arabic commentary on the Hippocratic *Oath*, presented by Magdelaine and Mouton. Yet, my team and I also had a surprise for the delegates. Previously, scholars had accepted the attribution to Palladius of a commentary on the *Aphorisms* that survives only partially in a privately owned Arabic manuscript.[22] Yet during our weekly reading class when we perused this commentary, made available to us through the kindness of Hinrich Biesterfeldt, who shared his preliminary edition with us,[23] we realised that the Arabic text contains misunderstandings that cannot have occurred in Greek and therefore must be an Arabic work incorporating Greek translated material rather than a Greek commentary translated into Arabic.[24] In other words, the commentary is

17 Fortuna (2018).
18 Martínez Prieto (2017).
19 Barry (2018), Batten (2018), Dalen (2017a, 2017b).
20 See now Carpentieri, Mimura (2017), Mimura (2017a, 2017b), and Karimullah (2017, 2018).
21 For details of our outputs and further research emanating from the project, see Pormann, Karimullah (2017).
22 See Biesterfeldt (2007), who initially discovered this text.
23 See https://doi.org/10.3927/52131856 [accessed 13 March 2020].
24 See Pormann et al. (2017).

not by Palladius and was not originally written in Greek, even if it incorporates a lot of material from late antique Alexandria.

This volume stands in a long tradition of proceedings of *Colloques Hippocratiques* that have been published over the last 46 years.[25] Yet, the overview above already shows that the present volume differs from previous ones in a number of ways. Perhaps the most notable is that all the papers published here are in English. Previous meetings were organised in many different countries by different colleagues and appeared with different publishers. They all brought some of the best Hippocratic scholarship in multilingual form: articles appeared in French, German, Italian, Spanish, as well as English, and the editors did not try to impose linguistic unity. The approach taken here is a different one. The organising committee of the fifteenth *Hippocratic Colloquium*, consisting of Véronique Boudon-Millot, Philip J. van der Eijk, Jacques Jouanna, David Langslow, Amneris Roselli, and me, met on 10 September 2014 and decided that papers could be given in any language during the oral presentations, but that the publication would be in English. This compromise had been suggested by Jacques Jouanna to accommodate my desire to make this volume as accessible as possible, notably to undergraduate students in Manchester and the wider English-speaking world, many of whom do not read languages other than English. Thus the choice of English was motivated by the target audience: we wanted to reach not just the experts, but also students, and interested scholars from other fields who want to get an impression of what is happening in Hippocratic studies. The foremost authority in the field, Jacques Jouanna, only writes in French, but some of his works have thankfully been translated into English (as well as other languages).[26] Therefore, this choice of English is not motivated by linguistic hegemony, but rather accessibility and practicality.

25 Université des sciences humaines de Strasbourg (1975), Joly (1977), Grmek and Robert (1980), Lasserre and Mudry (1983), Baader and Winau (1989), Potter, Maloney and Desautels (1990), López Férez (1992), Wittern and Pellegrin (1996), Garofalo, Lami, Manetti, and Roselli (1999), Thivel and Zucker (2002), van der Eijk (2005b), Horstmanshoff (2010), Jouanna and Zink (2014), and Dean-Jones and Rosen (2015).

26 See Jouanna (2012). (My own preference for reading Jouanna in French does not just stem from the fact that for many years, French was my first foreign language, but also from my attending his lectures on Sophocles' *Ajax* during the academic year of 1990–1991 as an undergraduate in Paris. During one of the lectures, he even asked me about a reading in the Oxford Classical Text edition of Sophocles by Hugh Lloyd-Jones and Nigel Wilson, which had just appeared and which I had brought to class. It was rather an intimidating experience to be singled out like that by the *grand maître*, but I still remember it vividly today.)

Moreover, this volume is intended to be a companion to the recent *Cambridge Companion to Hippocrates* (if you forgive the pun).[27] Both the *Cambridge Companion* and the present volume are, in a way, the result of the ERC project on the Arabic commentaries on the Hippocratic *Aphorisms*. Whereas the *Companion* aims at providing and easy access to the topic of Hippocratic studies, the present volume can serve to illustrate some of the best recent scholarship in this area in an accessible format. It is for this reason that I have worked particularly hard at harmonising the style of the contributions and to make them as accessible as possible. To be sure, some contributions will be more difficult for the novice than others, but collectively, they illustrate the kind of scholarly debates that the Hippocratic Corpus provokes today. In the *Companion*, I provided some guidance about style and references, and its conventions have been followed here, as well.[28]

The Manchester *colloque hippocratique*, and the present volume that arises from it, would not have seen the day, were it not for the help and support of many individuals and institutions. The original idea goes back to Jacques Jouanna, who asked me informally during the 2012 Paris meeting whether I would be willing to host the next; I immediately agreed most enthusiastically and the final panel of the meeting voted to hold its fifteenth iteration in Manchester. I would like to record my gratitude to Monsieur Jouanna and the other members of the *comité scientifique*, as well as the authors who contributed papers here. I know full well that things have taken longer than they should have, and the *Cambridge Companion* (to which many of the present authors also contributed) is only a feeble excuse for the delays. The authors also put up with more editorial interference than is customary in these sorts of publications, and again, I thank them for their forbearance.

When organising the conference and editing this volume, I was also able to draw on the help of the *Aphorisms* project team, not least Dr Michelle Magin, the project administrator, who did so much to make the colloquium not just an intellectual, but also a culinary and social success; the then doctoral students and now Drs Rosalind Batten, Elaine van Dalen, and Samuel Barry; and the postdocs Drs Taro Mimura, Kamran Karimullah, and Nicolà Carpentieri. The University of Manchester, the School of Arts, Languages, and Cultures, and especially the Graduate School all provided an extremely congenial institutional environment, and the last also a wonderful space in which to meet.

27 Pormann (2018).

28 Pormann (2018), xvi–xx.

Finally, none of this work would have been possible without the support of our external funders, first and foremost the European Research Council, but also the British Academy and Leverhulme Trust, who supported this meeting through a small grant, as well as the Maison Française d' Oxford, who facilitated the travel of some of the delegates coming from France.

My gratitude also goes out to my commissioning editor at Brill, Giulia Moriconi, and to the editors of the series *Studies in Ancient Medicine*, who accepted this book for publication (as well as my very first book, Pormann 2004a). Moreover, I would like to record my admiration for the superb work done by my production editor at Tat Zetwerk, Arianne Moerland, who had to overcome significant difficulties when typesetting not only the Latin and Greek, but also Syriac, Arabic and Hebrew. Philip J. van der Eijk, the editor in charge of the present project, went through the whole manuscript with great attention to detail and saved me from many an error. He also served on the organising committee of the Manchester colloquium, and I therefore owe him a special debt of gratitude, which I would like to record here.

In 2018, the *colloque hippocratique* took place in Rome, and in October 2021, it will come to Munich, celebrating nearly fifty years of Hippocratic scholarship. The papers published here and the recent surge of publications on all things Hippocratic, including popular culture,[29] show that the interest in Hippocrates and the works attributed to him continues to grow. We can also discern here a trend to take greater account of the 'Eastern' or 'Oriental' legacy of Hippocrates and the Hippocratic corpus, particularly of the Syriac and Arabic evidence that has only recently begun to come into clearer focus. Likewise the field of studying the exegetical modes employed to elucidate the meaning of the Hippocratic text is now firmly established, although much remains to be done—after all, we still do not have critical editions of most of the Galenic commentaries on Hippocrates, not least that on the *Aphorisms*, perhaps the most influential of them all.[30] Therefore, it can only be hoped that the present volume (as well as the 'companion' *Cambridge Companion to Hippocrates*) will open up new areas of research and stimulate scholars to close many of the gaping holes that still remain in our understanding of the intellectual world that is Hippocrates.

29 See e.g., King (2019).

30 The commentary on book 6 has recently appeared in the Corpus Medicorum Graecorum (Savino 2020a); and those on books 5 and 7 are in preparation.

CHAPTER 1

Reflections on Hippocratic Commentary

Elizabeth Craik

1 Preamble

This short introductory paper, a lightly revised and slightly extended version of that presented at the colloque, has few pretensions.* It ranges very widely but its coverage is uneven in depth. It may, however, serve as an appropriate introduction to the more detailed papers that follow. In the first part of the paper, the rationale of editorial choice is examined, with particular reference to the history of the commentary tradition. In the second part, it is suggested that the distinction between commentary and critique is somewhat artificial and proposed that the new term 'quasi-commentary' may be applied to many works of many periods, not generally classified as commentaries; examples of these are given and, in conclusion, a brief sketch of typology is essayed.

2 Questions of Rationale in the Exegetical Tradition

The writing of commentary involves a series of choices, foremost being choice of works for exegesis, choice of topics for emphasis, and choice of length or detail in exposition. In all of these, prospective readership is an important determinant and authorial self-presentation tends to play some part. The rationale for choice in the writing of commentaries tends to be taken for granted, rather than examined. We are all conditioned by our own place and time. But all of us who have written commentaries are aware of certain reasons for our own choices, even if we seldom declare them.[1]

* I am very grateful to Peter E. Pormann for organising a rich conference programme, to David Langslow for valuable reactions to this paper, and to Mathias Witt (see below with note 19) for generous information about his prior work on Galen's complex approach to commentary.

1 For my part, I remark that I seem to gravitate towards unusual or neglected—and rather difficult—works: I chose Euripides' *Phoenician Women* rather than a more familiar play; then the Hippocratic *Places in Man* in preference to *Ancient Medicine* or the ubiquitous *Oath*, followed by the relatively unknown *Anatomy*, *Vision* and *Glands*. The brevity of these three may have been an attraction (but both *Phoenician Women* and *Places in Man* are unusually long). As to choice of topics for emphasis and choice of length or detail in exposition, my main

© ELIZABETH CRAIK, 2021 | DOI:10.1163/9789004470200_003

In this paper, commentators' choice of work or works is a recurrent concern; the reasons for and the purposes of writing commentaries are closely related questions. The power of a bandwagon effect is a recurrent topic. The situation is paralleled in attitudes to Greek tragedy. Why are there so many modern productions of Sophocles' *Antigone* and Euripides' *Bacchae*? Of course, these plays are perceived as 'good' or 'important' and viewed as having a perennial 'relevance' to the human condition; but they are also plays that have become popular choices, and so, through general familiarity with previous interpretations, have become easier for directors to produce and stage, and for audiences to appreciate.

Among Hippocratic works, *Aphorisms* has had an enduring popularity over the centuries. *Epidemics* too was long elevated and its clinical insights valued; an old popular view held that *Epidemics* represented the practice of Hippocrates' prime and *Aphorisms* the reflections of his old age. The veneration accorded *Aphorisms* continued as late as the nineteenth century.[2] This is due primarily to its perceived value as a teaching aid and pithy *vademecum* but it may be asked why this collection (often somewhat allusive and obscure) is valued to the exclusion of the collection *Coan Prognoses* (generally, by contrast, clear and well-organised). In early printed collections of Hippocratic works, *Aphorisms* was sometimes known as '*Lex* (the law)', somewhat confusingly. Incidentally, we may wonder why the Hippocratic *Oath* is so much valued and the comparable *Law* so little. One more example may be given: there is no obvious reason why *Prorrhetic* 2 was traditionally neglected in comparison with the similar and much-studied *Prognostic*.[3]

Then since Littré's influential favour, putting *On Ancient Medicine* at the beginning of his monumental edition, it has had more than its fair share of commentaries.[4] It is evident that there is an enduring imbalance in the tradition: certain Hippocratic texts have been strongly favoured and others largely, or even completely, neglected. To some extent, this bias stems from the perceived importance of certain aspects of medical theory (such as professional ideals) and practice (such as prognostic skills and therapeutic method) on the

---

interest has been language and expression rather than medical content. There is a place for Hippocratic works in the regular Classics syllabus, and at a conference on commentaries it is appropriate to plead that more commentaries be written to make these texts accessible.

2 *Aphorisms*, designated the 'Sacred Volume', is extensively eulogised in Adams (1849) at 52 and 685–696.

3 There is, however, at least one excellent eighteenth century commentary containing 'annotations, critical and explanatory' on the two works combined: Moffat (1788).

4 Festugière (1948) and Schiefsky (2005) stand out.

part of medical commentators writing for a medical readership; but other reasons can be isolated also in different ages. In the early modern period, after the fundamental anatomical and physiological discoveries and insights of Harvey and Aselli, such Hippocratic works as *On Places in Man*, *On Bones* and *On Glands* seemed to acquire a new relevance and appeal, as they put forward theories of fluid components and action in the body (see further below). In more modern times, with the advent of women's studies as an academic subject, there was a new interest in Hippocratic gynaecology; in this the vast body of material in *On Diseases of Women* was rather selectively quarried, while the short tract *On Diseases of Girls* became disproportionately popular.[5]

Hippocratic commentary began early. Thanks to Galen, we know the names of many of his predecessors in a long exegetical tradition. Among them Baccheius (c. 270–200 BC) can be singled out as an important early figure, an éminence grise in the later tradition. According to Galen, Baccheius, well known for his importance in lexicography, made significant contributions to the commentary tradition also; among his works were commentaries on *Aphorisms* and on *Epidemics* 6. In addition, it appears on Galen's authority that he had a serious interest in anatomy: he disseminated views expressed in public lectures (ἀκροάσεις) on the important topic of the pulse, vessels and heart.[6] This type of publication may reflect a didactic activity broadly similar to that of the great early modern pioneers in anatomical and physiological research: like them, Baccheius was operating in a climate of extraordinary scientific research and discovery.

Erotian's Hippocratic lexicon (dated to the age of Nero through its dedication to the imperial physician Andromachus and so about a century before Galen) sketched a classification of the Hippocratic works. In this, *On Fractures*, followed by *On Joints*, was placed at the head of the group comprising surgical works. These highly technical works had already attracted specialised commentators and have long continued to do so. About 100 BC, or a little later, Apollonius of Citium wrote an outstanding commentary on *On Joints*, illustrated by diagrams. Galen's commentary on *On Joints* was his longest and most full. And in the nineteenth century the Hippocratic surgical works still attracted specialist exegetical interest.[7]

5 See especially King (1998).

6 Galen, *On the Differences of the Pulses*, 8.732 and 749 K.; *Commentary on Hippocrates' 'Epidemics' 6*, 17a.794 K.; *Commentary on Hippocrates' 'Surgery'*, 18b.631 K.; and *Medical Definitions* 19.408 K.

7 On Apollonios see Schöne (1896); Kollesch and Kudlien (1965); for Galen, *Commentary*

Galen has his own peculiar rationale and his subsequent influence is one significant element, justly recognized by its prominence in the programme and proceedings of this conference.[8] Galen, more perhaps than anyone before or after, had an equally strong motivation in philological and philosophical interests on the one hand and medical exigencies on the other. He knew his Plato and Aristotle as well as his Hippocrates and had a deep understanding of Ionic Greek vocabulary and idiom. Galen's aim to elucidate and to clarify Hippocratic texts is undeniably fulfilled and if he hoped for the notice of posterity, he surely succeeded. But as to contemporary readership, though pupils and colleagues are frequently named we may be sceptical over the common *topos* that a commentary was undertaken in response to the request of a 'friend': Galen is ever self-conscious and self-promoting. Also, much of his commentary is vitiated by personal polemic. There is a marked tendency to superimpose his own ideas on Hippocratic texts; thus he favours works that seem to express humoral theories similar to his own and fancifully identifies expressions of supposed teleological slant, in line with his personal interpretation.[9] Galen's own professed purpose in writing is to interpret obscurities in the Hippocratic account, which he finds not imperfect but merely incomplete, and his averred aim is to follow the Hippocratic method. It is typical of Galen's general view of himself as the supreme Hippocratic heir that he frequently asserts rather than argues his point. Although he does cite some passages to substantiate his stance of adherence to the Hippocratic model, on the whole he takes a uniform and monolithic view of 'Hippocrates' and quotes simply to fit his current purpose.[10] Galen's view of a monolithic Hippocrates prevailed. And in the coincidence between views expressed in the commentaries and views appearing elsewhere we can see the same elements of 'quasi-commentary' as those traced below in early modern writers.

The editorial work of Dioscurides and Artemidorus Capito served as a stimulus to the exegetical activity of Galen and many others. In the same way, the publication of Calvus' translation of all the Hippocratic works into Latin (1525) and the Aldine Greek *editio princeps* of Asulanus (1526) gave an immediate impetus to scholar-physicians seeking to interpret and to better the text of these first works. Here we may note that a careful translation can often itself

on Hippocrates' 'On Joints', 18a.300–767 K.; for the nineteenth century Petrequin (1877 and 1878). On the early commentary tradition see Ihm (2002), 262–263.

8 On Galen as commentator see, in general, Smith (1979) and Flemming (2008); on Galen's exegetical method see Curtis (2015).

9 See Craik (2017).

10 E.g., in *Usefulness of the Parts* 3.15 (17.21 K.).

serve as a rudimentary commentary. Calvus' Latin translation is frequently illuminating in its renderings, indicative of the text followed as well as the interpretation intended.

Cornarius (1500–1558) claimed in his edition (1538)—preceded by production of individual works, including *Airs, Waters and Places* and *Winds* as well as *Prognostic* and *Aphorisms*—to have improved on the Aldine; it has been demonstrated that he made changes in part by adopting Galenic readings, in part by consultation of additional manuscripts. Cornarius did not offer a translation with his edition (1538) but later added a Latin translation, for the benefit of Greekless doctors (1546). Cornarius innovated in the use of helpful subdivisions in the text, but the full organisation of the text in numbered sections, greatly facilitating ease of reference, was generally accepted only after the work of van der Linden (1665).

Foesius (1528–1596) in the main reprinted Cornarius' text, though with some independent source material, but suggested many changes in translation: whereas Cornarius' main contribution was textual, Foesius' was primarily exegetical. Foesius' unrivalled knowledge of medical Greek, evident already in *Oeconomia* (1588), pervades his editorial work (1595). There are short notes on each text, but Foesius' main commentary, in the form of long and somewhat prolix notes, is printed at the end of his volumes. This labyrinthine format often challenges the orientation of the reader, in a way not unlike that of today's CUF Budé texts, with notes both on the page and at the end of the volume.

Prior to Foesius, Zwinger (1533–1588) was an important and uniquely fascinating commentator (1579). In the first place, he selected twenty-two works for translation and comment. Then the layout of his commentary is remarkable: there are short, frequently exceptionally perceptive, verbal comments. These notes, however, are presented not sequentially but in a diagrammatic format intended to illumine the structure and argument of each work: the commentary is 'illustrated by diagrams (*tabulis illustrata*)'. Zwinger offered a similar analysis of the ten books of Aristotle's *Nicomachean Ethics* and the method is perhaps more suited to philosophy than to medicine. Zwinger's choice of works displays his interests in theoretical rather than the practical medical content: *Art*; *Ancient Medicine*; *Law*; *Oath*; *Physician*; *Decorum*; *Precepts*; *Flesh*; *Sevens*; *Generation*; *Nature of the Child*; *Seven-Month Child*; *Eight-Month Child*; *Nature of Man*; *Airs, Waters and Places*; *Winds*; *Nutriment*; *Places in Man*; *Glands*; *Regimen in Acute Diseases* 1–3; *Regimen in Acute Diseases* 4 (*On Dreams*); and *Use of Liquids*. Zwinger was following the 'méthode spatiale' pioneered by Pierre de la Ramée (Petrus Ramus, 1515–1572) in which the arts were methodically analysed with use of summaries and headings and above all with diagrammatic arrangement, rather than simply presented in verbal exposition. Zwinger's method illustrates an alliance between mathematical and medical thinkers, not uncommon in other places and at other times; his work was little emulated but much cited.

The prominence of *Aphorisms* in the early commentary tradition was overwhelming: critics vied to provide further interpretations of the text, frequently in conjunction with the commentary on it by Galen, occasionally with reference to the commentary of Oribasius. There was a longstanding and much repeated convention that with the Hippocratic text was printed the commentary of Galen, or very occasionally that of Oribasius: commentary by proxy was so perpetuated in the long-standing practice of echoing in agreement or disagreement the interpretations of one's predecessors.[11]

A few original contributions may be noted also. John Caius (1510–1573, who had been a friend of Vesalius at Padua) essayed a conjectural reconstruction of a putative lost Hippocratic work on anatomy involving the conjunction of several works transmitted separately: *Anatomy*, *Bones*, *Heart* and *Glands*.[12] In the course of his argument, Caius made pertinent remarks on the common content and expression of these works, annotating in full details of the text. Other doctor-scholars too chose to focus on particular works that engaged their interest. A few early editions with vestigial commentary are here noted: Jean de Gorris (1505–1577) *On Generation* and *On the Nature of the Child* (1545); Adrien L'Alemant (1527–1559) *On Winds* (1557); Étienne Gourmelon (1538–1593) *On Nutriment* (1572); all have a marked philosophical bent. A less slight work, and an important corrective to the protracted focus on *Aphorisms*, is an edition of *Coan Prognoses* produced by Jacques Houllier (d. 1562); later, this was republished considerably augmented by admiring followers (1576).

3 Commentary and Quasi-Commentary

Commentary, regarded now as a distinct genre, was not always so, though anachronistically we tend to forget this. Galen used the descriptive term *hypomnḗmata* ('notes') in a wide-ranging way, generally but not always distinct from his use of *syngrámmata* ('connected work', 'treatise'). Paul of Aigina subtly employed exegetical skill in presentation of material, partly straight borrowing more or less verbatim, partly abridgement and only occasionally elaboration; his proem evinces a clear view of his own rationale and achievement. The

11 For Oribasius, see Johannes Winter von Andernach, also known in the Wellcome catalogue and other sources as Johann Guenther, or Guinter von Andernach (1505–1574) in 1533.

12 Caius (1570).

scholarly physicians of the fifteenth and sixteenth century applied a range of terms interchangeably to works we might regard loosely as commentaries. Title pages announce a contribution as *liber commentariis illustratus*, as *commentaria*, as *expositio*; a work is presented *cum interpretatione et commentariis* or *brevi enarratione* and an author is described as *interprete et enarratore*.[13] But certain aspects and characteristics of the commentary could, then as now, be readily identified.

The canonical form of the commentary is sequential and systematic and the format is governed by the use of the lemma, in that words, phrases, sentences or segments are selected and excerpted for comment. The material selected to serve as lemma varies greatly in length and character. In layout, one of two methods is usually followed: entire commentary follows entire text; or sections of commentary follow sections of text. Similarly, where a translation is given, this may be laid out in its entirety or in sections facing or following the relevant sections of text. Although the basic structure is constant, there is much variation in slant and in style as well as in detail. The simple general intent is to clarify the content of the chosen text.

There is, of course, a distinction to be made between a complete commentary, discussing a complete text sequentially, and a partial commentary, discussing only selected passages from a text. In the reception of Hippocratic texts, however, a major part is played by (as I designate them) 'quasi-commentaries'. Certain pervasive features of these 'quasi-commentaries' replicate regular features of complete commentaries: in content, citation of the views of others, often polemical or with obvious parti pris; in form, extensive use of the lemma. It has been demonstrated that material presented by Galen in his *Therapeutic Method* (books 3–6) is replicated, in closely aligned form, in his subsequent commentaries on Hippocratic surgical texts. It has been argued further that the first represents an informal 'synthetic' type of commentary, directed at beginners, and the second a more formal 'lemmatic' type, intended for advanced learners; and thus that Galen employs two 'steps' of commentary, each having a distinct didactic function.[14]

It is, however, in the seventeenth century that the quasi-commentary really flourished. For several decades as physicians wrestled with the new discoveries relating to body fluids—not merely blood and chyle or lymph but all fluids, ranging from nasal mucus and sweat to semen and breast milk—certain pas-

---

13 See for example L'Alemant (1557); Gourmelon (1572); Houillier (1576).

14 See Witt (2012). It may be noted that a somewhat similar approach to aspects of 'synthetic' commentary in Galen's oeuvre appeared in some contributions at the meeting. The term 'quasi-commentary' seems to meet a need.

sages in certain Hippocratic texts, viewed as key, became over and over again the subject of comment. Body fluids, like the various 'humours' of Hippocratic physicians, were central in medical theory. The work of William Harvey (1578–1657) on the circulation of the blood (*de motu cordis et circulatione sanguinis exercitatio*, 1628) and that of Gaspare Aselli (ca. 1581–1626) on the lymphatic vessels (*de lactibus sive lacteis venis dissertatio*, 1627) received a quick response from Jean Pecquet (1622–1674), Jean Riolan the younger (ca. 1577–1657) and others, such as Anton Deusing (1612–1666), all attempting from their knowledge of Hippocratic texts to rebut or corroborate the latest anatomical and physiological advances. These dissertations or monographs on medical topics focus closely and repeatedly on particular Hippocratic passages; Riolan's view was that 'Hippocrates conceived, Harvey discovered and he (Riolan) corrected'. The commentator's practice of commenting on predecessors' comments is pervasive. Similarly, the letters of Walaeus (Jan de Wale, 1604–1649) base their response to these fundamental medical questions on Hippocratic analysis.

And in the medical faculties of every prestigious university, professors gave courses of lectures on medical topics based on Hippocratic doctrine and involving close study of particular texts, especially *Aphorisms* and *Prognostic*. Guerner (Werner) Rolfinck (1599–1673), who at Jena made practical innovations in the teaching of anatomy and by introduction of a botanic garden, wrote a commentary on *Aphorisms* (1662) and in his lectures cited Hippocratic texts with immense erudition. In all these activities there was active ongoing interaction in a relatively small intellectual community operating in an increasingly international world. The activity of Baccheius in Alexandria evinces the same impetus from medical research to philological exegesis, the same combination of pedagogy and publicity.

In conclusion, I return to van der Linden (1609–1664). The complete Hippocratic commentary, published posthumously by his son (1665), is well known. In addition, van der Linden displayed an unrivalled mastery of literature relating to the great anatomical and physiological discoveries of the age, both in terms of the original presentations and of subsequent reactions to them. He published magisterial collections of the most seminal papers, notably in a beautiful volume published by Blaeu in Amsterdam (1645). Further, he produced a wide-ranging work of his own on physiology, replete with Hippocratic citation and, tellingly, with appropriate Hippocratic quotation as the starting point of each successive chapter (1653). In all his publications, there was a strong focus on detailed exegesis of Hippocratic texts. There is the same wrestling with philological detail in passages excerpted from texts; the same citation or discussion of, and polemic against, earlier views (frequently those of Zwinger), all in a style close to that of commentary.

Towards the end of his life came an important series of *exercitationes*, professedly the work of students but effectively reflections of the master's doctrine and each concluding with a summation replete with reflections on significant questions: *27 Hippocratic exercises about blood circulation* (*Hippocratis de circuitu sanguinis exercitationes XXVII*) (1659 etc.). The format was a presentation by a named author followed by the master's response; the fourteenth *exercitatio* is the work of one Lucas Walckier.[15] The series was recognised as a standard authority by the immensely erudite doctor-philologist D.W. Triller (1695–1782) in the magisterial *Opuscula medica* (1766–1772).

Finally, I mention *Discussion and Advice on Menstrual Migraine* (*de hemicrania menstrua historia et consilium*) (1660, 2nd ed. 1668), a short piece dedicated to the *serenissima princeps* Sophia Margaretha of Brandenburg-Solms (1634–1664): an attempt to explain and advise on menstrual headaches affecting sometimes the left sometimes the right side of the head. The *serenissima princeps* was married at the age of eighteen to Albrecht von Brandenburg-Ausbach; she died at the age of twenty-nine, having in the intervening years had five children. Perhaps it is surprising that she was free from pregnancy for long enough to notice menstrual problems. As a dissertation on an aspect of period pain the work is useless; as a collection and exegesis of Hippocratic passages on the character and action of the blood it is remarkably full and authoritative: the quasi-commentary at its best.

4 Typology

Quasi-commentaries take various forms, most common being dissertations, letters and lectures: monographs with a learned agenda, correspondence notionally personal but in truth open and intended for publication, and sequences of pedagogic instruction for learners. Like Socrates' companions, we may have described characteristics rather than reached a definition of the quasi-commentary. But there is no doubt that an open minded examination of the rich tradition will reveal many further examples.

15 The fourteenth *exercitatio* is the only one I have traced (University Library, Leiden).

CHAPTER 2

Asclepiades of Bithynia as Hippocratic Commentator

David Leith

Asclepiades of Bithynia is probably one of the least well known Hellenistic commentators on the Hippocratic Corpus. He is more readily recognised as a leading figure in the transference of Greek medicine to Rome, as an important Rationalist precursor of Methodism, as a vociferous critic of the Empiricists, or as a proponent of a perplexing corpuscular theory of matter. Indeed, he is often seen as *anti*-Hippocratic, an impression that is certainly encouraged by Galen's extensive polemics. His in-depth and sustained engagement with the Hippocratic Corpus has accordingly not received much attention, though it evidently represented a significant part of his output. Undoubtedly, too, this relative lack of attention is due partly to the very poor nature of the surviving evidence, even when compared with that for other Hellenistic commentators, who have hardly fared well.[1] Another possible reason is that he stands somewhat apart from the Alexandrian tradition of Hippocratic exegesis. The glossaries and commentaries that seem to have been produced primarily by members of the Herophilean and Empiricist medical sects belonged to the finest tradition of Hellenistic scholarship, but it remains very difficult to find a place for Asclepiades in relation to this. Living in the later second and early first century BC, Asclepiades' medical career began in the area of the Hellespont, moving on to Athens and ending of course in Rome, but there is no evidence, and no good reason to believe, that he ever went to Alexandria. Yet he was certainly closely familiar with, and critical of, the writings of Erasistratus, and his disputes with the Empiricists reveal to some extent the medical authorities he felt he needed to overcome.

Our sources explicitly refer to only three commentaries by Asclepiades, on the treatises *Surgery*, *Aphorisms* and *Epidemics* 1 respectively.[2] In this paper, I shall go through the meagre reports on the three attested Asclepiadean commentaries, with a view to forming a basic picture of their nature and aims. I

1 See especially von Staden (2006).

2 For the first two commentaries, see Vallance (1993), 709; Ihm (2002), 72–73. The evidence for the *Epidemics* 1 commentary has appeared since; see below.

© DAVID LEITH, 2021 | DOI:10.1163/9789004470200_004

shall consider what kinds of exegesis he engaged in, what his particular concerns and purposes might have been, what picture he had of the figure of Hippocrates, as well as how he stood within the Hellenistic commentary tradition more broadly. The limited nature of the evidence naturally permits only very provisional and impressionistic answers to these questions, but there is room for at least some speculation.

Before looking at the testimonia on individual commentaries, it is worth considering a report on the overall scope of Asclepiades' exegetical project on the Hippocratic Corpus. An offhand remark made by Galen refers in general terms to the extent of Asclepiades' coverage, when compared with other Hellenistic exegetes. In his own *Commentary on Hippocrates' 'Surgery'*, Galen lists four older commentators on this particular treatise, but comments also on their wider output. These four are the early Herophilean Baccheius of Tanagra, the Empiricists Zeuxis and Heraclides of Tarentum, and finally Asclepiades, which places him in distinguished company.[3] Unfortunately, however, the passage is corrupt where Asclepiades is mentioned. The sole authoritative witness to the text is the manuscript P, which reads as follows:[4]

> τέτταρες δέ εἰσιν αὐτῶν, δύο μὲν εἰς ἅπαντα Ἱπποκράτους βιβλία γεγραφότες ὑπομνήματα Ζεῦξίς τε καὶ Ἡρακλείδης, οὐκ εἰς πάντα δὲ Βακχεῖος Ἀσκληπιάδης †δισσολόγιστα†.
>
> There are four of these (previous interpreters): two, Zeuxis and Heraclides, who wrote commentaries on all of Hippocrates' writings; and Baccheius Asclepiades, (who wrote commentaries) not on all †...†.

The asyndeton in P between the names Baccheius and Asclepiades is awkward, and the Aldine prints καὶ here to join them, but keeps the corrupt δισσολόγιστα. Chartier's edition, on which Kühn's text is based, also has καὶ linking the names, but offers the more meaningful adjective δυσλόγιστα at the end of the sentence. Nonetheless, it remains difficult to construe this with the rest of the sentence, though in the Latin translation in Chartier's edition, a conjunction was added

3 For Baccheius, see von Staden (1989), 484–500; for Zeuxis, ibid. 481–482, with Deichgräber (1965), 209; for Heraclides, Deichgräber (1965), 172–202, and Guardasole (1997).

4 Galen, *Commentary on Hippocrates' 'Surgery'*, preface (18b.631–632 K.), here according to Paris, Bibliothèque nationale de France, MS 1849 fonds grec, fol. 175^{v}, lines 27–29 (http://gallica.bnf.fr/ark:/12148/btv1b10721651b/f358.item.zoom [accessed 13 November 2018]). I am very grateful to Ivan Garofalo for sharing with me his provisional edition of the relevant passage.

to give sense: '... at non in omnes, sed obscuros Baccheius, et Asclepiades (... but Baccheius and Asclepiades did not (write commentaries) on all, but (only) the obscure ones)'.[5] Ivan Garofalo, however, has suggested an emendation that seems much more satisfying, being palaeographically closer to P's reading, and avoiding the asyndeton problem without positing an omission. In place of δισσολόγιστα, he proposes δ' εἰς ὀλίγιστα, to give the following:

> τέτταρες δέ εἰσιν αὐτῶν, δύο μὲν εἰς ἅπαντα Ἱπποκράτους βιβλία γεγραφότες ὑπομνήματα Ζεῦξίς τε καὶ Ἡρακλείδης, οὐκ εἰς πάντα δὲ Βακχεῖος, Ἀσκληπιάδης δ' εἰς ὀλίγιστα.
>
> There are four of these (previous interpreters): two, Zeuxis and Heraclides, who wrote commentaries on all of Hippocrates' writings; Baccheius, (who wrote commentaries) not on all; and Asclepiades, (who wrote commentaries) on very few.

Galen would thus be listing the Hellenistic commentators in descending order of the number of Hippocratic commentaries they composed.[6] The emended text would indicate that Asclepiades was regarded as among the most important of the older commentators on *Surgery*, but that his coverage in regard to the rest of the Hippocratic Corpus was very limited, and he made no attempt at comprehensiveness.

The 'very few' commentaries that Galen seems to have referred to here could easily have included more than the three for which we have direct evidence, and we need not assume that our surviving evidence is representative of his output; indeed, the evidence for his commentary on *Epidemics* 1 has surfaced only very recently from a papyrological source.[7] Nor need we assume that Galen was familiar with all of Asclepiades' Hippocratic commentaries. He never mentions, for instance, the commentaries on *Aphorisms* or *Epidemics* 1, only ever referring to that on *Surgery*, which he does in the context of his own commentary on that work.[8] It is also worth noting in this context that there is a

5 Similarly, von Staden (2006), pp. 17–18, note 12, very tentatively suggests the addition of ⟨ἀλλὰ τὰ⟩ to the Greek before δυσλόγιστα in Kühn's text.

6 On the question of what Galen might have meant by 'all of Hippocrates' writings', see von Staden (2009), 153–155.

7 For Zeuxis, for example, said by Galen to have commented on 'all' Hippocratic treatises, we have evidence for commentaries on only seven (including *Surgery*): see von Staden (2006), 30–40.

8 Galen's failure to mention Asclepiades' commentaries on *Aphorisms* and *Epidemics* 1 is not in itself surprising, given his tendency to mention by name few, if any, earlier exegetes

striking coincidence between Asclepiades' known commentaries and those of Baccheius the Herophilean, with whom Asclepiades is here closely associated.[9] The only three commentaries that we know Baccheius composed are almost identical to the attested Asclepiadean commentaries: similarly *Surgery* and *Aphorisms*, but *Epidemics* 6 instead of *Epidemics* 1. It is tempting to wonder whether these treatises in particular (taking *Epidemics* 1–7 as a single group) were among the most popular subjects of Hellenistic Hippocratic exegesis.

1 *Surgery*

Despite his reference in the above passage to a plurality of Asclepiadean commentaries, as noted above Galen only ever mentions by name the *Commentary on Hippocrates' 'Surgery'*, which he claims he used as a source for his own commentary on this work, along with those of the other Hellenistic exegetes. It had not generally been Galen's practice to consult such older commentaries. His purpose in doing so in this particular context was to discover ancient readings predating the more recent copies of Hippocratic works, in particular those deriving from the editions by Artemidorus Capito and Dioscorides, that had imported into the text a range of bold conjectures.[10] Thanks to his reports, together with a single testimony from Erotian, Asclepiades' *Commentary on Hippocrates' 'Surgery'* is the one for which we have most evidence.

Galen discusses Asclepiades' comments explicitly in a further four passages within his commentary proper. From these, we know that Asclepiades gave his views on the correct form of the Hippocratic work's title, along with analysis of what exactly it was intended to refer to.[11] He also discussed variant readings in two short passages from *Surgery* 4 and 11. In the first, Galen himself admits

in his own commentaries on those Hippocratic works: they are among the commentaries he characterised as not being composed for a general audience, and generally refrain from engaging explicitly with the early exegetical tradition; see von Staden (2009), 135–144, esp. 141–144.

9 For Baccheius' Hippocratic commentaries, see von Staden (2006), 16–25, correcting earlier attempts to uncover evidence also for commentaries on *Epidemics* 2 and 3, and on *Nature of the Child*. Smith (1979), 146, claims that Baccheius wrote no commentary on *Surgery*, but he seems unnecessarily sceptical about Galen's statements; see von Staden (2006), 18–19.

10 See Smith (1979), 145–148; Manetti and Roselli (1994), 1546; von Staden (2006), 18–19, and id. (2009), 147–148.

11 Galen, *Commentary on Hippocrates' 'Surgery'* 1.5 (18b.666 K.): 'θαυμάζω δὲ Ἀσκληπιάδου τὴν μὲν κατ' ἰητρεῖον (P: ἰητρίην Kühn) γραφὴν φυλάξαντος, σημεῖον δὲ αὐτὴν οἰομένου περὶ τῶν αὐτῶν κατὰ τὸ ἰατρεῖον. τὸ γὰρ κατ' ἰητρείην ἐστὶ τούτου σημαντικόν, οὐ τὸ κατ' ἰητρεῖον, ἵνα τις ἰατρεῖον τῶν νόσων ἰατρείην ἀκούσῃ (I am surprised at Asclepiades, since he preserves the

his own uncertainty about the correct reading, and mentions, as possible interpretations, two emendations that had been suggested by Asclepiades and by Heraclides of Tarentum.[12] In the second, Asclepiades is cited for his awareness of a variant reading, which Galen approves, at least in part, because of its antiquity.[13]

It is noteworthy that Asclepiades' views are often recorded alongside the views of other Hellenistic commentators on the same and similar questions, and it seems very plausible that Asclepiades himself was engaging directly and explicitly with earlier commentators, revising and correcting previous interpretations. In fact, Wesley Smith has argued that Galen had access only to Asclepiades' commentary, and that all his reports on earlier commentators must derive from it.[14] While it is a possibility that Galen was using only a single source for all these Hellenistic commentators, there is little evidence to support it, but even if it were true, it is more likely on chronological grounds that it would have been Heraclides of Tarentum's commentary that Galen was using, rather than Asclepiades'.[15] Certainly the papyrus discussed below, preserving part of a commentary on *Epidemics* 1, shows that Asclepiades' commentaries were engaged with directly by his successors, and there is no reason to doubt that Asclepiades similarly positioned himself in relation to previous Hippocratic scholarship.

Galen's most detailed report from Asclepiades' commentary comes from a discussion of another passage within section 11 of the Hippocratic text:[16]

---

reading *kat' iētreîon*, but thinks that it means "concerning the same things in the surgery". For *kat' iētreíēn* means this, not *kat' iētreîon*, so that one would understand "surgery" as "curing of diseases".)'

12 Galen, *Commentary on Hippocrates' 'Surgery'* 1.22 (18b.715 K.), concerning *Surgery* 4 (3.286 L.): Asclepiades is reported to have read νοῦσος δέ, δι' ἣν καὶ βλάπτονται τοῖς ἐν γενετῇσι ἢ ἐν τροφῇ εἴθισται … etc., where Galen's Hippocratic lemma (18b.713 K.) had νοῦσος δὲ δι' ἣν καὶ βλάπτονται, οἷσιν ἐν γενετῇσι ἢ ἐν τροφαῖς εἴθισται.

13 Galen, *Commentary on Hippocrates' 'Surgery'* 2.30 (18b.810–811 K.), concerning *Surgery* 11 (3.310.4 L.): 'γέγραπται δὲ διχῶς ἡ λέξις ἥδε, κατά τινα μὲν τῶν γραφῶν 'ὅριον τοῦ μάλιστα' καὶ ταύτην γε ὁ Ἀσκληπιάδης οἶδε τὴν γραφήν, ἐν ἄλλοις δὲ 'οὔτε ὅριον τοῦ μᾶλλον τὸ συμψαύειν' καὶ ἔστιν ὥσπερ ἀμείνων, οὕτω καὶ παλαιοτέρα ἡ διὰ τοῦ 'μάλιστα' (This text is written in two ways: in some copies (it is written) *hórion toû málista*—Asclepiades at any rate knew this reading—, but in others *oúte hórion toû mâllon tò sympsaýein*, and the reading with *málista* is as superior as it is older)'.

14 Smith (1979), 145–148.

15 Manetti and Roselli (1994), 1616, think it likely that Galen had access to Asclepiades' commentary. Asclepiades appears to have died in the first decade or two of the first century BC (see most recently Flemming 2012), while Heraclides' *floruit* probably lay in the early first century BC (Guardasole 1997, 23).

16 *In the Surgery* 11 (3.308.6–310.1 L.).

> ἀναλελάφθαι δὲ ἢ κέεσθαι ἐν σχήματι ἀπόνῳ τῷ κατὰ φύσιν. ὧν δὲ ἂν ἀποστῇ τἀναντία.
>
> Let it be suspended and lie in a comfortable, natural configuration. Where there is *apóstasis*, the opposite.

Here most ancient commentators appear to have read the text as describing the appropriate way to bandage the patient when there is an *apóstasis* or suppuration through a lesion.[17] However, the transmitted text says that the opposite should be done when there is an *apóstasis*, but this made little sense of the previous description of what should be done in cases of *apóstasis*.[18] Some interpreters accordingly suggested that the negative μή should be added to the text, so that it read: 'Where there is no *apóstasis*, the opposite'.[19]

Asclepiades, by contrast, offered what appears to have been a novel interpretation, which exploited the ambiguity in the verb *aphístēmi* and its cognate *apóstasis*. Instead of taking it as referring to a kind of suppuration, and the correct way to bandage it, Asclepiades believed it must refer to the *apóstasis* of the bandage itself, that is, its separation or slippage from the part it was meant to bind. As Galen's quotation shows, he spelt out in considerable detail the required sense of the passage as he saw it:[20]

> Ἀσκληπιάδης δὲ ἐπὶ τῆς ἐπιδέσεως ἀκούων τούτων 'ὧν δὲ ἂν ἀποστῇ τὰ ἐναντία' τὴν ὅλην διάνοιαν εἶναι βούλεται· 'ἂν δὲ ἐπιδεῖν ἐν σχήματι, ἐν ᾧ μήτε ἀπόσφιγξις μήτε ἀπόστασις ἔσται, τοῦτο δ' ἐστὶν ἅπαν κατὰ φύσιν. ἐφ' ὧν δὲ ἂν ἡ ἐπίδεσις ἀποστῇ, ἐπὶ τούτων τἀναντία πρᾶττε, τουτέστιν ἐν τῷ ἐναντίῳ σχήματι τὴν ἐπίδεσιν ποιοῦ.' καὶ γράφει κατὰ λέξιν οὕτως· 'ἐν ᾧ σχήματι τοῦ μέρους ἐπιτιθέντος σχήματος ἐπίδεσμος ἀποστῇ, τῷ ἐναντίῳ τούτῳ σχήματι τὴν ἐπίδεσιν ποιοῦ. οἷον ἐκτεταμένου τοῦ ἀγκῶνος, ἐπειδὰν ὁ βραχίων καταδεθῇ, ὁ ἐπίδεσμος οὐ μένει, ἀλλ' ἀφίσταται, τοὐναντίον σχῆμα τῇ ἐκτάσει κατασκευάσας, ἐπεὶ δὲ τουτέστι κάμψας τὸν ἀγκῶνα, ἐπίδει πάλιν. ἐπεὶ κατὰ φύσιν μὲν σχῆμα τοῖς σκέλεσίν ἐστι τὸ ἐκτεταμένον, ἐὰν καὶ κεκαμμένων τῶν σκελῶν ἐπιδήσας ἐκτεῖναι κελεύσῃς, μεταβάντων τῶν μυῶν εἰς ἄλλους τόπους ὁ ἐπί-

17 Galen, *Commentary on Hippocrates' 'Surgery'* 2.29 (18b.802–805 K.).

18 *Surgery* 11; 3.306.8–9 L.: 'ἀφεστεῶτα μέν, ὥστε τὰ μετέωρα τῆς ἕδρης ψαύειν μέν, πιέζειν δὲ μή ([Close] a sinus so that the upper parts touch the base without pressing on it)'; trans. Withington (1928).

19 Esp. Galen, *Commentary on Hippocrates' 'Surgery'* 2.29 (18b.802 K.); Kühlewein (1902, p. 38, line 3) accepted the addition.

20 Galen, *Commentary on Hippocrates 'Surgery'* 2.29 (18b.805–806 K.).

δεσμος ἀποστήσεται ἀπ' ἐκείνων, ἀφ' ὧν μύες ἀπεχώρησαν, τὸ ἐναντίον σχῆμα τοῦ κατακεκαμμένου ποιήσας.'

Asclepiades understands these words, 'where there is *apóstasis*, the opposite', in reference to bandaging, and wants the whole meaning to be: 'Bandage in a configuration in which there will be no squeezing nor looseness—this is fully in accordance with nature. In cases where the bandaging is loose, do the opposite—that is, make the bandaging in the opposite configuration.' He writes verbatim as follows: 'In whatever configuration the bandage slips off the configuration of the part on which it is placed, make the bandage in the opposite configuration. For example, in a case where the elbow is extended, when the arm is bound, and the bandage does not remain, but is loose, having made a configuration opposite to the extension, that is, having bent the elbow, bind it once more. Since an extended configuration is natural for the legs, if you bandage when the legs are bent and then order (the patient) to extend them, when the muscles move to other positions the bandage will be distant from those positions from which the muscles departed, having made the configuration opposite to the bent one.'

An additional fragment from Asclepiades' commentary is preserved by Erotian, who refers to the work as being in a single book. The fragment contains a definition of the type of bandage called the *sképarnos*, literally 'adze', which is mentioned at *Surgery* 7.[21] This was a bandage suitable for the elbow or knee, forming a cross at the joint which allowed it to bend:[22]

σκέπαρνος· εἶδός ἐστι δεσμοῦ ὁ σκέπαρνος, ὅταν ὁ ἐπίδεσμος πλάγιος δεθῇ. μαρτυρεῖ δὲ Ἀσκληπιάδης ἐν τῷ Ἐξηγητικῷ τοῦ Κατ' ἰητρεῖον λέγων· 'ἔστι γὰρ ὁ σκέπαρνος, ὅταν ὁ ἐπίδεσμος ἐπιβάλλων αὐτὸς ἑαυτῷ καὶ χιεζόμενος κλάσιν τινὰ ποιῇ καὶ γωνίαν, οἷον ὅταν ὀρθόλοξος ἐπιδεθῇ'.

'Adze': the 'adze' is a type of bandage, whenever the upper bandage is tied obliquely. Asclepiades bears witness to this in his *Commentary on Hippo-*

21 *Surgery* 7 (3.290.7–292.1 L.): 'τὰ δὲ εἴδεα, ἁπλοῦν, σκέπαρνον, σιμόν, ὀφθαλμός, ῥόμβος, καὶ ἡμίτομον (As to kinds (of bandaging), simple, adze-like, very oblique, the eye, the rhomb, the half-rhomb', trans. Jones, with minor changes).'

22 Erotian, *Glossary* Σ 21; Nachmanson (1918), p. 78, lines 14–18; a different description is given at Soranus, *Fasc.* 53; Ilberg (1927), pp. 169–170, with pl. xiv 53.

> *crates' 'Surgery'* when he says: 'For it is the "adze" when the upper bandage, lying upon itself and forming a cross, makes a bend and an angle, as when it is tied crosswise.'

These various references seem to put it beyond doubt that the form of Asclepiades' work was that of a line-by-line, lemmatised commentary. Comprising a single book, it began with discussion of the work's title, and offered relatively lengthy entries paraphrasing and expanding upon the original text to elucidate its intended meaning, as well as definitions of specific terms. Galen also indicates that Asclepiades suggested emendations to resolve interpretative difficulties.

2 *Aphorisms*

We also know that Asclepiades wrote a commentary on *Aphorisms*. The sole surviving report comes from Caelius Aurelianus, from near the beginning of the third book of his treatise *On Acute Diseases*. It preserves Asclepiades' definition of *synánchē*, from book 2 of his commentary:[23]

> hanc diffiniens Asclepiades passionem secundo libro explanatorio Aphorismorum Hippocratis, 'synanche', inquit, 'est humoris fluor sive humectatio faucium vel summitatis ipsarum saepissime ex capite accidens.'
>
> Asclepiades, defining this disease in the second book of his *Commentary on Hippocrates' 'Aphorisms'*, says, '*Synánchē* is a flow or moistening of fluid in the throat or its upper part most often occurring from the head.'

Caelius cites the title of this commentary in a manner very similar to Erotian's reference to the *Commentary on 'Surgery'* just discussed: the Latin 'libro explanatorio' followed by the genitive might well represent the Greek ἐν τῷ Ἐξηγητικῷ as Erotian had it. Furthermore, as with the fragment of the *Commentary on 'Surgery'* quoted by Erotian, we have here a definition of an individual word found in the Hippocratic source text.[24] It is natural to assume that Asclepiades would have wished to provide a definition of *synánchē* at the *first* appearance

23 Caelius Aurelianus, *Acute Diseases* 3.1.5; Bendz (1990), 294.

24 It is worth noting that Asclepiades had a general interest in cataloguing medical knowledge by defining key terms, and composed a separate work entitled *Definitions*: cf. Caelius Aurelianus, *Acute Diseases*, 2.13.89, 3.19.188.

of the word, which comes in the third book of *Aphorisms*.[25] It seems reasonable to infer, then, that Asclepiades discussed the third book of *Aphorisms* in the second book of the commentary, suggesting a work of three to four books altogether.

A probable additional testimonium for this commentary, however, is recorded by Erotian. Under his entry for the lemma 'πόνοι σιτίων ἡγείσθωσαν' from *Epidemics* 6, Erotian claims that the word *pónos* is used in three different senses in the Hippocratic Corpus. In the third of these senses, according to him, it means 'harm (βλάβη)', and in support of this interpretation he cites *Aphorisms* 2.1; 4.470 L.: 'In a disease in which sleep produces *pónos*, it is fatal; but if sleep brings benefit, it is not fatal'. Erotian immediately observes that Asclepiades had failed to understand the required sense of the aphorism, and quotes him as saying: 'How can this be true, given that *pónos* occurs through intensification of perception, while sleep occurs through its slackening? (πῶς δύναται τοῦτο εἶναι ἀληθές, τοῦ μὲν πόνου κατ' ἐπίτασιν αἰσθήσεως γιγνομένου, τοῦ δὲ ὕπνου κατ' ἔκλυσιν;)'. Evidently Asclepiades was reacting to the first part of the aphorism, where sleep is said to 'produce *pónos*': according to the common understanding of *pónos* as 'pain', he thought the aphorism did not make sense, since sleep and pain are opposed (pain occurring through intensification of perception, and sleep the opposite). Erotian's criticism was apparently that Asclepiades failed to take account of the second half of the aphorism, which reveals that *pónos* here does not mean 'pain', but rather 'harm', since 'ὠφελέῃ (brings benefit)' is intended as the opposite of 'πόνον ποιέει (produces *pónos*)'. Given that this is a direct comment by Asclepiades on an individual aphorism, and that Erotian draws elsewhere on Asclepiades' commentaries (on *Surgery* specifically; see above), it seems likely that his commentary on *Aphorisms* was the source here, too. It is also interesting to see Asclepiades questioning the truth of the Hippocratic author's statement here.

3 *Epidemics* 1

New evidence from a recently published papyrus, P. Oxy. LXXX 5231, has revealed that Asclepiades also wrote a commentary on *Epidemics* 1, hitherto

25 *Aphorisms* 3.16 (4.492 L.): 'νοσήματα δὲ ἐν μὲν τῇσιν ἐπομβρίῃσιν ὡς τὰ πολλὰ γίνεται, πυρετοί τε μακροί, καὶ κοιλίης ῥύσιες, καὶ σηπεδόνες, καὶ ἐπίληπτοι, καὶ ἀπόπληκτοι, καὶ κυνάγχαι (The diseases which generally arise in rainy weather are protracted fevers, fluxes of the bowels, mortifications, epilepsy, apoplexy and *kynánchē*/angina)', trans. Jones (1931).

unknown. The papyrus in question is from Oxyrhynchus, and was copied in the late first or early second century AD. It held an unidentified commentary on *Epidemics* 1, which, given its reference to Asclepiades, must have been composed in the first century BC or the first century AD.

The structure of the commentary displays some interesting features. In the surviving section, consisting of remains of two columns of text, the passage under discussion is the second case history from the final part of *Epidemics* 1.[26] This case history records the illness and eventual demise of one Silenus. He was a young man of about 20 years of age, who apparently succumbed to fever after indulging in some drinking combined with too much exercise. He developed a very serious acute illness, and after eleven days of mental and physical suffering finally died. His case is the subject of the whole section of the commentary as we have it here. At the top of the first column of the papyrus, filling the first eight lines, we have the very end of a lemma containing the final part of the case history. This lists the symptoms which characterised the last two days of Silenus' illness, and adds a few concluding remarks on the case. Then, in the remainder of the first column, and in the first four lines of the second, the commentator offers some general comments, in particular his criticism of the way in which his predecessor Asclepiades discussed the case. Then in the second column, we have another lemma, but this contains the *first* part of Silenus' case history, including the introductory remarks on Silenus and the symptoms he experienced on the first day. That is, this second lemma contains a passage from *earlier* in the *Epidemics* than the passage in the first. The first lemma, therefore, will have contained the whole of Silenus' case history, on which the commentator first of all gave some general introductory remarks. Then came a more detailed section of the commentary, which perhaps commented on each successive day of the case individually: hence we have a reduplicated lemma in the second column, with the initial details of the case and the events of the first day, followed by what must have been the commentator's detailed analysis.

Immediately after the first lemma, our anonymous commentator begins with a critique of Asclepiades' discussion of the case history, and it seems overwhelmingly likely that the source of this discussion was likewise a commentary by Asclepiades on *Epidemics* 1. Here our commentator is marking out his own exegetical approach by contrasting it with the misguided commentary of a prominent predecessor.

26 *Epidemics* 1.13.2 (2.684–688 L.).

At least two distinct criticisms may be distinguished in what survives of the commentator's attack on Asclepiades. The first, which comes immediately after the lemma, runs as follows:[27]

> τὴν μὲν κατα]σ̣κευὴν τοῦ πά-
> θους καὶ τὴν καθ'] ἕκαστον αἰτίαν
> ὅσο]ν̣ ἐκ̣ τ̣[ῶν πα]ρακολουθησάν-
> τ]ω̣ν Ἀσκληπιάδης, ὡς ἔφη̣ν,
> συν]έγραψεν· ἡμῖν δὲ θεραπεί-
> αν] α̣ὐτὸ μόνον προθεμένοις
> εὑ]ρ̣εῖν δυσκολίαν εἰκότως πα-
> ρέ]χ̣ει τὸ πρᾶγ̣[μ]α̣· ἐπὶ μὲν γὰρ
> τῆς] ἐναργείας ἐνῆν πάντως
> τιν]ὶ μὴ σαφῆ τινα τῆς νόσου
> λόγ]ον λαβεῖν.
>
> Asclepiades, as I said, described the condition of the disease and the cause in each part, (insofar as these can be inferred from the) accompanying (symptoms). But to us, whose purpose is merely to find a treatment, the practice reasonably causes discontent. For as far as the manifest facts are concerned, it was certainly possible (for someone) to get an unclear account of the disease.

The commentator complains of Asclepiades' attempt to specify the precise nature of the disease whose symptoms the Hippocratic author recorded, and the cause underlying the different stages of the disease as it developed. It would seem then that Asclepiades engaged in what might be called a retrospective diagnosis of the Hippocratic case history. The anonymous commentator was not sympathetic to this approach. Rather, he believed that a general understanding of the disease could be achieved without reference to its causes and specific nature, and just on the basis of *enárgeia*, what is self-evident or manifest. Nevertheless the understanding of the disease achieved through *enárgeia* is acknowledged to be an unclear one. As we shall see, it seems to emerge later on in the passage that this lack of clarity is due to the Hippocratic author's account and what he has chosen to include, rather than any limitations associated with *enárgeia*.

27 P. Oxy. 5231, col. i 9–19.

Asclepiades developed a theory of matter which was based directly on Epicurean atomism. Thus he believed that the human body, as with everything in the universe, is made up of tiny imperceptible particles which are perpetually flying around in void space.[28] Asclepiades named his particles *ónkoi*, literally 'masses' or 'lumps', and in the structure of the human body the void spaces through which they move were referred to as 'pores'. As long as the motion of these *ónkoi* through the pores is balanced and unimpeded, health is maintained. But when they become obstructed and create a blockage, different diseases are produced, depending on where the obstruction is located.[29]

By a fortunate coincidence, Galen happens to have preserved some details of Asclepiades' account of the motions of the *ónkoi* in the different stages of the disease phrenitis, and it may give some flavour of Asclepiades' description of Silenus' disease. For Galen states in his own commentary on *Epidemics* 1 that Silenus' disease was almost identical to phrenitis, except that he suffered from heaviness of the head,[30] and it is conceivable that Asclepiades believed the disease actually was phrenitis. According to Galen, Asclepiades' account of the cause of phrenitis was as follows:[31]

إن الحمى المحرقة تحرق أغشية الدماغ، فيحدث من ذلك للحبيبات أن تذهب إلى الشيء اللطيف الأجزاء أو يكون ما يذهب منها أكثر ما يكون عدوا وأشده حركة دفعة؛ ويتبع ذلك وقوف الحبيبات في النقب، وعن هذا تحدث العلة المعروفة بالاختلاط. ثم أن ما دون الشراسيف يمتد إلى فوق بسبب الانجذاب إلى الشيء اللطيف الأجزاء. وإذا سعدت الحبيبات الكثيرة جدا وهاكّت الأجزاء اللاحجة، رجعت فطهرت. ثم أنها بعد ذلك تعود إلى المواضع الواسعة التي تصلح لقبولها، فيستطلق البطن بهذا السبب. وإذ كان الأمر على هذا، فقد ينبغي أن يتقدم حدوث الحمى الحارة وما يكون معها، ثم يتبع ذلك الاختلاط وانجذاب مواضع الشراسيف إلى فوق، ويتبع الاختلاط استطلاق البطن.

Burning fever inflames the cerebral membranes, and it results from this that the corpuscles/*ónkoi* make their way to the 'finely divided thing', or those of them which do so become extremely fast and violent in motion

28 See recently Leith (2009b) and (2012).

29 On Asclepiades' pathology, see Vallance (1990), 93–122.

30 Galen, *Commentary on Hippocrates' 'Epidemics'* 1.3.19 (17a.264 K.); Wenkebach (1936), 132–133.

31 Galen, *On Medical Experience* 28.3; Walzer (1944), p. 74, lines 3–12 (text), pp. 146–147 (transl.) with modifications.

> all at once; this is followed by a stoppage of the corpuscles in the pores, which causes the disease known as phrenitis [*iḫtilāṭ*]. Thereupon the hypochondriac region [*mā dūna l-šarāsīfi*] extends upwards, being attracted by the 'finely divided thing'. Now when the very numerous corpuscles rise and rub against the resisting parts, they are repelled and then become clean [*raǧaʿat fa-ṭahurat*]. After this they return to the roomy parts which are capable of receiving them, and for this reason the belly is loosened. Since this is the case, it is therefore necessary for the burning fever and its accompanying symptoms to come first, after which phrenitis follows, then the hypochondriac region [*mawāḍiʿ al-šarāsīfi*] is attracted upwards, and the phrenitis is followed by the loosening of the belly.

Phrenitis was conceived principally as a mental illness, so that in Asclepiades' system it was located in and around the membranes of the brain, as also in the diseases lethargy, mania and epilepsy.[32] But he also attempted to make this account of the disease capable of explaining some rather different symptoms, in particular the looseness of the bowels, which at first sight seems entirely unrelated to the mental illness. His goal was clearly to describe the underlying cause of the disease in a way which could account for a number of apparently unconnected and disparate symptoms: to show that both the mental impairment and the looseness of the bowels are actually part of a single unified and causally connected process. And of course this was all explained with reference to his quasi-atomistic theory of matter.

Now this combination of mental impairment and looseness of the bowels corresponds very closely to Silenus' symptoms. Thus on the first day Silenus' stools were copious, on the second they became even more copious, and then on the third there was a general intensification of the disease. This general picture seems to have continued on the eighth, ninth and tenth days, too. But Silenus' loose bowels were a symptom which took place along with his worsening mental condition, which started to deteriorate on the second day. Thus there are notable parallels between the Hippocratic case history and the account of phrenitis which Asclepiades gave according to Galen.

I suggest, then, that Asclepiades will have tried to explain all or most symptoms that Silenus suffered, in terms of a unified process of disease based on the motions of imperceptible particles through the body. On the subject of Silenus' mental illness and loose bowels, Asclepiades will have given an account much like the one Galen records. Asclepiades will presumably also have tried

32 Caelius Aurelianus, *Acute Diseases*, 1.pref. 6, 17, 20; Bendz (1990), 24, 30, 32.

to account for the other symptoms, such as pain in the loins, heaviness of the head, the tension which Silenus suffered in his neck and later his hypochondrium, and so on. I take it that this is the sort of analysis that the commentator objected to when he referred to Asclepiades' practice of describing the precise nature and cause of the disease and its associated symptoms. It is easy to see how anyone who did not subscribe to Asclepiades' theory of matter could find this explanation of Silenus' disease a pointless and frustrating diversion. Yet for Asclepiades and his followers such explanations presumably served to reinforce the explanatory power of his theory of matter.

The commentator also objects to Asclepiades' analysis of the periodicity of the disease, in particular the regularity of its periods of intensification and remission:[33]

ἀλλὰ οὖν παρο-
ξυσ]μ̣οῖς καὶ διαλείμμασιν
̣ ̣ ̣ ̣]ν̣[34] παρηκολούθησεν καὶ ἐ-
κεί]ν̣οις ⟨οἷς⟩ ἕκαστα τῶν προσαγο-
μέ]ν̣ων δυνησόμεθα παραμε-
τρ]ε̣ῖ̣ν· ἐν τούτοις δὲ τοῖς παρ̣ὰ
Ἱπ]ποκράτους εἰρημένοι[ς] ο̣ὐ-
δὲ]ν ῥᾳδίως τοσοῦτον εὑρ̣[εῖ]ν
ἐν]ῆ̣ν, ἀλλ' ὥσπερ ἐπιδρα̣[μ]ε̣ῖ̣ν̣
τι]ν̣ος βουλομένου τὰ χαλε-
πώ]τατα καὶ ἀνελόντα τὸν ἄν-
θρω]πον ἢ διηγήσασθα̣[ι] καθά-
ρῶς], τὰ κατὰ τὴν νόσον ἔοικε̣ν
̣ ̣ ̣ ̣ ̣]η[35] εἶναι.

However, he concentrated (too much?) on paroxysms and intervals and on those things ⟨by which?⟩ we shall be able to measure out each of the things that are prescribed. But in these things said by Hippocrates it was not possible to find anything so easily, but, as though someone wanted to run through the most serious (symptoms) and those which killed the man (i.e. Silenus) rather than to describe them clearly, the matters concerning the disease appear to be (unclear?).

33 P. Oxy. 5231, col. i 19–32.

34 Perhaps ἄγα]ν̣.

35 Perhaps οὐ σαφ]ῆ (cf. col. i 18).

Asclepiades apparently devoted considerable attention to working out the days on which the disease reached its peaks, that is the days on which its paroxysms fell, and accordingly also on the intervals in which the disease was relatively dormant.[36] The commentator's main criticism appears to be that Hippocrates simply did not record enough information about the case to permit the sort of analysis that Asclepiades undertook. He seems to be emphasising the brevity of the case history, and the fact that the Hippocratic author was very selective in the symptoms which he chose to record. The implication appears to be that there was much more information which could have been recorded; and this selectivity seems to have resulted in the unclear picture of the disease that the commentator remarked on earlier in the column, at i 18. Yet the information which *was* recorded, the commentator apparently insisted, was not complete enough to answer the kinds of questions that Asclepiades was asking.

We know from elsewhere that Asclepiades was intensely interested in the regularity of paroxysms as an indication of when to provide particular forms of treatment. Celsus refers to Asclepiades' views on the periodicity of disease, in the context of his attack on the Hippocratic theory of critical days. As Celsus says:[37]

> igitur sic aegros nutriebant, ut dierum inparium accessiones expectarent, deinde postea cibum quasi levioribus accessionibus instantibus darent, adeo ut Hippocrates, si alio die febris desisset recidivam timere sit solitus. id Asclepiades iure ut vanum repudiavit, atque in nullo die, qua par inparve esset, iis vel maius vel minus periculum esse dixit. interdum enim peiores dies pares fiunt, et oportunius post eorum accessiones cibus datur. … verum in his quidem antiquos tum celebres admodum Pythagorici numeri fefellerunt, cum hic quoque medicus non numerare dies debeat, sed ipsas accessiones intueri, et ex his coniectare, quando dandus cibus sit.

> Therefore they administered food to their patients as follows: they awaited paroxysms on odd days, and after that they gave food, as though slighter paroxysms were impending, insomuch that Hippocrates, when the fever ended on any other than an odd day, was accustomed to fear

36 The author of *Epidemics* 1 reports, for example, that all symptoms intensified (πάντα παρωξύνθη) on the third day (2.686.3 L.).

37 Celsus, *On Medicine* 3.4.12, 15, trans. Spencer (1935).

> that it would come back.[38] Asclepiades has justly attacked this as false, and he said that no day is more or less dangerous to patients for being even or odd. For sometimes even days are the worse, and it is more suitable to give food after paroxysms on these days. … But in these matters indeed the Pythagorean numbers, then quite famous, deceived the ancient physicians, since here also the doctor ought not to count days, but observe the actual paroxysms, and from these infer when food should be given.

Asclepiades felt that identifying the paroxysms of a disease was crucial for deciding when to prescribe food to the patient. Food should be given *after* the paroxysm, as it begins to abate.[39] This is the period in which the patient is most able to digest the food safely and without disturbance, for at this time there is least likelihood of a paroxysm recurring and interfering with the digestive process, which could have disastrous consequences for the patient's health. But Asclepiades thought it entirely mistaken to predict paroxysms based on a preconceived theory about critical days, as outlined in various treatises of the Hippocratic Corpus.[40] Asclepiades rejected this theory outright, and insisted that no day is more likely than any other to bring a paroxysm. Hence it is wrong to count the days, but the doctor must actually observe the paroxysms himself, free from any preconceived ideas about their regularity.

Asclepiades' critique of Hippocratic theories of critical days, as Celsus reports it, seems to have been focused primarily on statements to be found in *Aphorisms*. Celsus records a further series of arguments against various aphorisms concerned with critical days,[41] and it seems likely that these were similarly taken from Asclepiades' writings. So there is a strong likelihood that such criticisms might also have been found in Asclepiades' *Commentary on Aphorisms*. But since *Epidemics* 1 itself contains its own discussion of critical days, set out immediately before the case histories,[42] it does not seem implausible that Asclepiades could have included some critical remarks also in his commentary on this treatise, which would be fully in keeping with the close attention he paid to the regularity of paroxysms in commenting on the individual case histories.

38 Cf. *Aphorisms* 4.61 (4.524 L.).

39 Caelius Aurelianus, *Acute Diseases*, 1.14.110; Celsus, *On Medicine* 3.4.16.

40 See also Caelius Aurelianus, *Acute Diseases*, 1.14.109.

41 Celsus, *On Medicine* 3.4.12–15, which appears to refer to *Aphorisms* 2.23–24, and 4.71, and may have connections with *Coan Prognoses* 145 and 564.

42 *Epidemics* 1.12 (2.678–682 L.).

The final part of the papyrus column, from line 32 on, is difficult to interpret, since it is not immediately clear whether it refers to Asclepiades or Hippocrates.[43] Whoever its author was,[44] this commentary offers a tantalising insight into the nature of Asclepiades' own work. Asclepiades evidently engaged in a detailed analysis of the individual case histories, focusing on identifying the nature of the disease from which each patient suffered, and offering an account of the causes underlying the symptoms described by the Hippocratic author. He also attempted to isolate the paroxysms that the disease presented, as a prerequisite for effective treatment.

So Asclepiades appears to have imported his own medical theory into the exegesis of the Hippocratic source text. He was not thereby attempting to interpret Hippocrates in his own image, but rather to make sense of what was obscure in these ancient texts from his own privileged position of understanding. The medical reality of these case histories mattered, but Asclepiades offered his *own* account of this reality, moving well beyond the source text. Asclepiades did not limit himself to explanation of what the Hippocratic author meant or intended; his duties as a commentator were also to fill in the gaps with the benefit of his own up-to-date medical system.

The anonymous commentator, however, had a comparable sense of the incompleteness of the case histories, conceding that the account of Silenus' case gave an 'unclear' picture of his disease. Such acknowledged deficiencies of course justified the commentator's own project. But it is interesting to see both commentators apparently less sympathetic to what Galen regarded as Hippocrates' characteristic brevity, or *brachylogía*. On the other hand, the anonymous commentator disagreed with Asclepiades over how far one should go in

43 The mention at col. i 34–35 of the care, *epiméleia*, that Silenus underwent suggests that Asclepiades may have been meant, since there is almost no reference to treatment in the Hippocratic case history. It is not difficult to imagine that Asclepiades could have given a description of the therapies he would have recommended for Silenus on each day of his disease. Such an exercise, possibly involving a counterfactual imagining of how Silenus could have been saved, may well have prompted the commentator to remark on its unpleasantness (col. i 38–39). On the other hand, the reference to Silenus' care might just be a general one, implying only the regular visitation of the Hippocratic doctor, which may have included treatment that was just not mentioned in his account. The difficulties mentioned would then have arisen from what the Hippocratic author chose to exclude.

44 See intro. to P. Oxy. LXXX 5231: the only writer we know to have written a commentary on *Epidemics* 1 in the period between Asclepiades and the copying of the papyrus is Heraclides of Tarentum. As an Empiricist, Heraclides would have had excellent reasons to attack Asclepiades, and the nature of his criticisms themselves suggests an Empiricist perspective. However, there may well have been other commentaries on *Epidemics* 1 from the relevant period of which we know nothing.

attempting to elucidate and supplement what was recorded in *Epidemics* 1. For Asclepiades, someone with a proper understanding of disease, such as himself, could make sense of the medical reality behind the text, and use it to infer a range of details concerning the nature of each case history and its causes, as well as to map out its periodicity. For the papyrus commentator, by contrast, the discovery of proper treatment had to be remembered as the fundamental goal, and it seems to have been important *not* to imagine that one could go beyond what the limitations of the text allowed.

4 Other Commentaries?

There are two further testimonia which provide more tenuous links between Asclepiades and certain Hippocratic treatises, namely *Epidemics* 3 and 6. They are worth considering, but in my view do not establish that he wrote commentaries on the relevant works. In his *Commentary on Epidemics* 3, Galen observes that certain commentators found significance in details recorded by the Hippocratic author that others saw as purely incidental. One such detail was the ethnicity of the unnamed individual recorded first in the second batch of case histories in *Epidemics* 3:[45]

> ἐν Θάσῳ, τὸν Πάριον, ὃς κατέκειτο ὑπὲρ Ἀρτεμισίου, πυρετὸς ἔλαβεν ὀξύς, …

> In Thasus, acute fever seized the man from Paros, who lay sick past the temple of Artemis, …

Some commentators (in fact later identified as Sabinus)[46] believed that the patient's origin on Paros was meant to be relevant to the case. In support, they cited Asclepiades' clinical observation that phlebotomy is beneficial to those in Parium.[47] Caelius Aurelianus confirms that Asclepiades made this observa-

45 *Epidemics* 3.17.1 (3.102.13–14 L.).

46 See Galen, *Commentary on Hippocrates' 'Epidemics'* 3.3.76 (17a.744 K.); Wenkebach (1936), 165, lines 11–13; Raiola (2018), fr. 16b; for Sabinus, see now Raiola (2018), as well as the two articles by Raiola and Jouanna in this volume.

47 Galen, *Commentary on Hippocrates' 'Epidemics'* 3.3.76 (17a.737–739 K.); Wenkebach (1936), 161, line 14–162, line 8: 'περιέργως κἀνταῦθα πάλιν τῶν ἐξηγητῶν ἔνιοι τὴν πατρίδα τοῦ κατακειμένου φασὶν οὐκ ἀργῶς προσκεῖσθαι. καὶ γὰρ ὑπ' Ἀσκληπιάδου λελέχθαι τοὺς ἐν Παρίῳ μάλισθ' ὑπὸ φλεβοτομίας ὀνίνασθαι (Here once again some commentators make too much of the text in saying that the patient's homeland is not added redundantly, and that hence it was also stated by Asclepiades that people in Parium are especially benefited by phlebotomy.)'

tion in book 2 of his work *On Acute Diseases*, where the benefits of phlebotomy for pleurisy in Parium and the Hellespont were contrasted with its detrimental effects for the same disease in Athens and Rome.[48] Galen also refers to a similar observation in his treatise *On Medical Experience*, though there are certain discrepancies in that version.[49] Clearly Sabinus cited Asclepiades in his own commentary on *Epidemics* 3, but there is no reason to assume that his source was itself a commentary by Asclepiades on the same case history. As the testimonia in Caelius Aurelianus and Galen suggest, Asclepiades' observation may have been relatively well known, and it is not obviously related to the Hippocratic case history at all.[50] It could easily have been Sabinus who made the connection: the point he wanted to illustrate was apparently only that location could have an effect on treatment, which was why the Hippocratic author included the patient's ethnic. But Asclepiades' observation illustrates this irrespective of the locations or diseases involved.[51] While it is entirely possible that Asclepiades wrote a commentary on *Epidemics* 3, this testimonium does not constitute reliable evidence for its existence or its putative content.

Wenkebach (1936, 162, line 1) emends Παρίῳ to Πάρῳ against the unanimous manuscript tradition, but the evidence of Caelius Aurelianus (see following note) confirms that the manuscripts are correct.

48 Caelius Aurelianus, *Acute Diseases* 2.22.129–133; Bendz (1990), p. 218, line 18–p. 222, line 5: '*Asclepiades secundo volumine Celerum vel Acutarum Passionum pleuriticos phlebotomat, praedi⟨s⟩cens primo ab his qui in locis consistunt vel commorantur utrum regio adiutorium phlebotomiae permittat adhiberi. se enim vidisse testatur apud Athenas atque urbem Romam phlebotomia vexatos vel peius affectos esse pleuriticos, in Pario vero atque Hellesponto resumptos ac relevatos* (Asclepiades in Book 2 of *On Acute Diseases* phlebotomizes pleuritics, first discovering from those who reside or dwell in those places whether the region permits the therapy of phlebotomy to be prescribed. For he claims that he has himself seen that pleuritics in Athens and Rome were troubled or made worse by phlebotomy, while in Parium and the Hellespont they were relieved and got better.)'

49 Galen, *Medical Experience* 26.6; Walzer (1944), 142: 'Thus it happens that this is something which you, Asclepiades, alone profess. When you say: "I saw in Parium that the condition of a man attacked by phrenitis became worse on the application of blood-letting" (ويحصل أن هذا أمر تنتحله أنت خاصة يا أسقليبيادس، وإذا أنت قلت لي «إني رأيت في فاريون أن من أصابه الاختلاط وفصد له العرق كان أسوأ حالا») ...'.

50 Indeed, Asclepiades spoke about the city of Parium on the Hellespont, whereas the Hippocratic case history concerned a man from the island of Paros.

51 Note too Galen's emphasis, in his comment, on the lack of any mention of phlebotomy in the case history, which was the focus of Asclepiades' observation: Galen, *Commentary on Hippocrates' 'Epidemics'* 3.3.76 (17a.739 K.); Wenkebach (1936), p. 162, lines 2–4. Cf. Manetti and Roselli (1994), 1616.

A similar case is found in Galen's *Commentary on Hippocrates' 'Epidemics'* 6, where Asclepiades is mentioned again:[52]

> ἀνθρώπου ψυχὴ αἰεὶ φύεται ἄχρι θανάτου. ἢν δ' ἐκπυρωθῇ, ἅμα τῇ νούσῳ καὶ ἡ ψυχὴ τὸ σῶμα φέρβεται.
>
> μαντείας δεῖ μᾶλλον ἤ τινος μεθόδου, καθ' ἣν εὑρήσει τις, ὅ τι ποτε σημαίνειν βουληθεὶς ἔγραψε τὸ 'φύεται'. δύναται μὲν γὰρ ἀκούεσθαι καὶ ⟨ἀντὶ⟩ τοῦ "γεννᾶται", καθάπερ ὁ Ἀσκληπιάδης ὕστερον ὑπέλαβε, δύναται δὲ καὶ ⟨ἀντὶ⟩ τοῦ "αὐξάνεται", δύναται δ', ὥσπερ τινὲς ἤκουσαν, ἀντὶ τοῦ "διασῴζεται", τροφῇ καὶ ἀναπνοῇ χρωμένων ἡμῶν.
>
> *The soul of a man is always growing until death. If it is heated up together with the disease, the soul consumes the body.*
>
> It needs divination rather than a methodical procedure by which to discover what he wanted to get across when he wrote 'grows'. For it is possible to understand it as a substitute for 'is generated', as Asclepiades later thought. It is possible also (to take it) as a substitute for 'increases'. It is also possible, as some people have understood it, to take it as a substitute for 'is preserved', since we make use of nourishment and respiration.

Here Galen seems merely to be listing the various possible senses in which the soul might be said to grow (φύεσθαι). But it does not follow that each of these senses were originally proposed as interpretations of this particular passage of *Epidemics* 6, let alone in a commentary dedicated to that work. It seems plausible that in this case Galen was merely drawing indirectly on Asclepiades' theory of the soul as one potential way of cashing out the meaning, in contrast to interpretations which draw on competing theories of the soul.[53] Galen's point is that the meaning of the Hippocratic term will vary depending on what kind of psychology one adopts. Again, this is not compelling evidence for the existence of an Asclepiadean commentary on *Epidemics* 6, plausible as that might be on other grounds.

---

52 *Epidemics* 6.5.2 (5.314.14–15 L.), followed by Galen, *Commentary on Epidemics* 6.5.5 (17b.246 K.); Wenkebach (1954), 270.

53 Manetti and Roselli (1994), 1616–1617: 'Sia questa notizia sia la menzione della teoria che l'inspirazione serve alla generazione del pneuma psichico … si inquadrano nella trattazione della teoria asclepiadea dell' anima e non provengono necessariamente da un commento ad "Epidemie" VI.'

5 Asclepiades and Hippocrates

The evidence we have considered above raises the question of what Asclepiades' commentaries might reveal about his general attitude to the Hippocratic Corpus, and what sort of authority it might have held for him. It can be easy to associate ancient Hippocratic commentaries with an attitude that sought vindication for what Hippocrates said, that is, with the assumption that a correct interpretation of a Hippocratic text will be one that shows Hippocrates to have been right. But, as we have seen, Asclepiades was happy to reject some fundamental notions within the Corpus, such as the theory of critical days. His own corpuscular system, similarly, seems incompatible with the various humoral theories found in it, and he also rejected the idea that Nature had a basic tendency to restore balance and health.[54] We also saw above that Asclepiades could question the truth of certain Hippocratic aphorisms.

But this is not at all to say that Asclepiades is likely to have been critical *in general* of what he found in the Hippocratic Corpus. Undoubtedly Galen's attacks on Asclepiades have created a picture of anti-Hippocratism, but of course it is Galen's *own* image of Hippocrates against which Asclepiades is framed in his rhetoric. There is no sign in the surviving fragments of any polemical attitude on Asclepiades' part.[55] He appears concerned above all with exegesis, with making sense of what is to be found in the Corpus, and with conveying this as clearly as possible. He was elsewhere concerned to point out where paradoxical statements made by Hippocrates could in fact be confirmed clinically. An example is preserved by Oribasius, in which Asclepiades reports on two cases in which patients suffered hip dislocations without any obvious cause.[56] He explicitly cites the Hippocratic treatise *Joints* in support of

54 Caelius Aurelius, *Acute Diseases* 1.14.115, '*neque naturam aliud esse quam corpus vel eius motum. deinde inquit non solum prodest sed etiam nocet* (Nor is Nature anything but body and its motion. Then he says: it not only helps but also harms)'.

55 Cf. Flemming (2008), 331, 334.

56 Oribasius, *Medical Collections* 47.12; Raeder (1928), 256, lines 22–32: 'ἐκ τῶν Ἀσκληπιάδου τοῦ Βιθυνοῦ. ὅτι καὶ διὰ νόσον χρονίαν ἔξαρθροί τινες γίνονται. ὅτι χωρὶς φανερᾶς αἰτίας νοσησάντων χρονίως ἐκβαίνει τὰ ἄρθρα, δίδωσι μὲν καὶ Ἱπποκράτης μαρτυρίαν ἐν τοῖς Περὶ ἄρθρων, περιπέπτωκα δὲ κἀγῶ δυσίν, ἑνὶ μὲν ἐν Παρίῳ, ὃς οὔτε πληγεὶς οὔτε πεσών, ἀλγήσας δὲ τὸ σκέλος ἐξ ἀρχῆς καὶ κατακλιθεὶς ἐπὶ τρεῖς μῆνας, εἱλκύσθη καὶ ἐξέβαλε τὴν τοῦ μηροῦ κεφαλὴν εἰς τὸ ἔξω, δι' ὑπερβολὴν τῶν ἀλγημάτων τοῦτο παθών, ὡς νομίζω, ἑτέρῳ δὲ νεανίσκῳ τραγῳδοποιῷ τινι· καὶ γὰρ καὶ οὗτος ἄνευ φανερᾶς αἰτίας ἐξ ἰσχιάδος ἐξέβαλε τὸν μηρὸν ἔξω, τῆς σαρκὸς διὰ τὴν φλεγμονὴν ἐπισπασαμένης τὸ ἄρθρον καὶ ἐκ τῆς οἰκείας χώρας ἐκβαλούσης (From the works of Asclepiades of Bithynia. On the fact that some people suffer dislocations also because of chronic illness. To the fact that joints are dislocated without any obvious cause in those suffering from chronic illness, Hippocrates also bears witness in *On Joints*. I, myself, have

his experience, confirming the accuracy of Hippocrates' observation. Of course, this allows Asclepiades to advertise the comprehensiveness of his own clinical experience at the same time. The manner in which *Joints* is introduced in this quotation preserved by Oribasius does not suggest that it came from a commentary on the treatise, but it at least appears to reflect a broad respect for some of the clinical observations found in the Hippocratic Corpus.

Unfortunately, the surviving evidence offers only suggestive glimpses of how Asclepiades might have engaged with previous Hippocratic commentators. There can be little doubt that he was self-conciously working within the tradition of Hippocratic commentary that had developed within Alexandria since the third century BC. It is no accident that Galen referred to him alongside the Herophilean Baccheius and the Empiricists Zeuxis and Heraclides of Tarentum. And even if Galen, in reporting Asclepiades' comments on *Surgery*, does not explicitly tell us that these were presented as corrections of his predecessors' interpretations, the implication is nonetheless generally clear.

Yet we know almost nothing about the ways in which Asclepiades would have staked out his own position within this tradition. He certainly engaged in a sustained and comprehensive attack on the principles of the Empiricist sect, criticising among other things their claims to be able to manage without the use of reason.[57] We also catch a glimpse of Asclepiades criticising Herophilus' discussion of the problem of why round wounds heal more slowly, overturning his predecessor's solution before offering his own.[58] But Heinrich von Staden has shown that sectarian disputes were not necessarily one of the principal motivations for debate within the Hellenistic commentary tradition, although they certainly played a role.[59] Interpreting the Hippocratic Corpus became an arena of competition in its own right, to a certain extent disengaged from the primarily epistemological disputes between the sects.

---

also come across two cases, one being in Parium: he had not been struck, nor had fallen over, but he had pain in his leg from the start and had been laid up for three months; he was wrenched and dislocated the head of his femur outwards, suffering this because of excessive pain, as it seems to me. The other was a young tragic poet: he too dislocated his femur from the hip outwards without any obvious cause, but his flesh had pulled on the joint because of the inflammation and threw it out of its proper place'). Cf. *Joints* 55 (4.240.19–24 L.), in the section on dislocation outwards at the hip.

57 See especially Galen, *On the Sects* 5 (1.75 K.); *Medical Experience* 1–4 (Walzer 1944, 1–7); John of Alexandria, *Commentary on Galen's 'On the Sects'* 4rb70–4va64 (Pritchet 1982, 49–50, 52).

58 Cassius the Iatrosophist, *Problems* 1 (Garzya 2004, 35–36; Ideler 1841, 144–145).

59 Von Staden (2006), 27–28, 34, 43, 44–45.

Even if we cannot see how he responded to the work of his predecessors, the Oxyrhynchus papyrus of course offers a glimpse of how one of his successors reacted to *him*. He was evidently taken seriously enough to be repeatedly referred to in this commentary, which itself circulated widely enough to reach Oxyrhynchus in the first or second century AD. The anonymous commentator notes in this passage that he has discussed, and apparently criticised, Asclepiades' approach before, presumably in his comments on the first case history in *Epidemics* 1, suggesting a sustained and comprehensive critique. The commentators with whom Galen felt most obliged to engage seem to have belonged to the previous few generations, but clearly Asclepiades' impact on the tradition at the end of the Hellenistic period was greater than Galen's relative silence would suggest, even if Erotian mentioned him on only one occasion.

Asclepiades' work on the Corpus, then, need not reflect any particular investment in the figure of Hippocrates *per se*. There is no sign, for example, that he was attempting to construct an Asclepiadean Hippocrates.[60] Rather, the Hippocratic commentary had become contested territory for erudite doctors by the end of the Hellenistic period. It was a necessary area of expertise for a first-rate medical author, and a vehicle for establishing one's command of medical scholarship. Sectarian disputes will have provided some motivation, but the primary focus of polemic was the quality and plausibility of the interpretations themselves. As far as we can see, Asclepiades was using the Corpus to showcase the explanatory power of his own medical theory, and his mastery of the medical art in general. His relation with Hippocrates was evidently a highly complex one, but it is far from clear that Hippocratic medicine held any direct authority for him. But of course such conclusions are based on only a tiny surviving fraction of a once extensive body of work. The new papyrus fragment of a commentary on *Epidemics* 1 is another reminder of the sheer quantity of Hippocratic exegesis that has been lost.

60 Although the Empiricists' interest in the Corpus has often been interpreted by scholars as motivated by attempts to co-opt Hippocratic authority for their own approach to medicine, von Staden (2006), 44–45, emphasises how lacking the evidence is for this interpretation.

CHAPTER 3

Sabinus 'the Hippocratic': His Exegetical Method in the *Commentaries on Hippocrates*

Tommaso Raiola

Sabinus (first to second century AD) was one of the most influential Hippocratic commentators prior to Galen.[*,1] His works, as far as they have survived, consist of fragments from his commentaries on Hippocratic works. Our main source is Galen, who quoted Sabinus often in his own commentaries in order to discuss or reject Sabinus' interpretations. Sabinus had at least two pupils, Metrodorus and Stratonicus. As a young student, during his stay in Alexandria, Galen attended the lessons of the latter. The former, according to Galen, wrote commentaries similar to those of his teacher. Sabinus and his followers were referred to as 'Hippocratics' (Ἱπποκρατεῖοι), which in all likelihood, was what they called themselves.[2]

As far as we know Sabinus commented on *Aphorisms*; *Nutriment*; *Nature of Man*; *Airs, Waters, Places*; and the second, third and sixth book of Hippocrates' *Epidemics*. His works survived at least until the fourth century, since Oribasius, in his *Medical Collections*, seems to quote a long passage about climate directly from Sabinus; it was probably excerpted from a monograph dealing with the same subject of Hippocrates' *Airs, Waters, Places*.[3]

* The author is the principal investigator of the GALCOMM project (RBSI14283W) hosted by Università degli Studi di Napoli 'L'Orientale': the project is funded by the SIR 2014 Financial Programme. An edition of Sabinus' fragments and *testimonia* is now available: see Raiola (2018).

1 Sabinus' *floruit* is commonly placed in the first quarter of the second century AD, two generations before Galen, since he was the master of Stratonicus, one of Galen's teachers in Alexandria: see Galen, *On Black Bile* 4.12 (de Boer 1937, p. 78, lines 22–29); *Commentary on Hippocrates' 'Epidemics'* 6.5.14 (Wenkebach 1954, p. 287, lines 13–20 and p. 303, lines 12–14). On Sabinus, see Wellmann (1912); Gossen (1920); Deichgräber (1930), 25–29; Smith (1979); Manetti (1985); Manetti and Roselli (1994), 1607–1614.

2 See, for instance, Galen, *On Black Bile* 4.12 (de Boer 1937, p. 78, lines 22–24): 'ὕστερον δέ ποτε μετ' ἐνιαυτὸν εἷς τῶν ἐν Περγάμῳ διδασκάλων ἡμῶν Στρατόνικος ὄνομα, μαθητὴς Σαβίνου τοῦ Ἱπποκρατείου; Gal., *Commentary on Hippocrates' 'Epidemics'* 3.1.4 (Wenkebach 1936, p. 17, line 7): ἐπὶ δὲ τοὺς Ἱπποκρατείους ἑαυτοὺς ὀνομάσαντας ἐλθών τις ...' On the meaning of the adjective Ἱπποκρατεῖος in Galen, see Boudon-Millot (2015). On the 'ancient' Hippocratics, see Lloyd (1993) and Manetti (2014).

3 Oribasius, *Medical Collections* 9.15–21 (Raeder 1929, p. 15, line 30–p. 20, line 13). On this excerpt see Nutton (2000), and Raiola (2018), 136–150 and (forthcoming).

© TOMMASO RAIOLA, 2021 | DOI:10.1163/9789004470200_005

1 Sources

Due to the nature of Galen's quotations, it is always difficult to reconstruct the original opinion of the authors he quoted. In view of presenting and discussing the main aspects of Sabinus' works, the commentaries on *Epidemics* seem to offer a more productive starting point, since for this work we have a significant number of quotations. The amount and quality of this textual material allow us to draw a picture of Sabinus' exegetical method.

As we interpret Sabinus through Galen's quotations we should not forget that Galen himself is constantly in the middle, filtering and (sometimes) distorting the thought of his predecessor. This is precisely the reason why we always need to reconsider our first impression of what Galen says about Sabinus' exegesis (whether he praises or blames him). We need to evaluate Galen's reliability each time and compare passages dealing with similar themes. If we only consider Sabinus' commentaries on *Epidemics* we have some 60 texts, which is a sufficient sample size for our investigation.

Here, we will focus in particular on the fragments from the Commentary on Book 3. Here the Greek textual tradition is sometimes unreliable, and the editor Wenkebach (1936) often rewrote the corrupt or missing Greek text by effectively rendering back into Greek a German translation of a ninth-century Arabic translation. Therefore, where possible, the Arabic evidence has been taken into consideration.[4] We will also discuss passages from Galen's *Commentary on Hippocrates' 'Nature of Man'*,[5] and from Galen's commentary on *Epidemics* 6.[6] The abridged critical apparatus (when present) only records the interventions by the editors that are relevant to our purposes.

2 Sabinus' Wordiness

The first issue at stake is Sabinus' (supposed) wordiness, which Galen usually refers to as 'chattiness (*perilálēsis*)'. Our first case comes from the *Commentary*

4 See Pormann (2008) and (2012); and Vagelpohl (2014) and (2016), who edited the Arabic version of books 1 and 2. I would like thank Peter E. Pormann for enriching this paper with his readings of Ḥunayn's Arabic translation of Galen's commentary (based on Madrid, Escorial, MS Arab. 804).

5 Mewaldt (1914).

6 Wenkebach and Pfaff (1956). For the purpose of clarity and to promote discussion, I have printed the Hippocratic lemma prior to the text of the commentary in all cases.

on Hippocrates' 'Epidemics' 3.1.12 (Wenkebach 1936, p. 40, lines 7–19; lemma in 3.36.1 L.; Raiola 2018, F 12):

> Τεσσαρεσκαιδεκάτῃ ἀπύρετος, οὐχ ἵδρωσεν, ἐκοιμήθη, κατενόει πάντα.

> On day fourteen, he recovered from fever, he did not sweat, he slept, he perceived everything well.

> [...] εἴρηται μὲν οὖν περὶ τούτων ἐπὶ πλέον ἐν ἑτέροις, ἀλλὰ νῦν ἐν κεφαλαίοις ἅπαξ ἀρκείτω λελέχθαι περὶ τῶν ἀλόγως ἐπὶ χαλεποῖς νοσήμασιν *ἀπυρέτων* γενομένων· ὅσῳ γὰρ ἂν ὀλεθριωτέρων προηγησαμένων σημείων ἄμεινον ἔχειν δόξωσι, τοσούτῳ τὴν νόσον ὀλεθριωτέραν ἔχουσιν, ἅθ', ὡς οἱ περὶ τὸν Σαβῖνον εἰρήκασι, *λοχῶντος τοῦ νοσήματος ὥσπερ θηρίου τινὸς ἢ ἀνθρώπου πονηροῦ*· διάνοιαν γὰρ ἔχοντός ἐστι ζῴου τὸ λοχᾶν, ⟨ὅταν⟩[7] ἐξαίφνης ἐπιθῆται λάθρᾳ μὴ προσδοκῶσι τοῖς ἐνεδρευομένοις ὑπ' αὐτοῦ. **ἀλλὰ τὰ μὲν οὕτως εἰρημένα προσηκόντως ἄν τις ὀνομάσειε περιλάλησιν.** οὐδὲν γὰρ εἰπόντες ἐπιστημονικόν, ἀλλὰ περιλαλήσαντες μόνον οἴονται τὸ προκείμενον ἀποδεδειχέναι διὰ παραδείγματος οὐδὲν οὐδὲ τοῖς παραβαλλομένοις ὅμοιον ἔχοντός τι. καταλιπόντες οὖν αὐτοὺς αὐτοὶ συμπληρώσωμεν ἤδη τὰ προκείμενα.

وقد وصفت هذا وصفا بالغا في غير هذا الكتاب. وأنا واصف في هذا الموضع أيضا بإيجاز جملة رأس من يقلع عنه الحمى على غير قياس ما تقدم من شواهد حاله، بل تكون قد ظهرت فيه دلائل تدل على صعوبة علته، وأقتص على ذكر ذلك مرة واحدة، فأقول: إنه كلما كانت تلك الدلائل التي ظهرت قبل أدل على هلاك ثم حدثت حال توهم أنها حال صلاح وتماثل، كان من هذه حالة أقرب إلى الهلاك. وآل سابنس يقولون إن المرض في هذا الحال أكمن كأن المرض سبع من السباع أو إنسان سوء لأن الكمون إنما هو من فعل حيوان †يقعه وكرحى عفى نفسه† ثم يثب بغتة على الذي يكمن له وهو لا يشعر وما قيل ويقال على هذا الطريق بالواجب يسمى هذيان وذلك أنهم لم يأتوا فيه بعلم لكنهم أتوا بكلام لا معنى له ثم ظنوا أنهم قد بينوا الأمر الذي قصدوا لتبيينه بمثال إتوائه. وذلك المثال أيضا لشيء يشبه ما ثقلوا به شيئا. فأنا تارك أصحاب هذه الأقاويل وقاصد قصد استتمام ما قصدت له وأقول إلخ

7 ὅταν add. Wenkebach.

> Elsewhere, we deal with these matters more fully. May it now suffice to talk briefly about those who, during serious illnesses, recover from fever unexpectedly. In fact, the better they feel after dangerous symptoms appear, the more pernicious the disease is. For, as Sabinus and his followers[8] have said, *the disease lies in ambush like a wild beast or an evil man.* [Only] an animal endowed with thought can ambush: it suddenly and secretly attacks, and those who are ambushed will not expect it. But such words could be rightfully called chattiness. Indeed although they say nothing scientific but only chatter, they believe to have explained the passage in question through an example which has nothing to do with the topics discussed. Therefore, let us leave them and and accomplish what we have set out to do.

This case history of *Epidemics* 3 deals with Hermocrates—a patient affected by fever. On the fourteenth day, Hermocrates seemed to have completely recovered, but as Galen says a few lines beforehand, his recovery had no logical explanation. However, Galen writes that the most ignorant physicians hastily rejoiced at the patient's recovery, for they indeed believed that a remission of symptoms corresponded to a full recovery. Galen not only claims that the above inference is untrue, but he points out that Hippocrates himself indicated the causes of the apparent recovery of the patient: the inborn heat, the action of which on the affected parts is the source of the fever, is eventually weakened by the illness itself and results in a remission of fever and other symptoms.[9] Then Galen quotes Sabinus, criticizing his interpretation of the text not in terms of medical doctrine (likely because Sabinus did not make 'wrong' statements, like the others), but for what Sabinus said about the illness described as a wild animal suddenly attacking. The metaphor, according to Galen, is probably effective in illustrating the remitting illness, but is completely lacking in 'scientific' value. In this case, what Sabinus said is therefore useless 'chattiness', undeserving of neither Galen's attention, nor that of his students. The meaning of the word *perilálēsis* is better understood if we consider what Galen had written some pages before about the 'bad habits' of Hippocratic commentators:[10]

8 I chose to translate 'οἱ περὶ τὸν Σαβῖνον' with 'Sabinus and his followers', although the phrase οἱ περὶ followed by the accusative is also used to refer to a single person. For literature on this question, see Salanitro (1987); Radt (1988); Gorman (2001); Cohen-Skalli (2007); and Savio (2017).

9 *Commentary on Hippocrates' 'Epidemics'* 3.1.12; Wenkebach (1936), p. 39, lines 14–30.

10 *Commentary on Hippocrates' 'Epidemics'* 3.1.4; Wenkebach (1936), p. 22, lines 20–24.

ὅσοι δὲ τῶν ἐξηγουμένων ἀπόδειξιν οἷς λέγουσιν ἐπιφέρειν οὐ δύνανται, περιλαλήσαντες τοὺς ἀκροατὰς † ὑποστέλλουσι τῇ δόξῃ[11] τοῦ συγγραφέως, ἀξιοῦντες οἷς λέγουσι δι' ἐκεῖνον πιστεύεσθαι. καὶ διὰ τοῦτο μεταβαίνουσιν ἀπὸ ῥήσεων ἐπὶ ῥήσεις[12] οὐδ' οὖν οὐδὲ ταύτας οὐδέν τι συντελούσας τοῖς προκειμένοις.

وأما القوم الذين يرومون التفسير، وهم لا يقدرون أن يأتوا على ما يدعونه ببرهان. فإنهم يغمرون السامع بالخطب، ويريدون منه أن يقتصر على رأي واضع الكتاب واعتقاده، وأن يصدق أقاويلهم لموافقتها لقوله. ولذلك لا يزالون يأتون بحجة من كلامه بعد حجة ويطنبون في ذلك، حتى أنهم ربما أتوا بحجج من كلامه غير موافقة لغرضهم الذي قصدوا إليه.

Those, among the commentators, who are not able to support their words with demonstration, by chattering, defraud their disciples of the writer's opinion by asking them to trust their words. Therefore, they move from passage to next, although the passages are useless for the present topic of discussion.

Here, Galen does not attack the style of some commentators, but the way in which they performed their exegesis. He suggests that some of them try to mask their poor skills (and ignorance) through wordiness. They are told to accumulate sayings (probably trying to explain Hippocrates through Hippo-

11 'ὑποστέλλουσι τῆι δόξηι' is the reading of the two Greek manuscripts (L O); Wenkebach conjectured 'ἀποστεροῦσι τῆς δόξης' probably on the basis of Pfaff's German translation of the Arabic ('sie überschütteten den Hörer mit ihrem Geschwätz und wollten *ihn über die Meinung des Verfassers in Finsternes setzen*'). The Arabic, however, reads 'they douse the listener in discourses and *want him to restrict himself to the author's opinion* (*fa-innahum yaġmurūna l-sāmiʿa bi-l-ḫuṭabi wa-yurīdūna minhu an yaqtaṣira ʿalā raʾyi wāḍiʿi l-kitābi wa-ʿtiqādihī*)'; in other words, Ḥunayn understood Galen to have said that these incompetent commentators want their audience to be satisfied with an outline of Hippocrates' doctrine, without elucidating the philological details.

12 Wenkebach indicates this place as corrupt beyond repair, placing a crux after ῥήσεις. According to Pormann, there is no need to doubt the text, as repeating the negation for emphasis is nothing unusual in Greek, and the Arabic confirms the meaning: 'Therefore, they constantly and excessively bring argument after argument about his [sc. Hippocrates'] text, to the point that occasionally these arguments do not even agree with the aim that they have set themselves (*li ḏālika lā yazālūna yaʾtūna bi-ḥuǧǧatin min kalāmihī baʿda ḥuǧǧatin wa-yuṭnibūna fī ḏālika ḥattā annahum rubbamā ataw bi-ḥuǧaǧin min kalāmihī ġayri muwāfiqatin li-ġaraḍihimu llaḏī qaṣadū ilayhi*).'

crates). And, even if they exhibit extensive knowledge of Hippocrates' works, their pupils do not enjoy any benefit from their excess of words (*perilálēsis*): as they do completely cover the texts, they do not clarify them.

Going back to the case of Hermocrates, and leaving aside Galen's critical attitude, we must admit that Sabinus was not totally wrong. He was clearly aware that Hippocrates was warning about asymptomatic phases of the illness. Nonetheless, he failed to give a detailed explanation of the physical causes leading to such conditions.

We find the verb *perilaleîn* used again to describe Sabinus' exegesis in Galen's commentary on *Nature of Man* 13 (Mewaldt 1914, p. 82, lines 17–25; Raiola 2018, F 4; lemma in 6.64.15–18 L.):

> Ὁκόσα δὲ τῶν νοσημάτων γίνεται ἐξ ὀλίγου καὶ ὁκόσων αἱ προφάσιες εὔγνωστοι, ταῦτα δὴ ἀσφαλέστατά ἐστι προαγορεύεσθαι κτλ.
>
> Diseases which arise 'quickly' and whose causes are easy to discern are those whose history can be foretold with the greatest certainty.
>
> Τούτῳ μάχεσθαι δοκεῖ τὸ κατὰ τοὺς Ἀφορισμοὺς εἰρημένον· 'τῶν ὀξέων νοσημάτων οὐ πάμπαν ἀσφαλέες αἱ προαγορεύσιες οὔτε τῆς ὑγιείης οὔτε τοῦ θανάτου.' καὶ Σαβῖνος αὐτὸ πειραθεὶς λῦσαι περιελάλησε μέν, οὐδὲν δὲ εἶπε πιθανόν.
>
> This appears to contradict the words of the *Aphorisms*: 'for acute diseases, both the prognoses of healing and death are absolutely uncertain'. When Sabinus tried to solve this, he only chattered and said nothing plausible.

Here, Galen reports an apparent contradiction between this passage and *Aphorisms* 2.19. In the following, Galen says that this contradiction is due to Sabinus (and other commentators) misunderstanding the meaning of the adverbial clause 'quickly (*ex olígou*)', by interpreting it as an equivalent for 'acute and short-term (diseases)'. Galen's solution simply consists in giving a different interpretation: *ex olígou* corresponds to 'recent, newly appeared'. So, in Galen's opinion, the parallel between this passage of *Nature of Man* and *Aphorisms* is not correct. The two texts simply do not deal with the same subject. Being unable to explain what Hippocrates meant with the expression *ex olígou* in the passage of *Nature of Man*, Galen's Sabinus tried to hide his poor exegetical skills behind *perilálēsis*, that is, worthless accumulation of scholarly quotations. As a result, instead of throwing light on Hippocrates' words, the commentator added new ambiguities to the text.

3 Sabinus' (Lack Of?) Exegetical Depth

Sabinus and his pupils enjoyed great esteem in the eyes of Galen's contemporaries. In a large section (Wenkebach 1936, 10–26) of his Commentary on the third book of *Epidemics*, also known as 'Against the Bad Commentators', Galen points his finger at all of his predecessors, highlighting the faults and failings of their exegetical method and adding examples to support his judgment. Among the other commentators, Galen partially approves of the Empiricists, praising their loyalty to Hippocrates' text. On the contrary, he blames Lycus, totally condemning his interpretation of Hippocrates' doctrine, together with his misguided attempts to imitate the method of the Empiricists. After that, he inveighs against the Hippocratics, whose eminent members were Sabinus and his pupil Metrodorus. Their works, says Galen, were largely praised for their accuracy (ἀκρίβεια).[13] Then Galen adduces an example to demonstrate that their reputation for accuracy was undeserved, referring to the text of Sabinus' commentary on the first lines of *Epidemics* 3 about the well-known case of Pythion, a man seized with trembling that originated in his hands:[14]

> Πυθίων, ὃς ᾤκει παρὰ Γῆς ἱερόν· ἤρξατο τρόμος ἀπὸ χειρῶν.
>
> Pythion, who lived by the temple of Earth, was seized with trembling which began in the hands.
>
> οἱ τοίνυν περὶ τὸν Σαβῖνον καὶ τὸν μαθητὴν αὐτοῦ Μητρόδωρον, ἀκριβέστεροι δόξαντες εἶναι τῶν ἔμπροσθεν Ἱπποκρατείων, ὅμως καὶ αὐτοὶ φαίνονται μοχθηρῶς ἐξηγούμενοι πολλάκις τὸν Ἱπποκράτην. αὐτίκα γέ τοι κατὰ τὸν προκείμενον ἄρρωστόν φασιν αὐτοῖς ὀνόμασιν· 'ὥσπερ[15] ὁ σπασμὸς γίνεται καὶ ὑπὸ πληρώσεως καὶ ὑπὸ κενώσεως, οὕτως καὶ ὁ τρόμος μικρὸς ὢν σπασμὸς ὑπὸ[16] τῶν ἐναντίων ἀποτελεῖται.' […] φαίνονται δ' ἐν αὐτῷ τούτῳ πρῶτον οἱ περὶ τὸν Σαβῖνον ἐσφαλμένοι, μικρὸν σπασμὸν εἰπόντες εἶναι τὸν τρόμον. ὅλῳ γὰρ τῷ γένει διενήνοχεν ἀλλήλων τὰ πάθη ταῦτα.

13 We have another witness of the fame enjoyed by Sabinus among the broader public of intellectuals. Aulus Gellius, in his *Attic Nights* (3.16.8), enthousiastly praises Sabinus' commentary on *Nutriment*, before quoting one of his interpretations: '*Sabinus medicus, qui Hippocratem commodissime commentatus est* …'.

14 *Commentary on Hippocrates' 'Epidemics'* 3.1.4; Wenkebach (1936), p. 17, line 22–p. 18, line 8; Raiola (2018), F 11b.

15 ὥσπερ Wenkebach : ὡς γὰρ codd.

16 ὑπὸ Wenkebach : ἀπὸ codd.

وقد نجد آل سابينس ومطرودورس تلميذه على أنه نظر بهم أنهم أشد استقصاء ممن كان قبلهم من شيعة أبقراط يفسرون أشياء كثيرة من أقاويل أبقراط تفسيرا رديئا، من ذلك أن سابينس قال في قصة هذا المريض الذي كلامها فيه قولا بهذا اللفظ: «فكما أن التشنج يكون من امتلاء ومن الاستفراغ كذلك للرعشة إذا كانت إنما هي تشنج يسير وإنها تكون من هذين السببين المتضادين.» [...] وقد نجد آل سابينس قد غلطوا في هذا الباب أولا حتى قالوا إن الرعشة إنما هي تشنج يسير، وذلك أن هذين العرضين مختلفان[17] في الجنس بأسره.

> Sabinus, his pupil Metrodorus and their followers, who are considered more accurate than previous Hippocratics, appear nevertheless to have often badly interpreted Hippocrates. For example, in this case they had written that: 'As a spasm happens owing to both repletion and depletion, so trembling, which is a small spasm, is produced by (these) contraries.'. [...] From the start, Sabinus and his followers seem to be wrong in saying that trembling is a small spasm. These accidents wholly differ from each other according to their genre.

Sabinus is mentioned from the very beginning in Galen's commentary. In fact, he considers the Hippocratic word *trómos* as an equivalent for *spasmós*, which, according to Galen, clearly is a mistake due to ignorance. Galen explains that the two phenomena are completely different, although they are both natural movements. The first (*trómos*) is a voluntary movement; the second (*spasmós*) is involuntary. But this is not enough for Galen. He continues his merciless attack contesting other statements made by Sabinus. In particular, his explanation of *trómos* as due to an affection of the *stómachos*, suffering from a prolonged sexual abstinence.

Even if we cannot reconstruct the whole text, what survives here of Sabinus' exegesis is far from weak and inconsistent. In this case, Galen is not criticizing empty words, ineffective *perilálēsis*, but what appears to be a (though based on incorrect premises) complex and argued explanation of a difficult text.

Another passage reveals a somewhat reversed perspective, where Sabinus tries to distinguish the meaning of two adjectives, *ánaudos* and *áphōnos*:[18]

17 مختلفان corr.: مختلفين cod.

18 *Commentary on Hippocrates' 'Epidemics'* 3.3.78; Wenkebach (1936), p. 172, line 28–p. 173, line 4; Raiola (2018), F 18.

Σαβῖνος δὲ κατὰ ταὐτὰ τοῖς ἄλλοις τὸν μὲν οὐδ' ὅλως ἔχοντα φωνὴν οὐδεμίαν *ἄναυδον* εἰρῆσθαι νομίζει, τὸ δ' ἄφωνον ἐν ἴσῳ τῷ *ἀπόπληκτον* ὑπὸ τοῦ Ἱπποκράτους γεγράφθαι φησίν, ὥσπερ οὐ δυναμένου καλέσαι τὸν οὕτω διακείμενον ἀπόπληκτον. οὐ μὴν οὐδὲ τἆλλα τὰ κατὰ ⟨ταύτην⟩[19] τὴν διάθεσιν εἰρημένα συνᾴδει τῷ γεγονέναι τὸν προκείμενον ἄρρωστον ἀπόπληκτον.

أما سابينس فظن أنه عنى بـ «عدم الصوت» «السكتة»، وهو الفالج. كان أبقراط لم يكن[20] يقدر أن يقول مكان ما قال «عدم الصوت» «أسكت» أو «أصابه فالج». وسائر ما ذكر أيضا من قصة هذا المريض ليس بموافق لقول من قال إنه أصابه فالج.

Sabinus, in the same way as others, believes that the man who has no voice at all is named *ánaudos* and he says that *áphōnos* was written by Hippocrates with the same meaning of *apóplēktos*, as if Hippocrates was not able to call such a man *apóplēktos*. Absolutely nothing of what (is said) about this disposition agrees with the patient in question being *apóplēktos*.

The exegesis applies to the third case history after the *katástasis*, where the case of Pythion is described. Pythion was a man from Thasos who on the fourth day became *ánaudos*, *áphōnos*. It is clear that Sabinus considers two distinguished conditions (and so *ánaudos* means 'without voice', 'mute'; *áphōnos* would be instead a synonym of *apóplēktos*, i.e. 'paralysed', 'cripped'). Galen points out that Sabinus' interpretation conflicts with the exact meaning of the two words and that the two adjectives should be understood as a sort of hendiadys, where the former means 'unable to articulate' and the latter 'voiceless', that is, 'unable to emit any kind of sound' as Pythion was 'completely unable to emit sounds'. In this case, leaving aside Galen's bias, we can reasonably suppose that behind Sabinus' statements (reported by Galen in very concise terms) there was a discussion supporting his exegesis, however we cannot, obviously, make inferences on how deep and precise it was.

19 ταύτην add. Wenkebach.
20 [يكن] in margine.

4 Use of Sources (and *opsimathía*)

Sabinus, like almost every other commentator, relies on other authors in order to consolidate his interpretation of the Hippocratic texts. Galen usually blames him for his use of the sources. For example, in a passage which closely follows the commentary on the case of Pythion,[21] Galen does not consider the authorities invoked by Sabinus (Democritus and Epicurus) to be relevant:[22]

> ἀλλ' ἐκ τοῦ μηδὲν ὧν ἴσασι δύνασθαι σιγῆσαι συμβαίνει τοῖς ὀψιμαθέσιν[23] ἐναντιώματα λέγειν ἀκαίρως φλυαροῦσιν. τίς γὰρ ἦν ἀνάγκη γράφειν Δημόκριτον μὲν εἰρηκέναι μικρὰν ἐπιληψίαν εἶναι τὴν συνουσίαν, Ἐπίκουρον δὲ μηδέποτε μὲν ὠφελεῖν ἀφροδισίων χρῆσιν, ἀγαπητὸν δ', εἰ μὴ βλάψειεν; ἐπὶ γὰρ τῶν ἐξ ἀφροδισίων ἀμέτρων νοσησάντων ἐχρῆν εἰρῆσθαι τοὺς λόγους, οὐκ ἐπὶ τῶν ἐναντίως αὐτοῖς διαιτηθέντων. ἀλλ' ὅμως καὶ ταῦτ' ἔγραψαν οἱ περὶ τὸν Σαβῖνον, οὐκ αἰσθανόμενοι τῆς ἐναντιολογίας.
>
> إلا أنه قد يعرض †للمرمدة† من قبل أنهم لا يصبرون أن يمسكوا عن ذكر شيء مما يحسنونه أن يأتوا بأقاويل متناقضة ويأتون بالشيء من غير موضعه فيصير هذيانا. وإلا فما الذي اضطرهم إلى أن كتبوا في هذا القول أن ديمقراطس قال إن الجماع إنما هو صراع إلا أنه من الصراع خفيف وإن إبيقورس قال إن الجماع لا ينفع من حال من الأحوال والقصارى منه ألا يضر. وذلك أن هذه الأقاويل إنما كان ينبغي أن يقال فيمن مرض من إفراط استعمال الجماع لا فيمن كان مرضه من ضد ذلك وآل سابينس مع هذا قد كتبوا هذه[24] الأقاويل في قصة بوثيون من غير أن يشعروا تناقض أقاويلهم.
>
> Because people who learn late cannot to stay silent about any of the things they know, it so happens that they make contradictory statements and talk nonsense. Why was it necessary to write that Democritus said that sexual activity is a 'small epilepsy'; or to write that 'Epicurus considered sex to be of no benefit, though it is pleasant if it does not harm'? They should have spoken about illnesses that result from excessive sexual intercourse, and not about those who follow a regimen contrary to theirs. Yet,

---

21 The first patient of this name in *Epidemics* 3, see above, p. 57.

22 *Commentary on Hippocrates' 'Epidemics'* 3.1.4; Wenkebach (1936), p. 25, lines 2–9; Raiola (2018), FF 11–12.

23 On the meaning of ὀψιμαθία, see e.g. Theophrastus, *On Characters* 27.

24 هذه] coni.: هذا cod.

Sabinus and his followers wrote this as well without noticing the contradiction.

Sabinus wanted to demonstrate that the *trómos* suffered by Pythion was the consequence of an abnormal stimulation of the *stómachos* owing to sexual abstinence, but it seems that the authors quoted by Sabinus mentioned the excess of sexual activity, and not abstinence. As a result, Sabinus' erudition turns into *opsimathía* ('learning acquired late'). The quotations from two authorities, far from strengthening the argument, undermine Sabinus' reputation, making him 'speak out of turn (*légein akaírōs*)', that is, 'speak nonsense (*perilaleîn*)'.

What concerns us more is that Sabinus made use of doxographical material to support his interpretation of Hippocrates. Quotations from the philosophical tradition are also attested by a passage from Sabinus' commentary on *Nature of Man*. Here, we learn that Sabinus, in his commentary, connected a philosopher to each physical element:[25]

> Οὔτε γὰρ τὸ πάμπαν ἠέρα λέγω τὸν ἄνθρωπον εἶναι ⟨οὔτε πῦρ⟩[26] οὔτε ὕδωρ οὔτε γῆν.
>
> For I do not say at all that a man is air, or fire, or water or earth.
>
> [...] κακῶς μὲν οὖν καὶ ὁ Καπίτων ἐτόλμησε μεταγράψαι τὴν παλαιὰν ῥῆσιν, οὔκουν οὐδὲ τοῦτο προσθείς, ὡς ἐνεδέχετο τὸν πρῶτον βιβλιογράφον ἁμαρτεῖν ἀντ' ἄλλου γράψαντ' ἄλλο, κακῶς δὲ καὶ τῶν ἐξηγητῶν ἔνιοι κατεψεύσαντο Ξενοφάνους, ὥσπερ καὶ Σαβῖνος, ὡδί πως γράψας αὐτοῖς ὀνόμασιν· 'οὔτε γὰρ τὸ πάμπαν ἀέρα λέγω τὸν ἄνθρωπον, ὥσπερ Ἀναξιμένης, οὔτε ὕδωρ,[27] ὡς Θαλῆς, οὔτε γῆν, ὡς ἔν τινι Ξενοφάνης.' οὐδαμόθι γὰρ εὑρίσκεται Ξενοφάνης ἀποφηνάμενος οὕτως. ἀλλὰ καὶ ὁ Σαβῖνος αὐτὸς εὔδηλός ἐστιν ἐκ τῶν αὐτοῦ καταψευδόμενος, οὐχ ὑπ' ἀγνοίας ἐσφαλμένος· ἢ πάντως ἂν ὀνομαστὶ προσέγραψε τὸ βιβλίον, ἐν ᾧ ταῦτα ἀπεφήνατο· νῦν δ' οὕτως ἔγραψεν· 'οὔτε γῆν, ὡς ἔν τινι Ξενοφάνης.'
>
> Capito was wrong in daring to change the ancient reading [he omitted 'οὔτε γῆν'], and he did not even add that the first copyist possibly made

25 Galen, *Commentary on Hippocrates' 'Nature of Man'* 1.2; Mewaldt (1914), 15, lines 11–21; Raiola (2018), F 3. The lemma is 6.32.4–5 L.

26 οὔτε πῦρ add. Cornarius Mewaldt.

27 οὔτε πῦρ, ὡς Ἡράκλειτος post ὕδωρ add. Mewaldt.

> a mistake and wrote something else. Some of the commentators were also wrong in making false claims about Xenophanes, as did, for instance Sabinus, who wrote the following words verbatim: 'For I do not say at all that a man is air, as Anaximenes, or water, as Thales, or earth, as in some work by Xenophanes'. Indeed, one cannot find Xenophanes saying anything of the sort in any of his books. But Sabinus himself shows with his own words that he made a false claim rather than being mistaken out of ignorance. Otherwise, he would have mentioned by name the book in which Xenophanes had affirmed these things. Instead, he wrote: 'nor earth, as in some work by Xenophanes'.

This passage proves that Sabinus wrote a scholarly commentary and his exegesis was anchored to the authorities of the past. And, last but not least, we learn that in this case he probably was more respectful of the Hippocratic text than the 'innovator' Artemidorus Capito.

This conservative attitude seems to disappear in the commentary on *Epidemics* 6, where Galen regularly includes Sabinus among those who changed the text of the ancient manuscripts. Perhaps this is due to the remarkable obscurity of the text of this book which induced commentators to intervene more frequently in order to 'normalize' the text when it appeared completely unintelligible. The passage below is a clear example of this approach:[28]

> φλέβες κροτάφων οὐχ ἱδρυμέναι οὐδὲ χλώρασμα λαμπρόν.

> Blood vessels of the temples not relaxed, and no bright freshness (of the skin).

> οὔσης οὖν ἀσαφοῦς καὶ αὐτῆς ταύτης τῆς λέξεως, ἔτι μᾶλλον ἀσάφεια γίνεται προσκειμένου τοῦ 'λαμπρόν'. ἄπορον γὰρ εὑρεῖν ὅ τι ποτὲ βούλεται δηλοῦν ἐκ τοῦ γράψαι χλώρασμα λαμπρόν. καὶ διὰ τοῦτ' ἄρα πᾶσαν τὴν τοιαύτην ἀσάφειαν θελήσαντές τινες φυγεῖν τῶν ἐξηγητῶν ἔγραψαν 'οὐ χρῶμα λαμπρόν' ἀκούειν τέ φασι δεῖν ἐπὶ τοῦ κατὰ φύσιν τοῦ κάμνοντος χρώματος τὸ λαμπρόν, οὕτω δὲ καὶ οἱ περὶ τὸν Σαβῖνον διελέχθησαν.

> Because this word ('*chlṓrasma*') is obscure in itself, it becomes even more obscure by adding *lamprón* to it. In fact, it is not easy to understand what he wants to indicate by writing '*chlṓrasma lamprón*'. Therefore some com-

28 *Commentary on Hippocrates' 'Epidemics'* 6.2.18; Wenkebach and Pfaff (1956), p. 79, lines 23–29; Raiola (2018), F 22; lemma *Epidemics* 6.2.6.1; 5.280.2–4 L.

mentators wished to avoid such an obscurity and wrote 'no bright colour (*ou chrôma lamprón*)', and said that '*lamprón*' should be understood as referring to the natural colour of the patient. Sabinus and his followers reasoned that same way.

5 Attention Paid to Concurrent Causes

Sabinus paid great attention to all the information provided by Hippocrates about the social status of the patients—where they came from, the places where they lived, or fell sick. Sabinus probably considered this data important for the diagnosis and conveniently emphasized them in his commentary. Galen takes every opportunity to make fun of his rival about this exegetical technique:[29]

Τρίτος ἄρρωστος. Ὁ κατακείμενος ἐν τῷ Δεάλκους κήπῳ.

Third case. The man lying in the garden of Dealces.

Κἀνταῦθα πάλιν οἱ περὶ τὸν Σαβῖνόν φασι ⟨τὸν κῆπον⟩ προσκεῖσθαι συναίτιον τῆς νόσου γενόμενον τἀνθρώπῳ, καὶ γράφουσί γε κατὰ λέξιν οὕτως· 'διὰ τοῦτο γὰρ μήποτε καὶ τὸν κῆπον παρέθετο, κἀντεῦθεν τὴν ἀφορμὴν τῷ πυρετῷ γεγονέναι ὑπεμφαίνων.[30] οὐ γάρ ἐστι ποηφάγον ζῷον ὁ ἄνθρωπος, ὥστε τῇ ἀλλοκότῳ διαίτῃ ⟨χρώμενος⟩[31] δικαίως ⟨τὸν⟩[32] νεωτερισμὸν ὑπομένειν.' καὶ ταῦτα μὲν ἐκεῖνοι γεγράφασιν.

إن آل سابينوس قد قالوا في هذا الموضع أيضا إن أبقراط إنما ذكر في قصة هذا المريض المقفلة لأنها كانت سببا مقبلا على حدوث العلة التي حدثت به وكتبوا في ذلك قولا بهذه الألفاظ: «ولعله يتورانا ذكر المقفلة ليدل بذكرها على أن سبب مرضه إنما كان من قبلها وذلك أن الإنسان ليس هو من الحيوان الذي غذاؤه العشب فيجب إن كان ذلك المريض قد استعمل عند امتنانها الطبيعة أن تحدث به علة» فهذا ما كتب آل سابينس.

29 *Commentary on Hippocrates' 'Epidemics'* 3.1.19; Wenkebach (1936), p. 48, line 18–p. 49, line 1; Raiola (2018), F 13; lemma *Epidemics* 3.1; 3.38.7 L.

30 κἀντεῦθεν O : τοίνυν ἐντεῦθεν L. *Pace* Raiola (2018); I now reject Wenkebach's corrections '⟨ἵνα⟩ τὴν ἀφορμὴν τοῦ πυρε⟨τὸν αὐ⟩τῷ γεγονέναι ὑπεμφήνῃ' as unnecessary.

31 χρώμενος suppl. Wenkebach in lacuna.

32 τὸν add. Wenkebach.

> Here again Sabinus and his followers say that the garden is the concurrent cause of the disease by which the man was seized, and they write verbatim: 'so, maybe he (Hippocrates) added "the garden", indicating that the fever takes its origin from there. For man is not a herbivorous animal, and if he follows that unusual diet, of course and fittingly, he suffers from the change.' This is what these men wrote.

Sabinus stresses the importance of the place where the patient lay sick—a garden. In fact, he interprets this information in the sense that the man became sick due to his vegetarian diet. In what follows this passage, Galen (as usual) disapproves of Sabinus' interpretation, arguing that the mention of the garden is a matter of no importance for medical purposes given that, in all probability, the patient did not usually live there and even so, says Galen, there is no need to infer that a man, living in (or near) a garden, would be compelled to eat only herbs and vegetables. In addition, many other factors might have been the cause of the disease. Galen pointed out that origins of the illness could have come from the exhalations of certain herbs, or the noxious smells coming from the manure.[33]

There are several other examples of Sabinus' tendency to gain information about the habits of the patients and their conduct before the disease from the initial words in the clinical cases of *Epidemics* (where Hippocrates briefly indicates places, job, geographical provenience of the patient). Sabinus appears to be trying to connect this information to the aetiology of the illness, in order to show that Hippocrates reported them with the purpose of guiding the diagnosis.[34]

This method seems to be applied often, but not always. See, for instance, the following passage from Galen's commentary on Book 3 of *Epidemics*:[35]

> Δεύτερος ἄρρωστος. Ἐν Θάσῳ τὴν κατακειμένην παρὰ τὸ ψυχρὸν ὕδωρ κτλ.

> Second case. In Thasos, the woman who lay sick by the cold water …

> Ἄξιον ἐπισημήνασθαι, πῶς οὐδὲν εἶπον οἱ περὶ τὸν Σαβῖνον περὶ τοῦ παρὰ τὸ ψυχρὸν ὕδωρ, ἐνὸν αὐτοῖς εἰπεῖν, ὅτι διὰ τοῦτο καταψυγέντι τῷ γυναίῳ νοσῆ-

33 See *Commentary on Hippocrates' 'Epidemics'* 3.1.19; Wenkebach (1936), p. 49, lines 2–20.

34 This reconstruction of the pathology through biographical details had been connected to the tradition of literary biography by Manetti and Roselli (1994), 1608 and note 298.

35 *Commentary on Hippocrates' 'Epidemics'* 3.3.77; Wenkebach (1936), p. 167, lines 1–6; Raiola (2018), F 17a; lemma *Epidemics* 3.17; 3.108.5 L.

σαι συνέβη. πολλῷ γὰρ ἦν τοῦτο πιθανώτερον τῶν εἰρημένων εἴς τε τὸν Πάριον ⟨τὸν⟩[36] παρὰ τῷ Ἀρτεμισίῳ καὶ τὸν ἐν τῷ κήπῳ κατακείμενον καὶ τὸν παρὰ τῷ τείχει[37] κατοικοῦντα.

قال جالينوس إني لأعجب كيف لم يقل آل سابينس شيئا في هذا الماء البارد الذي ذكر أبقراط. وقد كان يمكنهم يقولون إن تلك المرأة إنما عرض لها المرض من قبل أن ذلك الماء يبردها تبريدا شديدا فإن هذا القول [...][38] كان في المقفلة[39] وفي الآخر الذي كان في جانب هيكل أرطميس والآخر الذي كان مسكنه إلى جانب السور.

It is worth pointing out why Sabinus and his followers said nothing about the words 'by the cold water', although it was possible for them to say that the woman fell sick, because she got cold. This would have been much more plausible than what was said about the man from Paros who lay near the temple of Artemis, about that man who lay in the garden, or about the one who lived close to the wall.

Galen notes that Sabinus did not try to attribute the origin of the disease to the place where a woman lived (i.e. close to 'cold water'), although in this particular case that kind of interpretation was possible. This argument from silence seems to be somewhat ungenerous, but informs us that Sabinus was not systematic in the application of such a kind of exegesis, adapting his reasoning to the examined context.

6 Conclusion

This concise overview was meant to show some of the features of Sabinus' commentaries on Hippocrates. It is now possible to draw some conclusions from the passages we discussed. First, Sabinus carefully investigated all information provided by the text he commented on. In a few words, according to Sabinus, if Hippocrates had written something, he surely did it on purpose. This likely explains the great attention paid by this commentator to the places and to the

36 τὸν add. Wenkebach.
37 καινῷ ante τείχει add. Wenkebach sec. Hipp.; deest in codd. et vers. Arab.
38 The rest of the last line is illegible.
39 كان في المقفلة is a tentative reading of the manuscript.

geographical origin of the patients, from which he tries to reconstruct their way of life. Second, Sabinus quoted ancient authors with an apparent preference for philosophers. This sometimes led to *opsimathía* as Galen called it, but it is indicative of a scholarly commentary. Third, Sabinus was prone to use a florid style, not lacking in metaphors. His notes were rich in examples and he built wordy, long-winded sentences. These two aspects probably made Sabinus' commentaries popular among learned people, as attested by Gellius and Palladius.[40] Fourth and last, he surely was, in the eyes of his contemporaries, a highly valued commentator. Even Galen, who rebuts Sabinus every time he can, often seems to build his exegesis (especially that on *Epidemics*) on the refutation of Sabinus' opinions, whose commentaries were probably among the standard works in the field of Hippocratic studies when Galen wrote his own commentaries. This is indirectly confirmed by Galen himself in a passage from *On the Order of My Own Books*. Sabinus is here, somewhat to our surprise, among the commentators who Galen recommended to his pupils, to replace the commentaries he had not yet written.[41] But, since Sabinus' commentaries are far from being perfect, they must always be read in light of his own doctrine, as Galen remarks a few lines above:[42]

> ἄμεινον γὰρ ἔγνωσαν (*scil.* τὴν Ἱπποκράτους γνώμην) οἱ περὶ Σαβῖνόν τε καὶ Ῥοῦφον· ὁ δ' ἐν ταῖς ἡμετέραις πραγματείαις προγεγυμνασμένος ἱκανὸς καὶ τὰ τούτων κρίνειν καὶ φωρᾶσαι τά τε καλῶς ὑπ' αὐτῶν εἰρημένα καὶ εἴ που τύχοιεν ἐσφαλμένοι.
>
> Sabinus, Rufus and their followers understood (Hippocrates' thought) best. He who has been trained in our books beforehand is easily able to evaluate their statements and to detect both what is well said and the things they failed to understand.

40 For the quotation in Gellius see above, note 13. The adverb used by Gellius to describe Sabinus' exegesis, *commodissime*, means at the same time 'neatly', 'properly', 'skilfully' and indicates great appreciation: Gellius uses it only one more time, in a hendiadys with *aptissime*, to describe Cicero's translation of Theophrastus (see *Attic Nights* 1.3.9). Palladius the Iatrosophist (sixth century AD) records an interpretation made by Sabinus to book 6 of the *Epidemics*, describing his exegesis by the adjective *asteióteros*, comparative of *asteîos* ('polite', 'refined', 'elegant'): see *Commentary on Hippocrates' 'Epidemics'* 6.3.7; Dietz (1834), vol. 2, p. 80, lines 10–11.

41 *Order of His Own Books* 3.6; Boudon-Millot (2007), p. 98, lines 6–14.

42 *Order of His Own Books* 3.11–12; Boudon-Millot (2007), p. 99, lines 5–9; Raiola (2018), test. 11b.

These words, coming from a bio-bibliographical text, may offer a perspective which is more objective or, at least, less influenced by polemical issues. Seen in that light, Sabinus' commentaries, far from being perfect, appear to be reliable and tools worth reading which are suitable for students but probably not for experts.

CHAPTER 4

Galen as Commentator of Commentaries: The Case of the Hippocratic *Epidemics* 1 and 3

Jacques Jouanna

There is a remarkable contrast between the role previous commentators play in Galen's commentary on *Epidemics* 1 and on *Epidemics* 3.[*, 1] The numbers speak for themselves: in his commentary on *Epidemics* 1, Galen only cites one proper name (Quintus, first century AD), whilst in his commentary on *Epidemics* 3 he quotes fourteen.[2] This contrast becomes even more striking if we consider that the treatises *Epidemics* 1 and 3 are two separate parts of one and the same treatise attributed to Hippocrates.[3]

Beyond the striking difference in the number of quotations from earlier authors, Galen is himself conscious of doing something new, and explains it at the beginning of his commentary on *Epidemics* 3: first, Galen is above all a witness and critic of the commentators who have preceded him; second, he also provides information about and justifications for his own commentary. We are thus dealing with two exegetical modes: Galen comments not only on the commentaries of other scholars, but also on his own ones. We shall examine these two aspects in turn.

---

* I would like to express my profound gratitude to Peter E. Pormann and Elaine van Dalen for expertly translating this contribution into English. Pormann also helped establish the Greek text by providing a provisional edition of the Arabic translation of Galen's commentary for all the passages from *Epidemics* 3.

1 I have already devoted an essay to the contrast between these two commentaries offering a comparison of the three last patient records of *Epidemics* 1 and the three first patient records of *Epidemics* 3 (Jouanna 2015). This essay was analytical and more oriented on questions of structure and finalising the text, whereas the present article is more concise and deals with the commentators themselves; these two approaches complete each other.

2 For Galen's commentaries on *Epidemics* 1 and *Epidemics* 3, see the two editions by Wenkebach and Pfaff (1934) and Wenkebach (1936). The key study on Galen's commentaries remains Manetti and Roselli (1994), who discuss *Epidemics* 1 on pp. 1540–1542 and *Epidemics 3* on pp. 1552–1553.

3 For unity of the two books, see Jouanna (2016), xii–xxvii.

© JACQUES JOUANNA, 2021 | DOI:10.1163/9789004470200_006

1 Galen as Commentator of Commentaries by Other Exegetes of Hippocrates: the Commentaries on *Epidemics* 1 and 3

First of all, we should have a look at the names that Galen mentions in his commentaries on *Epidemics* 1 and 3. They are presented chronologically in the list below followed by the number of times they are mentioned:[4]

Epidemics 1 (ed. Wenkebach 1934):

1. Quintus (1st c. AD): 6 times (p. 6, lines 7, 11, 19; p. 17, lines 3, 18; p. 52, line 26).

Epidemics 3 (ed. Wenkebach and Pfaff 1936):

1. Mnemon of Side (3rd c. BC): 8 times (p. 77, lines 19 [based on a conjecture], 22; p. 79, lines 4, 16, 18; p. 80, line 7; p. 87, line 7; p. 157, line 11).
2. Zeno, the Herophilian (2nd c. BC): 19 times (p. 75, line 25; p. 76, line 24; p. 77, lines 6, 14, 16, 23; p. 86, lines 7, 16, 21; p. 87, lines 2, 3, 12; p. 89, line 22; p. 91, lines 16, 21 [based on a conjecture]; p. 92, lines 5, 10, 17; p. 93, line 5).
3. Zeuxis (2nd c. BC): 4 times (p. 78, line 29; p. 79, line 2; p. 169, line 9 [based on a conjecture]; p. 176, line 18)
4. Apollonius Empiricus (2nd c. BC): 2 times (p. 86, line 22; p. 91, line 16 [based on a conjecture]).
5. Apollonius Biblas, son of Apollonius Empiricus: 2 times (p. 87, line 2; p. 91, line 16 [based on a conjecture]).
6. Asclepiades of Bithynia (2nd/1st c. BC): 1 time (p. 161, line 19).
7. Heraclides of Erythrae (1st c. BC): 1 time (p. 80, line 16).
8. Heraclides of Tarantum (1st c. BC): 6 times (p. 80, line 15; p. 87, line 14; p. 88, lines 1, 6; p. 89, lines 9, 14, 23).
9. Quintus (1st/2nd c. AD): 6 times (p. 14, line 13; p. 17, line 1; p. 21, line 26; p. 59, lines 15, 16, 18);
10. Sabinus (1st/2nd c. AD): 17 times (p. 17, line 22; p. 18, line 6; p. 21, line 24; p. 23, line 28; p. 25, line 9; p. 40, line 11; p. 48, line 18; p. 72, lines 13, 17; p. 154, line 18; p. 165, line 11; p. 166, lines 6, 13; p. 167, line 1; p. 169, line 6; p. 172, line 28; p. 176, line 18).
11. Metrodorus (2nd c. AD), pupil of Sabinus: 1 time (p. 17, line 22).
12. Lycus of Macedonia (2nd c. AD): 11 times (p. 14, lines 5, 13; p. 15, lines 9, line 18; p. 16, lines 1, 5, 23; p. 17, line 7; p. 21, line 26; p. 59, line 14; p. 154, line 14).

4 This list draws on data provided by Anastassiou, Irmer (1997–2012), vol. 1, pp. 215–216, vol. 2.1, pp. 229–230.

13. Aephicianus (2nd c. AD): 1 time (p. 59, line 17).
14. Satyrus (2nd c. AD): 1 time (p. 59, line 17).

This list would on its own be enough to demonstrate the sharp contrast between *Epidemics* 1 and *Epidemics* 3 as regards previous authorities.

The only predecessor whom Galen mentions in both his commentaries is Quintus, a physician from Pergamum who lived slightly earlier than Galen in the late first or early second century AD, and who commented on the *Epidemics* in his lectures. Galen mentions Quintus in his commentary on *Epidemics* 1 in order to reproach him for not having retained essential parts of Hippocrates' text, namely the possibility to give a prognosis of diseases based on location and time of year.[5] In his commentary on *Epidemics* 3, Galen also mentions him in relation to the first patient Pythion, which proves that Quintus not only commented on *Epidemics* 1, but also on *Epidemics* 3. Galen then clarifies the source of his disciple Lycus' commentary, explaining that he adopts comparisons already made by Quintus between *Epidemics* 3 and *Prorrhetics* 1.[6] That the network of Galen's predecessors in *Epidemics* 3 is more ample than in *Epidemics* 1 is therefore obvious straight from the beginning, since Galen quotes a commentator who quotes another commentator.[7]

To avoid losing sight of the larger picture, we must first evaluate the chronological span of the fourteen names mentioned by Galen in his commentary on *Epidemics* 3: they range from the Hellenistic period at the end of the third century BC to Galen's own time in the second century AD; in other words, they span more than four centuries. They form a truly exceptional group, which we can only understand fully, when we examine what organisational principle Galen followed when mentioning them. It is possibly to class them into two categories corresponding to two major approaches in Galen's commentary on *Epidemics* 3: first, Galen points out flaws in previous commentaries; and second, he explains the so-called 'characters' (χαρακτῆρες), signs at the end of the patient records, normally written in groups of five letters.[8] It turns out that some commentat-

5 On Quintus as a commentator of Hippocrates, see Grmek and Gourevitch (1994) 1501–1510 (including a translation of the main passages of *Epidemics* 1 in which Quintus is mentioned) and Manetti and Roselli (1994), 1580–1581.

6 Ed. Wenkebach (1936), p. 14, lines 12–14.

7 We cannot agree with Grmek and Gourevitch (1994, 1510) that Galen tells us in his commentary on *Epidemics* 3.1.4 (ed. Wenkebach and Pfaff 1936, pp. 14, 17) that 'Quintus knew and used Lycus' commentaries'. On the contrary, Lycus attended Quintus' lectures (see Wenkebach 1936, p. 59, line 15–16). On Lycus, see Manetti and Roselli (1994), 1582–1588, especially note 197, which contains further reading.

8 Galen himself highlights these two aspects of his commentary through two concise digressions: one about 'those who explain badly (περὶ τῶν μοχθηρῶς ἐξηγουμένων)' (Wenkebach

ors specialised in the explanation of these characters, differing from those who commented on the whole treatise. These 'character specialists' happen to be the oldest commentators. They are the first seven on the list above, except for Asclepiades of Bithynia (nr. 6).

These oldest predecessors of Galen allow us to go as far back as possible into the history of the text of *Epidemics* 3, from the third to the first century BC. Galen believed that it was Mnemon of Side who added the characters at the end of the patient records in *Epidemics* 3, either in a copy of the Great Library of Alexandria (which he would have borrowed as a reader), or in a manuscript that he would have brought himself. Galen derived this information from the first book of Zeuxis' commentary on *Epidemics* 3.[9] This was probably also the book on which Galen based his famous description of the shipment of the manuscripts of the Greek tragedians Aeschylus, Sophocles and Euripides from Athens to Alexandria.[10] Zeuxis commented on all the characters at the end of each patient record in *Epidemics* 3.[11] Even more often than Zeuxis, Galen cites a work on the characters by Zeno, the Herophilian.[12] He also mentions his opponents (οἱ ἀντιλέγοντες τῷ Ζήνωνι).[13] Among them, he lists the empiricist Apollonius who wrote a treatise on the characters in which he refuted Zeno, and to whom Zeno replied in person. The debate was continued by the son of Apollonius, Biblas, who published a work on the characters which appeared after Zeno's death. One of the issues at stake in this debate was the authenticity of the characters. The dispute centred around the meaning of the first character present in all patient records, the famous pi written with an additional central line, which can be interpreted as 'πιθανόν (it is probable that)'.[14] According to Zeno, the characters derived from Hippocrates, but the empiricists disagreed with this.

Let us now discuss the second group of Galen's predecessors, those who commented badly on *Epidemics* 3. These commentators, who are listed in the second part of the list presented above, lived closer to Galen in chronological terms. Galen most frequently cites the three commentators Quintus (6 times), his pupil Lycus (11 times), and Sabinus (17 times), the most frequently men-

1936), p. 10, line 9–p. 26, line 33), the other about 'about the "characters" added to each of the patients' [records] (περὶ τῶν προσγεγραμμένων χαρακτήρων ἑκάστῳ τῶν ἀρρώστων)' (Wenkebach 1936, p. 27, line 1–p. 28, line 27).

9 Wenkebach (1936), p. 78, line 29.

10 Wenkebach (1936), p. 79, line 23–p. 80, line 19.

11 Wenkebach (1936), p. 169, line 9 (based on a conjecture); p. 176, line 18.

12 First attested in Wenkebach (1936), p. 75, line 25.

13 Wenkebach (1936), p. 77, line 14.

14 Wenkebach (1936), p. 91, line 20–p. 92, line 2.

tioned commentator in the commentary on *Epidemics* 3. In addition to these, Sabinus' pupil Metrodorus is also cited once. In his work *On the Order of My Own Books*, Galen lists Quintus and Lycus among the most important commentators of Hippocrates before him. Here, he condemns both of them for 'not having understood Hippocrates' thought.'[15] He continues saying that 'Sabinus and his followers, as well as Rufus and his followers, have understood it better.' Yet, in this work Sabinus is classed among the inferior commentators, whilst Rufus is not mentioned.

I shall discuss Sabinus in more detail, because many of his passages are quoted word for word in Galen's commentary on *Epidemics* 3, which does not happen in the case of the other commentators.[16] Sabinus is the first commentator whom Galen challenges in his commentary on the first patient, Pythion. Confusingly, Galen here gives an anonymous quotation (Wenkebach 1936, 11, 2 ἑνός), but much later reveals the name of the author in an oblique fashion.[17] We can, however, be sure that this anonymous quotation derives from the beginning of Sabinus' commentary on the first patient of *Epidemics* 3, Pythion, who lived by the Temple of the Earth:[18]

> … ὧν ἑνὸς παραγράψω τὴν ῥῆσιν αὐτοῖς ὀνόμασιν, ἵνα μή τις οἰηθῇ με καταψεύδεσθαι τἀνδρός· 'τὸ μέντοι τῆς Γῆς ἱερὸν τὸ τῆς Δήμητρος λέγει. παρείληφε μὲν ⟨τοῦ⟩το τὸ ἱερὸν μήποτε ὑπὲρ τοῦ δεῖξαι τὴν αἰτίαν, ἀφ' ἧς ⟨ὁ⟩ τρόμος τῶν χειρῶν καὶ τὸ νοσεῖν αὐτῷ ἐγένετο, ὡς τῇ ⟨…⟩ διὰ τὴν ἐποχὴν τῶν ἐπιμηνίων γενομένην, ὡς εἰκός, διὰ τὴν τοῦ μορίου ἀργίαν. καὶ πάλιν ἐν τῷ ἕκτῳ ἱστορεῖ, τἀνδρὸς ἀποδήμου γενομένου, ἀργευσαμένην τῷ μορίῳ τὴν γυναῖκα ἀναληφθέντων τῶν ἐπιμηνίων εἰς τὸ στόμα φῦσαι πώγωνα. καὶ τί γὰρ ἄλλο ἢ ἀνδρωθῆναι τὴν γυναῖκα; οὕτως οὖν καὶ Πυθίων ἀποσχόμενος συνουσίας διὰ τὴν πρὸς μόνον ἐπιμέλειαν τὸ ἱερὸν ⟨τὴν⟩ νόσον ὑπομένει.'

وأحد أنواع التفسير الرديء النوع الذي استعمله قوم في تفسير ما وصف من أمر هذا المريض.[19] وأنا واضع كلام واحد واحد منهم بألفاظه، كيما لا يظن في أني تقولت على ذلك

15 3.11 (ed. Boudon-Millot 2007, p. 99, lines 5–6).

16 See Manetti and Roselli (1994), 1607–1614, especially note 289 containing further literature. See now Raiola (2018).

17 Whilst Sabinus' name appears for the first time a little further on (Wenkebach 1936, 17, line 22), there is evidence of it at the beginning of the commentary on the third patient, as I shall show below.

18 Wenkebach (1936), p. 11, lines 3–14; the Arabic is edited according to Madrid, Escorial, MS 804 árabe, fol. 135[a], lines 1–10; Raiola (2018), F 11a.

19 مريض coni.: مرض E.

الرجل. وهذا قوله بألفاظه: قال «إن أبقراط إنما عنى بهيكل الأرض ديميطر. وخليق أن يكون إنما ذكر الهيكل كيما يبين السبب الذي منه عرض لهذا المريض رعشة اليدين ومنه كان مرضه. وإنما امتناعه كان من القساء [؟]. فقد قال في المقالة الأولى أيضا إنه عرض لماليديا التي كانت تسكن عند هيكل إيرا مرض من احتباس الطمث. ويشبه أن يكون ذلك الاحتباس إنما كان لتعطل الرحم. وذكر أيضا في المقالة السادسة امرأة[20] غاب زوجها عنها. فلما تعطل منها الرحم، تراقى دم الطمث إلى فيها[21]، وأنبت لها لحية، ومالت إلى طبيعة الرجل. وكذلك أيضا بوثيون لما امتنع من الجماع لتجديده التقيد في الهيكل عرض له ذلك المرض.»

I will transcribe a passage by one of them [the commentators] in his own words, so that nobody will think that I am slandering this man: 'He [Hippocrates] calls the 'Temple of the Earth' 'Temple of Demeter'. He possibly (μήποτε) mentions this temple to demonstrate the cause why his hands shook and he became ill:[22] *his abstinence was caused by hardness.*[23] *He also said in the first book of the Epidemics that Melidia, who lived near the Temple of Hera, became ill* because her menses were retained, probably because of the part [of the body, i.e., the womb] was idle. He also discussed in the sixth book a woman whose husband was absent. Since her womb was idle, menstrual blood ascended to her mouth, so that she grew a beard. What else is this than a transformation into a man? Likewise, when Pythion abstained from sexual intercourse because he was solely concerned for the temple,[24] he also suffered this disease.'

By quoting this lengthy passage, Galen wants to avoid being accused of misrepresenting the thought of the commentator whom he is about to critique.

20 امرأة coni.: مرأة E.

21 فيها] coni. (τὸ στόμα): بدنها، E.

22 The Arabic version shows that we most likely have here an omission because of a homoeoteleuton ('saut du même au même'); I have supplied the lacuna from the Arabic translation, here put in Italics. Wenkebach filled this lacuna with the following Greek text, but it omits the first sentence and also suggests a confidence about the Greek that can hardly be justified: 'Μελιδίᾳ τῇ κατὰ τὸ πρῶτον τῶν Ἐπιδημιῶν γεγραμμένῃ, ἣ κατέκειτο παρὰ τὸ τῆς Ἥρας ἱερόν'.

23 The reading of the word '*qasā*' (hardness)' is uncertain.

24 The Greek construction 'διὰ τὴν πρὸς μόνον ἐπιμέλειαν τὸ ἱερὸν' with the hyperbaton 'μόνον … τὸ ἱερὸν' is harsh, although retained by Wenkebach in his text. The Arabic has 'because he renewed his adherence to the temple (*li-taǧdīdihī l-taqayyuda fī l-haykali*)', which might suggest that there is a textual problem here.

Galen criticises this part of Sabinus' commentary for the causal relation established between the patient's location and the cause of his disease. According to Sabinus, Pythion abstained from sexual relations because he lived close to the Temple of the Earth. He believed that his sexual abstinence resulted in a state of plethora which caused his hands to shake as well as various other symptoms. Galen disagrees with this suggested aetiology. For one would have to assume a similar relation of cause and effect in all the other cases where one knows where the patient lives, which is impossible. Galen continues with a long argument against the explanation of the different symptoms as resulting from a state of plethora caused by a lack of sexual relations. In this argument, he attacks Sabinus and his followers by name (five times).[25] Galen castigates his adversaries for using a more confident tone in their conclusion than in their initial position. He then returns to the suggested relation between place of abode and absence of sexual relations to refute it with a new argument: the proximity of the Temple of the Earth does not mean that the patient was a priest or servant of the goddess, and even if he was, this does not imply that he would have remained chaste, as in the case of the cult of Artemis or Athena.[26]

That Sabinus was undoubtedly the author of this passage is proven by the way in which Galen introduces a new criticism of Sabinus when he begins his commentary of the third patient, who lived in the garden of Dealces.

> And here Sabinus and his followers again (πάλιν) say that the garden is mentioned as the secondary cause (συναίτιον) of the disease in the case of this person.[27]

The use of the adverb 'πάλιν (again)' clearly refers to the preceding passage in which Pythion's disease is explained by the closeness of the Temple of the Earth.

After this, Galen gives another exact quotation from Sabinus' commentary, saying:

25 Throughout the commentary of this first patient record, the author explicitly critiques other interpretations of Sabinus (Wenkebach 1936, p. 17, line 22 οἱ τοίνυν περὶ Σαβῖνον καὶ τὸν μαθητὴν αὐτοῦ Μητρόδωρον; p. 18, line 6 οἱ περὶ Σαβῖνον; p. 21, line 24 τοῖς δὲ περὶ τὸν Σαβῖνον; p. 23, line 28 οἵ γε περὶ τὸν Σαβῖνον and p. 25, line 9 οἱ περὶ τὸν Σαβῖνον).

26 This remarkable testimony on the question of the chastity of priests seems not to have been known to specialists of greek religion.

27 Wenkebach (1936), p. 48, lines 18–20; Raiola (2018), F 13.

> … and they write verbatim: 'so, maybe he (Hippocrates) added "the garden", indicating in veiled terms (ὑπεμφαίνων) that the fever takes its origin from there. For man is not a herbivorous animal, and if he follows that unusual diet, of course and fittingly, he suffers from the change.'[28]

This is another literal quotation like the first.[29] Since the two passages are quoted so precisely, they reveal some of the characteristics of Sabinus' style. In one of them, Sabinus uses the word μήποτε in the sense of 'maybe', which is uncommon in Galen, as Daniela Manetti and Amneris Roselli already remarked in their key work on Galen's commentaries on Hippocrates.[30] One should also note the use of the rare compound verb ὑπεμφαίνω in the sense of 'to indicate in veiled terms.' It captures Sabinus' method as a commentator who wants to bring out what he believes is implicit in Hippocrates' text. Sabinus thinks that the patient's place of abode specified by Hippocrates is an important medical detail in case of both the first and the third patient. According to him, the garden is one of the causes of the disease (συναίτιον).[31] The patient who lived in the garden followed a vegetarian diet which became harmful for him.

Galen formulates three lengthy objections against Sabinus' commentary. First, Hippocrates says that the patient was lying in the Garden of Dealces; this does not mean that he lived there when he was healthy.[32] Second, a man who lives in a garden does not necessarily eat grass constantly, like a herbivorous animal.[33] Third, if one wanted to establish a relation between the garden and the disease, there would be another explanation which Sabinus ignored, namely the inferior air coming from the canals where excrements were dumped, as well as the inferior smell of certain plants.[34]

In a similar vein, Galen inveighs against Sabinus for drawing too far-reaching conclusions from the patient's origin, as he had done in the case of the first patient mentioned after Hippocrates' nosological constitution, namely 'the Parian (τὸν Πάριον)'. Galen employs the same rhetorical strategy that he has

28 For a fuller quotation of this passage, see Raiola in this volume on pp. 63–64.

29 To introduce these two quotations, Galen repeatedly insists on their literality. In the case of the first quotation, he does so using the expression 'αὐτοῖς ὀνόμασιν (with his own words)' (Wenkebach 1936, 11, line 3); and here, with the expression κατὰ λέξιν.

30 Manetti and Roselli (1994), 1608, n. 297.

31 Wenkebach (1936), p. 48, line 19.

32 Wenkebach (1936), p. 49, line 1.

33 Wenkebach (1936), p. 49, lines 5–6.

34 Wenkebach (1936), p. 49, line 11.

used from the very beginning against Sabinus: he first quotes a commentary passages, and only later reveals that he has been talking of Sabinus. This is the beginning of the commentary on this patient:[35]

> Περιέργως κἀνταῦθα πάλιν τῶν ἐξηγητῶν ἔνιοι τὴν πατρίδα τοῦ κατακειμένου φασὶν οὐκ ἀργῶς προσκεῖσθαι. καὶ γὰρ ὑπ' Ἀσκληπιάδου λελέχθαι τοὺς ἐν Πάρῳ μάλισθ' ὑπὸ φλεβοτομίας ὀνίνασθαι. ἄτοπον δ' ἐστὶ μηδὲν εἰρηκότος Ἱπποκράτους ἐνταῦθα περὶ φλεβοτομίας, διὰ τοῦθ' ἡγεῖσθαι προσγεγράφθαι τῷ κάμνοντι τὸ τῆς πατρίδος ὄνομα. πολὺ δ' ἀτοπώτερον οἱ οὕτως ἐξηγούμενοι ποιοῦσιν, ὅτι μηδ' ἐζήτησάν ποτε, διὰ τί φλεβοτομίας ἅπαξ ὁ Ἱπποκράτης ἐμνημόνευσεν ἐν τοσούτοις ἀρρώστοις, ὅπερ ἡμεῖς ἐσκεψάμεθα.
>
> قد عبث أيضا قوم من المفسرين في قصة هذا المريض فقالوا إن أبقراط لم يتذكر أهل بيت هذا المريض باطلا،[36] لكنه لما ذكر ذلك لأن أسقليبيادس قال إن أهل باريون انتفعوا خاصة بالفصد. ومن الشَنِـع أن يكون أبقراط لم يذكر في قصة هذا المريض شيئا من أمر الفصد لتوهم أن أبقراط إنما ذكر أمر هذا المريض للعلة التي ذكروا. وأشنع من هذا ما فعله من فسر هذا التعبير أنهم لم يطلبوا في حال من الأحوال ويبحثوا عن السبب الذي من أجله لم يذكر أبقراط في أقاصيص المرضى على كثرة عددهم وقد بحثت[37] في ذلك
>
> Again, some commentators redundantly say that the home of the bedridden man is not added in vain. In fact, [they say] that Asclepiades said that those who live in Paros benefit the most from phlebotomy. Yet since Hippocrates has not spoken about phlebotomy here, it is absurd to think that this is the reason that the patient's home was mentioned in addition to his name. It is even more absurd that the commentators who think in this direction have not enquired why Hippocrates has only mentioned phlebotomy once in his discussion of so many patients; we, however, have looked into this.

Galen only reveals the identity of the commentator in question a few pages later when he states that 'what Sabinus has said about the home of this patient, I have mentioned previously.'[38]

---

35 Wenkebach (1936), p. 161, line 18–p. 162, line 6; Raiola (2018), F 16a.
36 باطلا] coni. واطلا E.
37 الذي ... بحث] in margine.
38 Wenkebach (1936), p. 165, lines 11–13.

Certainly, we can only agree with Galen's position and his critique of the wrongful connection made by Sabinus between place and patient. We must, however, also emphasise that Sabinus' position on the natural environment's influence as a secondary cause of disease was not unique among the commentators on *Epidemics* 3 before Galen. In fact, in the case of the second patient before the constitution, Hermocrates who lived near the New Wall (*Epidemics* 3.1.2), a debate formed among the commentators who believed that the environment influenced the disease itself. Some posited that the quicklime used during the construction of the remparts had a harmful effect, whereas others were of the opinion that the disease resulted from lack of fresh air, as the new remparts blocked it.[39]

Galen does not mention any of these commentators by name, but Sabinus was one of them. We find proof of this later, when Galen expresses his surprise, not without irony, at the fact that Sabinus has not made a connection between the place and the disease of the patient who lived near the cold water fountain. This is the second patient after the nosological constitution. Galen's spiteful remark reads as follows:[40]

> It is worth pointing out why Sabinus and his followers said nothing about the words 'by the cold water', although it was possible for them to say that the woman fell sick, because she got cold. This would have been much more plausible than what was said about the man from Paros who lay near the temple of Artemis, about that man who lay in the garden, or about the one who lived close to the wall.

The 'one who lived close to the wall' is a direct reference to the second patient before the constitution, Hermocrates, who lived near the new defence wall.

Another example of an important quotation of Sabinus is found with respect to the seventh patient before the fourth constitution (*Epidemics* 3.1.7). It involves an explanation of an unclear symptom, namely 'elevated respiration (πνεῦμα μετέωρον)', which is rejected by Galen. This quotation of Sabinus reads as follows:[41]

---

39 Wenkebach (1936), p. 29, lines 8–16. It remains unclear which of these explanations—the stench of the quicklime or the lack of fresh air—should be attributed to Sabinus. I have tentatively suggested that the quicklime is the more likely explanation, but this remains only a hypothesis (Jouanna 2015).

40 Wenkebach (1936), p. 167, lines 1–6; Raiola (2018), F 17a; the passage is also quoted in Raiola's article on pp. 64–65.

41 Wenkebach (1936), p. 72, line 12–18.

> φαίνεται δὴ τὸ πνεῦμα μετέωρον οὐκ εἶναι σαφές. ἀμέλει Σαβῖνος ὑπὲρ αὐτοῦ κατὰ τήνδε τὴν λέξιν ἔγραψε· 'μετέωρος δ' ἦν ἡ ἀναπνοή, τουτέστιν ἄκρᾳ τῇ ῥινὶ ἀνέπνει, διὰ φλεγμονὴν τῆς ἀρτηρίας, κλειομένης τῆς εὐρυχωρίας καὶ μηκέτι δυναμένης τῆς ὁλκῆς τοῦ πνεύματος εἰς τὸν πνεύμονα γενέσθαι.' ἀσαφὴς δ' ἐστὶ καὶ ἡ αὐτοῦ τοῦ Σαβίνου ῥῆσις, ὡς ἐξηγητοῦ πάλιν ἑτέρου δεῖσθαι.
>
> فأقول إن مما ليس معناه بأبين قوله «إنه كان نَفَسه عاليا». ولذلك قد رام سابينوس شرحه، فقال بهذا اللفظ: «وكان نَفَسها عاليا يعني أنها إنما كان يتنفس بطرف أنفها. وذلك أن مجرى قصبة الرئة كان قد انسد بالورم الذي كان فيه. فلم يكن ممكنا[42] أن يكون اجتذاب هذا التنفس إلى الرئة.» وهذا الكلام أيضا من سابينس غامض غير بين حتى يحتاج أيضا إلى مفسر آخر يشرحه.
>
> It seems that the phrase 'elevated breathing' is not clear. Sabinus of course wrote about this, the following being an exact quotation: '"The breathing was elevated" means that he breathed in through the upper part of the nose, because of an inflammation of the windpipe, so that the free passage was closed and the bulk of the breath could no longer reach the lungs.' This explanation of Sabinus himself, however, is unclear and requires another commentator [to explain it].

Galen uses the same formula to introduce the quotation, emphasising that it is quoted literally (κατὰ τήνδε τὴν λέξιν). Galen's critique of Sabinus' explanation involves a clever play on words aimed at refuting the usefulness of Sabinus' commentary. Hippocrates' phrase may not be clear (οὐκ εἶναι σαφές), but nor is Sabinus' own (ἀσαφὴς … ἡ τοῦ Σαβίνου ῥῆσις), to the point that the commentator Sabinus requires another commentator to explain his explication. Galen assumes this role of second commentator. He is therefore in this case a commentator of a commentator of Hippocrates in the true sense of the word. Only after commenting on Sabinus does he provide his own interpretation of Hippocrates' phrase, which differs from that of Sabinus. And there are other quotations in this book.[43]

These examples constitute a web of references to Sabinus' commentary which allows us to confirm that Galen had access to a continuous copy of Sabinus' commentary on *Epidemics* 3, from which he could quote. Galen cri-

---

42 ممكنا] corr.: ممكن E.

43 Wenkebach (1936), p. 40, lines 11–12; p. 154, lines 18–19; and p. 173, line 1.

ticised in particular Sabinus' tendency to over-interpret the Hippocratic text by creating a direct relationship of cause and effect between environment and disease. Galen does not, however, limit his criticism of Sabinus to this, but also takes him to task for his interpretation of particular phrases. Here, Galen continues to quote directly from Sabinus' commentary. I shall adduce Galen's longest quotation from Sabinus as an example. The former rebukes the latter for how he interpreted the symptom 'he passes an oily urine (οὔρησεν ἐλαιῶδες)' in the record of the Parian. This is Galen's second criticism of Sabinus' commentary on this patient:[44]

> Σαβῖνος τοίνυν 〈ἃ μὲν〉 περὶ τῆς πατρίδος τοῦ κάμνοντος τοῦδε εἶπεν, ἔμπροσθεν ἐπεσημηνάμην· ἃ δὲ περὶ τοῦ ἐλαιώδους οὔρου, νῦν ἐρῶ, διαφέρει γὰρ οὐκ εἰς μικρὸν ἡ περὶ τούτου θεωρία. γράφει δὴ περὶ αὐτοῦ κατὰ λέξιν ὧδε· 'τὸ οὖν ἐλαιῶδές τινες χολὴν ὠχρὰν[45] λέγουσιν· ἀλλ' οὐκ ἔστι χολή, ἐπεὶ οὐδ' ἂν πάνυ ἦν ὀλέθριον· πολλάκις γὰρ ἀπαλλάσσεται χολὴ καὶ οὐδὲν παραλυπεῖ. ἕτεροι δὲ λέγουσι νεύρων καὶ ὀστῶν καὶ χόνδρων εἶναι τηκεδόνα, ἅπαντα γὰρ ταῦτα τούτου εἶναι τοῦ χρώματος. πεπλανημένοι δ' εἰσὶν οὗτοι οἱ τὸ χρῶμα τὸ ἐλαιῶδες ὅμοιον ὀστοῖς καὶ χόνδροις καὶ νεύροις φάσκοντες εἶναι. οὔτε γὰρ τοσαύτη γε παράτασις ἐγένετο τῆς ζωῆς τῶν στερεῶν ἀναλυομένων (ἑκατοστῇ γὰρ καὶ εἰκοστῇ ἀπέθανεν), οὔτε ἀπέθανέ τις τοιοῦτον οὐρήσας. καὶ μήποτε διὰ τοῦτο ἀνεγράφη ὁ ἄρρωστος, ἵνα δείξῃ διὰ τούτου ὅτι οὐ χρὴ προσδοκᾶν θάνατον ἐλαιώδους ἀπουρηθέντος, ἀλλὰ καὶ χρόνον τινὰ δυνατὸν διαρκέσαι, ἔπειτα τελευτῆσαι, ὥστε οὐδὲν ἦν ἐλπίσαι[46] σωθήσεσθαι ὑπερβεβηκότα τὴν ὀξύτητα.' ταῦτα προειπὼν ὁ Σαβῖνος ἐφεξῆς γράφει· 'τί οὖν ἐστι τὸ ἐλαιῶδες; ὥσπερ τῷ ἔξω πυρὶ τροφή ἐστι τὸ ἔλαιον, οὕτω καὶ τῇ ἡμετέρᾳ φύσει πυρὶ ὁμοιουμένῃ τὸ στέαρ τῶν λαμβανομένων πεσσόμενόν ἐστι τροφή. τὸ οὖν ἐλαιῶδες οὖρον ἡ τροφή ἐστι τῆς φύσεως καὶ δηλοῖ ἀσιτεῖν τὴν φύσιν καὶ διὰ τοῦτ' ἄρ' ἀποθανεῖν, ὅτι μὴ τρέφεται ἡ φύσις. ἐχρόνισε δ' οὗτος εἰκότως διὰ τὸ μοῖραν καὶ μὴ πᾶσαν φέρεσθαι[47] τῆς

44 Wenkebach (1936), p. 165, line 11–166, line 19.

45 Wenkebach added '〈εἶναι〉' after ὠχρὰν, justifying it with the Arabic version ('sec[undum] Ḥ[unaynum] supplevi et correxi'), but the Arabic does not suggest the addition of εἶναι; it simply reads 'Some people say that the oily urine *is from* yellow bile (*Ammā al-bawlu l-duhnīyu fa-qad qāla qawmun innahū mina l-mirrati l-ṣafrā'i*)', where the 'is from' can imply that it 'belongs to' or is 'caused by' yellow bile. The Greek phrase λέγειν τί τι ('to call something something') is perfectly all right.

46 ὥστε οὐδὲν ἦν ἐλπίσαι is the reading of L; Wenkebach rewrote the Greek here on the basis of the Arabic as rendered into German, but, again, Pfaff's translation proved to be unreliable. The Arabic has: 'There was no hope that he could be saved after he had passed the sharpness (*wa-mā kānat turǧā lahū l-salāmatu lammā taǧāwaza l-ḥadda*)'.

47 Wenkebach corrected this into ἀφαιρεῖσθαι, but the reading of the manuscripts φέρεσθαι

φύσεως τροφήν.' αὕτη μέν ἐστιν ἡ τοῦ Σαβίνου ῥῆσις ἀξιοῦντος, ὥσπερ τὸ ἐκτὸς τοῦτο πῦρ ὑπὸ τοῦ ἐλαίου τρέφεται, οὕτω καὶ τὸ ἐν ἡμῖν θερμόν, ὥστ' ἔλαιόν ἐστι ποτέον τοῖς βουλομένοις ἑαυτοὺς ἀναθρέψαι, πρὸς τὸ κατὰ χρόαν μὲν καὶ σύστασιν ἐοικέναι τὸ ἐλαιῶδες οὖρον τῷ ἐλαίῳ, μήτε δὲ κατὰ τὴν λιπαρότητα μήτε κατὰ τὴν ὀσμὴν ἢ τὴν γεῦσιν. ἄξιον οὖν θαυμάσαι τῶν τὰ μὲν ἀλλότρια κακῶς ἐξελεγχόντων, ἀπερισκέπτως δὲ τὰ δόξαντα ἑαυτοῖς γραφόντων.

وقد وصفت فيما تقدم ما قاله سانيس في بلدة هذا المريض. وأنا واضف الآن ما قاله في البول الدهني، فإن النظر في هذا الباب عظيم الفروق. وقد كتب سابينس هذا بألفاظه هذا القول: «وأما البول الدهني فقد قال قوم إنه من المرة الصفراء. وما[48] هو من المرة، لأنه لو كان من المرة، لما كان يدل على الهلاك دلالة قوية جدا. وذلك أن المرة قد يتخلص صاحبها كثيرا من غير أن يناله منها مكروه. وقد قال قوم آخرون إن البول الزيتي يكون من ذوبان العصب والعظام والغضاريف لأن هذه كلها من هذا اللون. وقد غلط هؤلاء من قبل أن اللون الزيتي ليس بموافق للون العظام والغضاريف والعصب، ولا كانت تطول مدة حياة ذلك المريض مع تحلل أعصابه الأصلية. وذلك أنه إنما مات من بعد مائة وعشرين يوما. ولعله إنما أثبتت قصة هذا المريض حتى يتبين بها أنه لا ينبغي أن يتوقع الموت لمن يبول بولا دهنيا، لكنه قد يمكن أن يلبث مدة طويلة ثم يموت. وما كانت ترجى له السلامة لما تجاوز الحد.» فلما ودع سابينس هذا القول كتب بعده هذا القول الآخر: «فينبغي أن يخبر ما هو هذا الشيء الدهني. فأقول إنه كما أن الدهن غذاء لهذه النار الخارجة كذلك الطبيعة إذا كانت خطيرة البال إنما غذاؤها الشيء الدهني الذي تأخذه من الخبز وسائر ما يؤكل. والبول الدهني إنما هو غذاء الطبيعة، ويدل على أن الطبيعة لا تغتذي؛ وبالواجب طالت مدة حياة هذا المريض، لأنه إنما كان يخرج من غذاء الطبيعة البعض لا الكل.» فهذا قول سابينس الذي رام أن يخبرنا فيه أنه كما أن هذه النار الخارجة تغتذي من الدهن كذلك الحرارة الغريزية التي فينا. فقد ينبغي إذاً لمن أراد أن يملئ بدنه من الغذاء وينعشه به أن يشرب الزيت شربا مع أنه قد يمكن أن يكون يشبه الزيت في لونه وقوامه ولا يكون مثله في الدسونة ولا في الرائحة ولا في طعم. وإني لأعجب ممن كشف

---

is supported by the Arabic: 'because only part of nature's nourishment came out, not all (*li-annahū innamā kāna yaḫruğu min ġiḏā'i l-ṭabī'ati l-ba'ḍu lā l-kullu*)'. In other word, the translator took the genitive 'τῆς φύσεως' to go with τροφήν, the subject accusative of the accusative and infinitive construction.

48 وما] coni.: أو ما E.

خطأ قول غيره فيبلغ من ذلك الغاية وإذا جاء إلى ما يدعي هو وصفه من غير نظر ولا بحث ولا عيب لنفسه.

I have previously shown what Sabinus has said about the home of this patient; I shall now discuss what he has said about the oily urine, because the opinions about this differ considerably. About this, he wrote the following verbatim: 'Some say that oily [urine] is yellow bile; however, it is not bile, for that would not have been entirely deleterious. For bile is often purged and does not cause any additional damage. Others say that it is the dissolution of the tendons, bones and cartilages, because all these things have that colour. Yet those who claim that the oily urine is similar in colour to bones, cartilages and tendons are wrong. Actually, life could not have lasted so long, if the solid [parts of the body] had [really] been dissolved; for the patient died on the hundred twentieth day, nor did anybody die after having passed this urine. Perhaps (μήποτε) this is why this patient was included, to show by means of this symptom that one should not expect death immediately when oily urine is emitted, but that it is possible for the patient to last for a while and then die [later], so that one should not hope that the patient can be saved once he is past this amount of bitterness.' After he said this, Sabinus wrote: 'Then what is the oily (urine)? Just as oil nourishes outside fire, so does the fat of ingested food once digested also nourish our nature, which resembles fire. Thus the oily urine is nature's food. [When it is secreted,] nature is deprived of food. Therefore, death ensues, because nature has not been nourished. This patient has lasted possibly for a longer, because only part of nature's food, not all of it, was taken [away].'

This is what Sabinus said: he thinks that just as fire is fed by oil, so the heat within us [is fed by oily urine]. Therefore, those who want to feed themselves up need to drink oil. Moreover, oily urine resembles oil in terms of its colour and composition, but not in terms of fattiness, smell or taste. One therefore has to be surprised that those who wrongly criticise the opinions of others write down their own opinions without scrutiny.

The length of this quotation allows us to form an opinion of Sabinus' commentary independent of Galen's own interpretation. The third occurrence of μήποτε in the sense of 'maybe' constitutes an interesting use of vocabulary.[49] Moreover, Sabinus employs the method of beginning by examining two previous interpretations without mentioning his predecessors by name. Then

49 Wenkebach (1936), p. 166, line 2.

Sabinus provides his own personal explanation. This proves that the technique of critical commentary predates Galen, even if Sabinus' anonymous polemic contrasts with that of Galen, who does mention the names of previous commentators. We should also appreciate the clarity and conciseness of Sabinus' exposition as he finishes his criticism and continues with a comparison between internal physiology and external appearance. His commentary is a work of rational medicine.[50]

Finally, we need to ask why Galen decided to give this commentator such an important place in his commentary on *Epidemics* 3. Sabinus was not an isolated commentator, he had pupils. One of these, Metrodorus, is mentioned in the commentary on *Epidemics* 3. Metrodorus in turn also had his own pupils.[51] Was Sabinus perhaps a member of a medical sect? In *Der Kleine Pauly*, Fridolf Kudlien denies this possibility.[52] His claim is somewhat surprising, since Galen, in his commentary on *Epidemics* 3, associates Sabinus with the sect of the Hippocratics. Indeed, having blamed those who call themselves the Hippocratics for suggesting explanations that do not only diverge from Hippocrates but also from the factual truth,[53] Galen continues arguing the following:[54]

> οἱ τοίνυν περὶ τὸν Σαβῖνον καὶ τὸν μαθητὴν αὐτοῦ Μητρόδωρον, ἀκριβέστεροι δόξαντες εἶναι τῶν ἔμπροσθεν Ἱπποκρατείων, ὅμως καὶ αὐτοὶ φαίνονται μοχθηρῶς ἐξηγούμενοι πολλάκις τὸν Ἱπποκράτην.

> وقد نجد آل سابينس ومطرودورس تلميذه على أنه نظر بهم أنهم أشد استقصاء ممن كان قبلهم من شيعة أبقراط يفسرون أشياء كثيرة من أقاويل أبقراط تفسيرا رديئا.

50 Galen had to critique Sabinus' opinion. There must, however, be a lacuna of unknown length after ἀναθρέψαι and before πρὸς τὸ κατὰ χρόαν μὲν κτλ. (Wenkebach 1936, p. 166, lines 15–16). This lacuna has not been suggested until recently. What can be restored from Galen's argument from what remains is that he had to invalidate the analogy created by Sabinus between oil and oily urine by showing that while such a comparison works for colour and substance, it does not for smell, taste and grease. He had to preliminarily give his opinion on those of Sabinus' criticisms which he viewed as inferior (cf. Wenkebach 1936, 166, line 18 τῶν τὰ μὲν ἀλλότρια κακῶς ἐξελεγχόντων) before refuting his personal opinions which he judged as thoughtless (cf. Wenkebach 1936, p. 166, line 19 ἀπερισκέπτως δὲ τὰ δόξαντα ἑαυτοῖς γραφόντων).

51 Wenkebach (1936), p. 17, line 22.

52 Kudlien (1972): 'Über die Schulzugehörigkeit des S[abinus] ist nichts auszumachen.' Sabinus is also called Hippocratic in Galen, *On Black Bile* 4; 5.119.7 K., which was already noticed by Wellmann (1912), 9–10. With respect to Sabinus as a Hippocratic, see also Boudon-Millot (2015), 382.

53 Wenkebach (1936), p. 17, lines 12–21.

54 Wenkebach (1936), p. 17, lines 22–25.

> The followers of Sabinus and Metrodorus, although they are known to be more exact than the Hippocratics who preceded them, have nonetheless often commented on Hippocrates in an obviously wrong way.

Galen here clearly classifies Sabinus among the Hippocratics. Despite the progress Sabinus and his followers were able to make, compared to their predecessors, they did not manage to earn Galen's approval. The latter had, in fact, every interest in criticising the Hippocratics, who, like himself, claimed to be followers of Hippocrates. In this way he could prove that he was unaffiliated with a sect that must have seemed so close to him in they eyes of outsiders. As we know, Galen never ceased to assert his independence from the sects.

2 Galen, Commentator of His Own Commentaries

The originality of Galen as a commentator of Hippocrates in *Epidemics* 3 does not only result from the way in which he talks about previous commentators. It also derives from the constant comments that he makes in the first person singular and plural about his own commentary. One of the characteristics of Galen, at least in his commentary on *Epidemics* 3, is that he is a consistent commentator of himself.

In order to understand the way in which Galen continues to intervene within his own commentary, we will preserve the distinction made by Galen himself at the beginning of his analysis of the first patient in the form of two concise digressions; one related to the inferior commentators, and the other to the so-called 'characters', mysterious groups of letter symbols, at the end of the patient records. In this section, I follow Galen's structure by first treating the way in which he justifies his study of inferior commentators. I will discuss his treatment of the characters at the end. Galen's discussion of the characters is a hardly surprising innovation which is absent in the commentary on *Epidemics* 1 because of the differences in the source text of the commentaries. This innovation is nevertheless most revealing of Galen's challenges as a commentator.

Galen begins his first digression, about inferior commentators, with a long argument in the first person in which he clearly exposes the essential difference between his position as a commentator in *Epidemics* 1 and 3:[55]

55 Wenkebach (1936), p. 10, lines 10–25.

Ἐγὼ μὲν ᾤμην ἄμεινον εἶναι τὰ πολλῷ χρόνῳ ζητηθέντα μοι καὶ μετὰ κρίσεως ἀσφαλοῦς εὑρεθέντα μόνα γράφειν, ἄνευ τῶν εἰς τοὺς κακῶς ἐξηγησαμένους ἐλέγχων. ἐπεὶ δ' ἔνιοι μὲν διὰ τὸ μηδ' ὅλως πεπαιδεῦσθαι κατὰ μηδὲν τῶν παιδείων μαθημάτων, ἔνιοι δὲ καὶ φύσει νωθροὶ τὴν διάνοιαν ὄντες, ἀναγινώσκοντες ἐνίοτε παρά τισι τῶν γραψάντων ἐξηγήσεις ξένας, αὐτῷ τούτῳ μόνῳ τῷ ξένῳ συναρπασθέντες ἐπαινοῦσιν αὐτάς, διὰ τοῦτ' ᾠήθην ἄμεινον εἶναι κἂν ἅπαξ αὐτῶν που μνημονεῦσαι τῶν οὕτως ἐξηγουμένων, εἰρηκότος γε καὶ αὐτοῦ τοῦ Ἱπποκράτους· 'τὸ γὰρ ξενοπρεπὲς οὔπω ξυνιέντες[56] μᾶλλον ἐπαινέουσιν ἢ τὸ σύνηθες, ὃ ἤδη οἴδασιν ὅτι χρηστόν, καὶ τὸ ἀλλόκοτον μᾶλλον ἢ ⟨τὸ⟩ εὔδηλον.' ὅπως οὖν προειδότες οἱ τοῖς ἡμετέροις ὑπομνήμασιν ἐντυγχάνοντες, ὁποῖοι γοῦν τινες οἱ τρόποι τῶν μοχθηρῶν ἐξηγήσεών εἰσιν, γνωρίζειν αὐτοὺς δύνωνται, μακρότερον ἐνταῦθα περὶ πασῶν αὐτῶν ἔγνων γράψαι. καί μοι μηδεὶς ἀχθεσθῇ τῷ μήκει τοῦ λόγου, μέλλων ἔχειν αὐτὸν ἀεὶ βοηθὸν εἰς τὴν τῶν φαύλων ἐξηγήσεων διάγνωσιν.

قد كنت أرى أن الأجود أن أقصد إلى ما بحثت عنه واختبرته على طول المدة واستخرجته بالمحنة الوثيقة، وأقتص على ذكره من غير كشف خطأ من فسر تفسيرا درئيا. لكني رأيت قوما من قبل أنهم لم يتأدبوا بشيء أصلا من التعاليم التي يتأدب بها الأحداث وقوما من قبل أنهم أيضا مختلفون بالطبع ربما قرؤوا شيئا مما كتبه أصحاب التفاسير الغريبة، فكانت غرابة ذلك الشيء فقط هي التي تدعوهم إلى أن يحمدوا تلك التفاسير ويمدحونها. فلذلك رأيت أن من الأجود أن أذكر أصحاب هذه التفاسير، ولو مرة واحدة، وأنبه على رداءة تفاسيرهم. فإن أبقراط نفسه قد قال: «إن كثيرا من الناس يصير إلى الشيء المستغرب، وهو لم يفهمه بعد فيمدحه أكثر مما يمدح الشيء المألوف الذي قد عرفه وعلم أنه جيد؛ ويميل إلى الشيء الغريب البديع والملتبس أكثر من ميله إلى الشيء البين.» فكيما يتقدم فيعلم من قرأ تفاسيري مذاهب التفاسير الرديئة أي المذاهب هي فيصل إلى أن يقف ويعرفها، فإني قد رأيت أن أتكلم فيها كلما في هذا الموضع كلاما شافيا وليس ينبغي لأحد أن يستثقل كلامي وإن طال في هذا الباب لأنه يستفيد منه قوة يستعين بها دائما عل تعرف كل تفسير رديء.

56 Wenkebach supplies εἰ χρηστὸν after ξυνιέντες from the direct tradition, but the Arabic leaves little doubt that it did not have this addition; rather it simply reads: 'without understanding it yet (*wa-huwa lam yafhamhu baʿdu*)' rendering 'οὔπω ξυνιέντες'. Wenkebach was therefore probably right in assuming that Galen quoted from memory.

> I used to think that it would be better to write the things that I have researched for a long time and discovered with a steadfast judgment, without criticising those who have given bad explanations. Some people, however, have no knowledge whatsoever, not even of what children are taught; and others have a naturally sluggish intellect, so that when they sometimes read the strange explanations of certain commentators, they are beguiled by this strangeness and therefore praise them. For this reason, I thought that it would be better to mention those who comment in this way at least once, since Hippocrates himself said: 'They approve more of what is strange without even understanding it than of what is usual and of which they already know that it is useful; and they approve of the exotic more than the evident.' Therefore, I decided to write more extensively about all these things here, in order that the readers of my commentaries, having been warned in advance of what the ways of inferior commentaries are, may be able to recognise them. And nobody should be annoyed with me because of the length of my discourse, because he will always have them as an aid to recognise inferior interpretations.

While Galen sticks to a direct and personal style in his commentary of *Epidemics* 1, he changes this in *Epidemics* 3, where he decides to warn his readers against the inferior explanations of his predecessors. He feels the need to justify this change. To do so, Galen skilfully employs Hippocrates himself. He adopts a psychological remark from the author of *Fractures* and *Joints*[57] about the attraction of the exotic which fascinates men in order to warn his reader against appealing but false interpretations.

In this first comment, we recognise three instances in which Galen clearly confirms his decision to give a new orientation to his commentary of Hippocrates: 'I thought that it would be better (ᾤμην ἄμεινον εἶναι)', 'I thought (ᾠήθην)', and 'I decided (ἔγνων).' When Galen later revisits his justification of a criticism that he has levelled at Sabinus' comment on the third patient before the constitution, however, we surprisingly find a different explanation. After quoting Sabinus' passage which he is about to criticise, Galen says:[58]

> …, ἐπεὶ δ' ἐν τούτῳ τῷ ὑπομνήματι παρὰ τὴν ἐμαυτοῦ προαίρεσιν εἰς ἔλεγχον ἀλλοκότων ἐξηγήσεων ἐπείσθην τοῖς ἑταίροις γράψαι τινά, καὶ νῦν ὀλίγα προσθήσω ταὐτὸν εἶδος ἔχοντα.

57 Hippocrates, *Fractures* 1; 3.414.7–9 L.

58 Wenkebach (1936), p. 48, line 24–p. 49, line 1; the preceding quotation by Sabinus is quoted in Raiola's contribution on pp. 63–64.

> But since in this commentary, contrary to my own preference, I was persuaded by my students to write some words to refute the strange commentaries, I shall also add some remarks of the same kind here.

This explanation seems to be a contradiction. What has previously been presented as a personal decision now becomes a decision made under the pressure of his students. There has been a reversal. This new justification will be repeated and elaborated in the extensive introduction to book 2 of Galen's commentary, which ends with the following passage:[59]

> ἐγὼ μὲν οὖν τοὺς ἐν τῷ πρώτῳ καὶ δευτέρῳ[60] τῶν Ἐπιδημιῶν βιβλίῳ γεγραμμένους ἀρρώστους ἐξηγησάμην ἔμπροσθεν ἄνευ τῶν εἰς τοὺς μοχθηρῶς ἐξηγουμένους ἐλέγχων. ἐπεὶ δὲ πολλοὶ τῶν ἑταίρων ἠξίωσάν με καὶ ἐπ' ὀλίγων ἀρρώστων ἐπισημήνασθαι περὶ τῶν οὐκ ὀρθῶς ἐξηγουμένων, ἠναγκάσθην εἰς τρεῖς ἀρρώστους μόνους ἓν ἐξηγητικὸν βιβλίον ποιήσασθαι τὸ πρὸ τούτου. νυνὶ δ' ἡγοῦμαι πάλιν ἄμεινον εἶναι κατὰ τὸν αὐτὸν τρόπον ἐξηγεῖσθαι τοὺς ὑπολοίπους, ὅνπερ καὶ ἔμπροσθεν ἤδη τοὺς ἐν τῷ πρώτῳ τῶν Ἐπιδημιῶν ἐξηγησάμην. κινδυνεύω γὰρ εἰς ἕτερον ἐμπεσεῖν ἔγκλημα τῶν μισούντων μέγεθός τε καὶ μῆκος ὑπομνημάτων.

> وأما أنا فإني فسرت أقاصيص المرضى الذين ذكروا في المقالة الأولى والثانية أولا من غير أن أروم كشف خطأ من فسرها تفسيرا رديئا. فلما سألني كثير من أصحابي أن أوقفهم وأصف لهم ولو في قصص يسير من المرضى أمر تفسير من فسرها على غير الصوب، اضطروني إلى أن أكتب في قصص ثلاث مرضى فقط مقالة واحدة، وهي المقالة التي قبل هذه. وأما الآن فإني قد رأيت أن أجعل تفسيري لقصص سائر المرضى على طريق تفسيري لقصص المرضى الذين ذكروا في المقالة الأولى. وذلك أني لم آمن إن أفعل ذلك أن يلحقني لوم من وجه آخر من تقصص عظم الكتب وطولها.

> I have previously commented on the patients described in *Epidemics* 1 and 2 without criticising those who wrote inferior commentaries. But since many of my students thought it appropriate that I speak about the incorrect commentaries in the case of a few patients, I was forced to publish

59 Wenkebach (1936), p. 65, line 21–66, line 7.

60 Wenkebach athetised these two words, but they are present in the Arabic version ('and the second [*wa-l-ṯāniyati*]').

> one exegetical work about only three patients, the book before this one. But now I think it would be better to comment on the remaining patients in the same way, as I have already commented on those in *Epidemics* 1 previously. For I run the risk of being accused by those who hate the large size and length of treatises.

This passage reinforces Galen's explanation of his change of commentary technique as resulting from an external influence. While he earlier said he was persuaded by his students (ἐπείσθην τοῖς ἑταίροις), he now speaks of coercion (ἠναγκάσθην) exercised by many students (πολλοὶ των ἑταίρων). Faced with this coercion which made him write an exceptionally long argument about the first three patients of the list, with respect to the other patients he now expresses his wish to return to the old technique of commenting which he followed in his commentary on *Epidemics* 1, in order to avoid the criticism of long-windedness.

How is this promise fulfilled? Galen's return to his old technique is clearly visible in his discussion of the next three patients, patients 4, 5, and 6. However, in the case of patient 7, a rather short record of a woman with angina who dies on the fifteenth day, the commentary returns to being extremely long and detailed, filling 12 pages for a lemma that is only nine lines long.[61] Surprisingly, it includes rather precise references to the beginning of Sabinus' commentary that serve as a critique of his interpretation of one of the symptoms, 'elevated breathing.'[62] Galen kept his promise to return to his previous method for only three patients in his commentary.

The length of the argument devoted to this seventh patient does not only result from the return to criticising inferior commentators although he promised not to do this, but also from the importance of this patient for the question of the so-called 'characters' at the end of the patient records. The characters only begin to appear in the manuscripts and oldest commentaries from this seventh patient onwards.[63] This transition allows us to examine the way in which Galen introduces and justifies his commentary on the characters. We must note, however, that the importance of the characters and letters at the end of the patient records has already been discussed by Galen from the first patient record onwards, for although the oldest characters only appear from the seventh record onwards, they were later extended to the earlier records as well, as can already be found in Dioscorides' edition.

---

61 The lemma can be found in Wenkebach (1936), p. 71, lines 14–21; the commentary in Wenkebach (1936), p. 72, line 1–83, line 13.

62 Wenkebach (1936), p. 72, line 12–p. 74, line 16.

63 Wenkebach (1936), p. 46, lines 19–24.

Having described the five characters at the end of the first record, that of Pythion (ΙΠ Π ΟΥ Μ Υ), Galen asks two questions about these characters in first person plural:[64]

> ζητεῖν οὖν ἠναγκάσθημεν, ὅ τί ποτε σημαίνουσιν οἱ χαρακτῆρες οὗτοι, μετὰ τοῦ μηδὲ γινώσκειν ἡμᾶς, εἴθ' Ἱπποκράτης ἦν ἤ τις ἄλλος ὁ γράψας τὰ τοιαῦτα καθ' ἕκαστον τῶν ἀρρώστων. ἀλλὰ καὶ τοῦτο αὐτὸ ζητεῖν ἀναγκασθέντες ἐνοήσαμεν, 〈ὡς,〉 εἰ μέν, ὥσπερ ἐν τούτῳ τῷ βιβλίῳ τοὺς τοιούτους χαρακτῆρας εὑρήκαμεν, οὕτω κἀν τοῖς ἄλλοις ἅπασι τῶν Ἐπιδημιῶν ἐφαίνοντο προσγεγραμμένοι τῇ διηγήσει τῶν συμβάντων τοῖς ἀρρώστοις, ἴσως ἂν ἦν εὔλογον ὑφ' Ἱπποκράτους αὐτοῦ προσγεγράφθαι φάναι. μήτε δ' ἐν τοῖς ἄλλοις βιβλίοις αὐτῶν εὑρισκομένων, ἀλλὰ μηδ' ἐν αὐτῷ τῷ τρίτῳ διὰ πάντων ὁμαλῶς τῶν ἀντιγράφων, ὑποψία τις εὔλογος εἰσῆλθεν οὐχ ἡμᾶς μόνον, ἀλλὰ καὶ τοὺς πρὸ ἡμῶν ὑπό τινος αὐτοὺς προσγεγράφθαι τάχα μὲν ἐπιτρίβοντος τοῖς μαθηταῖς, ἵν' ἔχῃ σαφηνίζειν ὥς τι μέγα τὸ καθ' ἕκαστον αὐτῶν δηλούμενον, ἴσως δέ τινος αὐτῷ μόνῳ πεποιημένου τῆς καθ' ἕκαστον ἄρρωστον ὠφελείας 〈ἢ ἀπωλείας〉 ἐπιτομήν.

فاضطررنا بسبب ذلك أن نبحث وننظر على ماذا تدل هذه الأحرف مع أنا لا نعلم أيضا هل أبقراط هو المثبت لهذه الأحرف أو غيره في قصة كل واحد من المرضى. ولما اضطرنا الأمر إلى البحث عن هذا، توهمنا أنه لو كان كما توجد هذه[65] الأحرف من سومة في هذه المقالة في أقاصيص المرضى كذلك توجد في سائر مقالات كتاب إفيذيميا، ولا نجدها أيضا في هذه المقالة الثالثة منه بمتفقة في جميع النسخ فإن ذلك قد وهمنا وهو موضع توهم أن ملحِقا ألحقها غير أبقراط. وما ذلك توهم توهمت أنا خاصة لكنه قد سبقني إليه من كان قبلي. ولعل الملحق لهذه الأحرف إنما أراد بإلحاقها الإغماض على المتعلمين حتى يجد السبيل إلى أن يفسر ويبين المعنى الذي يدل عليه كل واحد من تلك الأحرف، فتوهم أنه قد أتى بفائدة عظيمة. ولعل الملحق لها لم يذهب إلى هذا لكنه إنما أراد بها أن يرسم لنفعه خاصة جملة من أمر كل واحد من المرضى مما كان به انتفاعه أو هلاكه.

We have been forced to research what these characters mean, even though we do not know whether it was Hippocrates who added them for each of the patients, or someone else. But, we were forced to research

64 Wenkebach (1936), p. 27, lines 13–27.

65 add. E الأحرف من سومة في هذه ex dittographia.

> this. If the characters appeared in all the other books of the *Epidemics* as additions to the case histories of the patients, just as we have found them in this book, then perhaps it would have been reasonable to assume that they were added by Hippocrates himself. Yet, since they do not occur in the other books nor in the same way in the manuscripts of the third book [*Epidemics* 3], not only we ourselves but also our predecessors began to suspect that perhaps they were written by someone to waste the students' time,[66] so that he would be able to show that something significant is revealed by each one of them; or perhaps as a personal summary of what is useful or harmful for each patient.

When one sees with how much insight Galen speaks about his research on the characters, which he clearly divides into two parts, one about the meaning of the characters, and the other about the question of their origin, one is inclined to compliment him. Besides questioning their meaning, he is also interested in the characters' origin. In relation to this second question, we must approve of the way in which Galen argues that these characters cannot derive from the author, but must have been added by a later scholar. Modern philological discoveries reinforce Galen's argument by determining that the lists of patients at the beginning of *Epidemics* 3 is the continuation of that at the end of *Epidemics* 1, something unknown in Galen's time. The absence of the characters at the beginning of the list at the end of *Epidemics* 1 contrasts with their presence at the end of the list at the beginning of *Epidemics* 3. This implies that the characters present in the records at the end of the list were added after the accidental separation of the original list into two independent parts.

But what surprises us is the way in which Galen formulates his own research of these characters. He does not announce it with passion and enthusiasm. Rather, he calls it research under coercion, or better, under renewed coercion, as Galen finds it necessary to justify himself. He twice uses the formula 'we have been forced to research (ζητεῖν οὖν ἠναγκάσθημεν, and ζητεῖν ἀναγκασθέντες).'[67] The final sentence of this discussion of the characters in the first patient record provides us with additional insights into Galen's mindset with which he seems

66 The expression 'ἐπιτρίβειν τινί' is used elsewhere by Galen in the sense of 'wasting someone's time'. The Arabic translator used a long circumlocution to render it: '… by adding them [the characters] he wanted to confuse the students to find a way to explain and elucidate the meaning indicated by each one of the characters. (… *innamā arāda fi-ilḥāqihā l-iġmāda ʿalā l-mutaʿallimīna ḥatta yaǧida l-sabīla ilā an yufassira wa-yubayyina l-maʿnā llaḏī yadullu ʿalayhi kullu wāḥidin min tilka l-aḥrufi.*)'

67 Wenkebach (1936), p. 27, lines 13 and 16.

to approach this field of research:[68] 'The sophists are admired as prophets by their students because of such commentaries [i.e. about characters].' Galen is reluctant, because certain commentators, whom he describes as 'sophists', obtain easy, poor quality success among their followers with regard to this futile subject. He does not want to resemble them.

This reluctance does nevertheless not prevent Galen from revisiting the meaning of the characters several times later on, gently forcing himself to satisfy the curiosity of his followers. I cannot discuss all instances where Galen revisits the question, or all the explanations he gives to justify them.[69] I shall, however, discuss the reference to book 2, which is part of the commentary on the seventh patient (before the constitution). Here, Galen points out that the question of the characters is not useful for the art of medicine, and therefore gives a new justification: it is the same justification which Galen had already given in book 1 in relation to the inferior commentators, namely the request made by his students. He writes that he shall accede to it, saying that 'I shall also say something about the characters once in this book (εἰπεῖν τί με καὶ περὶ τῶν χαρακτήρων τούτων ἅπαξ ἐν τῷδε τῷ βιβλίῳ).'[70] This discussion of the history of the characters began to occupy such a significant place that it led to an imbalance in the commentary, which obliged Galen to postpone his discussion of the climatic and nosological constitution, which he initially intended for book 2, to book 3.

Galen, however, uses this postponement to add an argument to the discussions related to the characters in the record of the eighth patient. He even includes a long final account in Zeno's and Apollonius' discussions of the famous character *pi* with three lines meaning 'πιθανόν (it is probable that)'. The way in which Galen justifies this last argument is indicative of the evolution of his position:[71]

> Ἐπειδὴ τὰ πλεῖστα τῶν κατὰ τὸ βιβλίον τοῦτο ταῖς ἀδολεσχίαις ἐχαρισάμεθα τῶν ἐξηγητῶν, οὐ χεῖρον ἂν εἴη καὶ περὶ τοῦ ⟨τὸ⟩ πιθανὸν ἐνδεικνυμένου χαρακτῆρος εἰπεῖν τι παραδείγματος ἕνεκεν. ἴσως γάρ τις θαυμάσει περὶ τοῦ μεγέθους τῶν βιβλίων, ὧν ἔγραψαν οἱ περὶ τὸν Ζήνωνά τε καὶ τὼ Ἀπολλωνίω. ἐὰν

68 Wenkebach (1936), p. 28, line 27.

69 He returns to this at the end of the second patient in this same book (1) and also further on in book 2 in his discussion of the seventh patient (Wenkebach 1936, p. 75, line 23–p. 80, line 19 and p. 81, line 22–p. 83, line 13), as well as the eight patient (ibid., p. 86, line 1–p. 91, line 9 and p. 91, line 10–p. 95, line 2).

70 Wenkebach (1936), p. 78, lines 5–6.

71 Wenkebach (1936), p. 91, 12–19.

> οὖν ἐφ' ἑνὸς χαρακτῆρος ἀκούσῃς πῶς κατὰ βραχὺ προῆλθεν αὐτοῖς εἰς μῆκος ἡ ἀντιλογία, γνώσῃ τε τὴν αἰτίαν τῆς μακρολογίας φυλάξῃ τε περιπίπτειν ταῖς τοιαύταις ⟨ἀδολεσχίαις⟩, ἐὰν νοῦν ἔχῃς.
>
> إني لما كنت قد وهبت أكثر هذه المقالة لهمر المفسرين، فلا بأس أيضا أن أقول شيئا من الحرف الذي معناه يشبه، لأجعل ذلك مثالا لغيره. فإنه لعل بعض أهل النظر يعجب من عظم الكتب التي[72] كتبها آل زينن وأبلونيوس الأول والثاني. فإن سَمِـعَ من أمر واحد من تلك الأحرف كيف تراقت بهم المغامرة[73] والخصومة قليلا قليلا إلى أن طالت، عَرَفَ السبب في طول كلامهم وإطنابهم، وحَذِرَ أن يقع فيما وقعوا فيه من الإطناب وتطويل الكلام، وإن كان معها عقل.
>
> Since in this book [the second book of Galen's commentary on *Epidemics* 3], we have mostly indulged the verbosity of commentators, it cannot harm also to say something about the character signifying 'persuasive' in order to give an example. For one may well be surprised by the large size of the books which the followers of Zeno and the two people called Apollonius have written. Therefore, if you hear how a controversy among them about one single character quickly descended into a long dispute, you will know the reason why their books are so long, and be careful not to succumb to the same verbosity, if you are sensible.

Of course, in the end, Galen says that it is for reason's sake that he provides this explanation. The pleasure (ἐχαρισάμεθα), however, that Galen admits that he gets from indulging the verbosity of commentators risks stifling this reason. Galen's ambiguous attitude as a commentator is surprising. He continues to indulge idle prattle by presenting the scholars' argument; he even employs the metaphor of a theatre with a play in three acts, the third of which will charm the spectators.[74] Galen turns something which has nothing to do with the subjects of the medical commentary into a fascinating spectacle about the subtleties of

72 التي] corr. الذي E.

73 المغامرة is a tentative reading.

74 Wenkebach (1936), p. 92, line 12 'κηλοῦσα τοὺς ἀκούοντας (charming the audience)'. The metaphor begins in 2.9 (p. 93, line 1 'τὸ μὲν δὴ πρῶτον μέρος τοῦ δράματος [the first part of the play]'); continues at p. 93, line 4 'ἐπὶ δὲ τὸ δεύτερον ἴωμεν καθέντες ἑαυτοὺς ἅπαξ εἰς τὸ δρᾶμα (let us for once dedicate ourselves and move on to the second act)'; and at p. 93, line 12 'ἐπὶ τὸ τρίτον μέρος ἀφίκεσθαι τοῦ δράματος ἀρέσαι δυνάμενον (it being sufficient to

language. We should recall what Galen said about the sophists at the beginning of his digression about the characters: 'The sophists are admired as prophets by their students because of such commentaries.' This makes clear that Galen transforms himself into a sophist himself to entice his students, at least during the metaphorical spectacle—even if he does not pretend to be a prophet—before he returns to his commentary on the last patients to conclude book 2 of his commentary.

This does not mean that Galen will not speak of the characters again in book 3. He will discuss them again with respect to two patients after the constitution. These are the following two passages:[75]

> ἄξιον δὲ θαυμάσαι καὶ πῶς οὐδὲν εἶπον οἱ περὶ τὸν Σαβῖνον εἰς τοὺς προσκειμένους χαρακτῆρας ἑκάστῳ τῶν ἀρρώστων, ὑπὲρ ὧν ἐγὼ μὲν ἱκανῶς ἐν τῷ δευτέρῳ τῶν ὑπομνημάτων διελθὼν οὐκέτι δέομαι μνημονεύειν αὐτῶν. ὅ γε μὴν ⟨Ζεῦξις⟩ ἐφ' ἑκάστου τῶν ἀρρώστων προχειριζόμενος ἐξελέγχειν πειρᾶται τὴν μοχθηρίαν τῶν ἐξηγησαμένων αὐτούς.
>
> إني لأعجب من آل سابينوس كيف لم يقولوا شيئا في هذه الأحرف الملحقة في أقاصيص هؤلاء المرضى. وقد وصفت الحال فيها في المقالة الثانية من كتابي هذا. فلست أحتاج بعد هذا الذي قلت فيها أن أذكرها. وأما زوكسيس فإنه يذكرها في قصة واحد واحد من المرضى، ويروم أن يكشف رداءة تفسير من فسرها وخطأهم[76] فيها.
>
> One can rightly be surprised at the fact that Sabinus and his followers have said nothing about the characters added to each of the patient records, which I have sufficiently discussed in the second book of this commentary, so that I do not need to discuss them further. Zeuxis examined [the characters] at each of these records and endeavoured to criticise the mistakes of those who have commented on them.

and

come to the third part of the play)'; it concludes at p. 94, line 19 'κάλλιον οὖν ἴσως καταπαῦσαι ἤδη τὸ δρᾶμα τριμερὲς γεγονός (it would perhaps be appropriate to end the play, as the three acts have been played)'.

75 Wenkebach (1936), p. 169, lines 6–11 (second patient after the constitution, at the end of the commentary); p. 176, lines 15–24 (fifth patient after the constitution, at the end of the commentary).

76 وخطأهم is a tentative reading.

> προσγέγραπται δ' ἐπὶ τῇ τελευτῇ κατὰ τὰ διεσκευασμένα τῶν ἀντιγράφων καὶ τούτῳ τῷ ἀρρώστῳ καὶ τῷ μετ' αὐτὸν πρότερον μὲν τὸ 'ὀξύ', μετ' αὐτὸ δὲ οἱ χαρακτῆρες, ὑπὲρ ὧν, ὡς ἔφην, οἱ μὲν περὶ τὸν Σαβῖνον ὀρθῶς φρονοῦντες οὐδὲν εἶπον, ὁ δὲ Ζεῦξις διελέγχει καθ' ἕκαστον ἄρρωστον τοὺς ἐξηγησαμένους μοχθηρῶς. ἀλλ' ἡμῖν ἔδοξε πάντα τὰ οὕτω προσγεγραμμένα παραλιπεῖν ἐν τῷ νῦν ἐνεστῶτι λόγῳ. γενήσεται γάρ, ἐὰν δόξῃ, βιβλίον ὅλον ἰδίᾳ τοῖς καὶ τὰ τοιαῦτα πολυπραγμονοῦσιν ἡδέως, ἐν ᾧ περὶ τῶν ἅπασι τοῖς ἀρρώστοις προσγεγραμμένων χαρακτήρων ὁ λόγος ἔσται. νυνὶ δ' οὐ προσήκει τοῖς χρησίμοις ἀναμειγνύναι τὰ ἄχρηστα.
>
> وقد نجد في آخر هذه القصة يلحق في النسخ المدخولة وفي آخر قصة المريض الذي بعد هذا أولا «حاد» ثم من بعده أحرف مثبتة. وقد أحسن أصحاب سابينوس كما قلت في إلغائهم ذكرها. وأما زوكسيس فإنه يروم في قصة كل واحد من المرضى أن يكشف خطأ من فسر تلك الأحرف. فأما أنا فإني قد رأيت أن ألغي ذكر جميع ما قد ألحق من هذا في الكتاب وإن رأيت أنه محتاج إلى ذكرها فسأفرد كتابا لذكرها لمن يجب البحث عن هذا ومثله أصف فيه من أمر جميع ما ألحق من الأحرف في أقاصيصها ولا المرضى وأما الآن فليس ينبغي أن أخلط بما ينتفع به ما لا ينتفع.
>
> At the end of the corrected manuscripts, the word 'acute' is added both to this patient record and to the one after it; and after this, the characters are added. As I have said, Sabinus and his followers judged correctly and said nothing about them. Zeuxis, however, refutes those who have written inferior commentaries in the case of each patient. Yet we decided to omit from the present discussion all those things that had been added. For, if need be, I shall produce a whole separate book for those who like to fuss over these things; it will discuss all the characters added to the patients' [histories]. But for now it is not appropriate to mix useful things with useless things.

The comparison between these two final comments leaves the reader perplexed. In both, Galen refers to Zeuxis and gives the same clues to the nature of his works. He also twice makes a judgement about Sabinus. At first, one has the impression that he criticises the latter for not discussing the characters in his commentary, as he contrasts this with his own discussion in book 2. In the second passage, however, Galen seems to adopt a rather different attitude: he approves of Sabinus' not discussing the characters in his commentary (they 'judged correctly [ὀρθῶς φρονοῦντες]'). He is, moreover, careful to mention his own discussion of the characters this time. Is there not a certain contradiction, or rather, a definite contradiction between the two passages? One could say that Galen returns to his true, uncompromising nature which seeks usefulness above all. Yet, at the same time, he does not want to ignore the voices of those who are charmed by the appeal of the mystery of the characters. Thus, he will treat his readers with a special work on all the characters of all the patients. This promise, made on the spur of the moment, does not seem to have been kept. Galen as commentator will keep to the right path, but he cannot avoid contemplating the idea of making detours in order to entice his readers.

In conclusion, we should mark the following essential points. First, there is a great contrast between Galen's two commentaries on *Epidemics* 1 and *Epidemics* 3. Second, compared to the commentary on on *Epidemics* 1, the innovations in the commentary on *Epidemics* 3 are twofold: one relates to a new element in the text, namely the presence of the character at the end of each patient record. The other is a methodological innovation of the way of commenting and involves the critique against inferior commentators.

One could add a third point: Galen is a commentator of his own commentary. The reasons that he gives for his innovations move between his personal decision and the urging of his followers. Galen is divided between his desire to enlighten his reader and to identify what is useful for the medical art; and his wish to entice and charm his reader by leaving the right path to embark on discussions of subtleties. These digressions are certainly useless for the medical art, but also so very precious for the history of the ancient polemics from the imperial period. Finally, it is useful to take part in the reconstruction of the Sabinus' Hippocratic commentary on *Epidemics* 3 by evaluating the fragments of this commentary preserved by Galen in his own commentary on *Epidemics* 3.

CHAPTER 5

New Fragments of a Commentary on *the Oath* Attributed to Galen

Caroline Magdelaine and Jean-Michel Mouton

On 17 October 1893, a fire destroyed the prayer hall of the Grand Mosque of Damascus during renovations of the roof.[1] The subsequent clean-up revealed a room that had been forgotten for centuries, situated at the south east of the building near the gate of Ǧayrūn. Having served as a depository for old papers in the second half of the medieval period, it was filled with documents such as receipts, sales and marriage contracts which had gone out of use, as well as private correspondence, incomplete Qur'ān copies, and snippets of religious manuscripts. The owners of these documents had not destroyed them after they had lost their purpose, but placed them here, undoubtedly because they contained the word 'God (*Allāh*)'.

The discovered documents were transported to Istanbul at the end of the Ottoman occupation of Syria. Only in the 1960's, however, were they examined for the first time, when Dominique and Janine Sourdel photographed, studied, and published the collection together with their students under the name 'papiers de Damas (Damascus papers)'. The most remarkable pieces of the collection known until recently were certificates of pilgrimage by proxy, collections of Abbasid Qur'ān leafs studied by François Déroche, and, most recently, several documents about the famous Sultan Saladin.[2]

The discovery presented here concerns twelve folios of a manuscript of particular interest to hellenists and historians of medicine.[3] They contain important fragments of a work previously considered lost: the *Commentary* on the famous Hippocratic *Oath*, which was attributed to Galen in the Arab world.

1 Al-Ḥāfiẓ (1989), 13.

2 Sourdel and Sourdel-Thomine (2006); Mouton et al. (2013), n. 2–7, pp. 13–15; and Mouton et al. (2015).

3 This discovery was first announced in September 2015: cf. Mouton and Magdelaine (2016).

© CAROLINE MAGDELAINE AND JEAN-MICHEL MOUTON, 2021 | DOI:10.1163/9789004470200_007

1 Background

Before presenting this new textual witness, we will provide a brief overview of the state of affairs of the text. The Hippocratic Oath, one of the most famous texts of the Hippocratic Corpus, is often considered to be the foundational work of medical ethics and deontology.[4] Galen, however, never quoted it, not even when he discusses ethical issues.[5] Likewise, Galen does not claim authorship of a commentary on the *Oath* in any of his bibliographic works, including the ninth chapter of *My Own Books*, where he lists the different treatises he has devoted to the exegesis of Hippocratic works.[6]

Moreover, the *Oath* only begins to be quoted in Graeco-Roman sources from the first century AD onwards by authors such as Scribonius Largus, a contemporary of Claudius (41–54), and the glossator Erotian, who lived under Nero (54–68) and put the *Oath* at the beginning of his last category of Hippocratic works related to the Art of Medicine.[7] Soranus of Ephesus (fl. ca. AD 100) links the *Oath* to the *Nature of the Child* in a passage which we will discuss later, and a papyrus dated to the second century lists it among works recommended for study at the beginning of a medical curriculum.[8] The other citations and references (Gregory of Nazianzus, Theodorus Priscianus, Marcellus, Olympiodorus) are significantly later.[9] Moreover, there is absolutely no reference to a commentary on the *Oath* written by Galen in any of these quotations.

The situation is rather different in the Middle East: apart from the recently discovered folios discussed here, numerous indications suggest that a Galenic commentary on the *Oath* circulated in that part of the world. For instance, the famous translator Ḥunayn ibn Isḥāq mentioned the *Commentary on the*

4 The literature on the *Oath* is extensive. Reference can be made to the bibliography begun by G. Fichtner, and after his death continued by his team in Berlin, available online at http://cmg.bbaw.de/online-publications/Hippokrates-Bibliographie_2017-12.pdf (nr. 14) [accessed 26 March 2021]. See also Anastassiou-Irmer (1997–2012), vol. 1, p. 320; vol. 2.1, pp. 289–291; and vol. 2.2, pp. 267–271. The date of the treatise remains the subject of intense scholarly debate, with opinions ranging from the fifth century BC to Hellenistic or later times (as argued by von Staden 2007, 424–466; all translations of the Greek text of the *Oath*, unless otherwise stated, are taken from this article). On the *Oath*, see now the authoritative edition of Jouanna (2018a), who dates it before Plato's *Protagoras* (pp. xxxvi–xlii).

5 In their survey of the Hippocratic quotations in the Galenic corpus, Anastassiou, Irmer (1997–2012, vol. 2.1) were unable to find a single reference to the *Oath*. About this conundrum, see Nutton (1993), 19; Jouanna (1996a), 214, and now also Jouanna (2018), cxxii–iii.

6 Boudon-Millot (2007), 160–161.

7 Anastassiou, Irmer (1997–2012), vol. 2.2, pp. 289–291.

8 *P.Oxy.* LXXIV 4970, ed. Leith (2009a).

9 Anastassiou, Irmer (1997–2012), vol. 2.2., pp. 267–271.

Oath first in his section on Hippocratic commentaries in his *Epistle* surveying Galenic works translated into Syriac and Arabic:[10]

> The commentaries on the Hippocratic *Oath*, in one volume. I have translated this text (from Greek) into Syriac while adding comments on difficult passages. Ḥubays[11] translated it to Arabic for Ibn al-Ḥasan Aḥmad ibn Mūsā.[12] It has also been translated (into Arabic) by ʿIsā ibn Yaḥyā.

As this report was written in AD 855, we know that the Galenic commentary must have been available to Ḥunayn by this date; moreover, Ḥunayn, an expert in all things Galen, does not doubt that this commentary was actually written by Galen.[13] After Ḥunayn, numerous medieval Arabic authors mention the text, while at times conveying extracts of the text itself. For instance, we find extracts in Saʿīd ibn al-Biṭrīq from ninth or tenth century, and in al-Birūnī during the eleventh century. Ibn Abī Uṣaybiʿa (d. 1270) transcribed the longest extracts of the text in his work *Essential Information about the Classes of Physicians* (*ʿUyūn al-anbāʾ fī ṭabaqāt al-aṭibbāʾ*).

The great Orientalist Franz Rosenthal (1956) collected fragments of the commentary and translated them into English, organised in three large sections: the origin of medicine; Asclepius; and the biography of Hippocrates. In this way, non-Arabic speakers gained access to this text for the first time. New fragments have since come to light, but none of these have provided any definitive information.[14] At the end of his study, Rosenthal (1956, 86) remained circumspect: he neither rejected nor accepted Galen's authorship, and dated the writing of the

10 Bergsträsser (1925), n. 87; Lamoureaux (2016), 94.

11 Ḥunayn's nephew.

12 The Banū Mūsā, of which Aḥmad was one, financed Ḥunayn's school to obtain translations of Greek authors; see Hill (1992), 639–640, and Micheau (1997), 167–170.

13 The case of this commentary is somewhat reminiscent of *How to Recognise the Best Physician*. Here too, there is no reference whatsoever to this work in Galen's Greek corpus, nor in his bibliographic works, nor is there any reference to the treatise in the Graeco-Roman world. We find numerous citations, however, in the Arabic world; an indication by Ḥunayn in his *Epistle* (n. 112), who does not express any doubt regarding its attribution to Galen, but, at the same time, does not include it in his lists of books that are not mentioned by Galen in *My Own Books*, nor of works that are falsely attributed to him; see Iskandar (1989), 13 and 27–30.

14 See Anastassiou, Irmer (1997–2012), vol. 2.2, pp. 267–271, especially the citations in al-Ruhāwī (end of the 9th century) and from Ibn Ǧulǧul (10th century). The passages from al-Ruhāwī have been used for the first time by Jouanna (1992), 247–251. For a more detailed study of these different sources, see Overwien (2009), pp. 84–86, and now also Jouanna (2018), cxxii–cxxxvi.

original Greek text anywhere between the second and the sixth centuries AD. Several later scholars on the commentary have revisited the question of Galen's authorship: some consider the attribution to Galen as plausible, whereas other reject it, and yet others refrain from giving their opinion.[15] The Arabic tradition of the *Oath* has been used as a complementary witness to enrich the edition of the Greek text of the treatise. Yet, the central question remains whether the narrative text of the *Oath* known in Arabic has resulted from an autonomous tradition or translation, or from a compilation of the lemmas extracted from the commentary.[16] We know of two complete Arabic translations of the *Oath* itself: the first is preserved by Ibn Abī Uṣaybiʿa, and the second has been transmitted in the *Selection from the Cabinet of Wisdom* (*Muntaḫab Ṣiwān al-ḥikma*) by Abū Sulaymān al-Siǧistānī (Dunlop 1979, pp. 77–78, lines 1609–1627). Strohmaier (1974) was the first to notice this second translation and considers it to be superior to the first. He also studied the relation between these two versions and the commentary and concludes they have been extracted from the lemmas in the original commentary, and therefore not do represent independent translations.

As it is impossible to cite all the scholarly work on the *Oath*, suffice it to mention the rich study by Vivian Nutton (2012b), in which he draws attention to this commentary, long neglected by classicists and historians of medicine. He demonstrates that irrespective of whether or not Galen was the author, it constitutes a very rich source. Moreover, Overwien (2009) focused on the Arabic readings of the *Oath*, its transmission in the Arabic world, and its relevance to the reconstruction of the Greek text.

2 Codicology and Palaeography

A codicological and paleographic study of the twelve folios found among the *Damascus Papers* provides a number of facts that illuminate the history of the

15 The commentary is classed among the pseudo-Galenic works by Ullmann (1970), p. 62, n. 111, and Sezgin (1970), p. 28. On the other hand, G. Strohmaier (1970, 1974) leans more towards an attribution to Galen, arguing that the author calls himself from Pergamum, and knew the cultural and local image of Asclepius well, while also relying on Ḥunayn's opinion. By contrast, Kudlien (1981, 119) challenged the text by pointing out that its author relates the invention of medicine to dreams sent by the gods and considered it incompatible with authentic Galenic concepts. Van Nuffelen (2014) returned to the question of Asclepius as he appears in the surviving fragments of the commentary, and attempted to minimise the gap between this text and Galen's otherwise known opinions. Van Nuffelen did not, however, comment on the authenticity of the commentary.

16 See Jouanna (1992), 235–251 and (1996b), 253–272.

manuscript. The folios have been preserved in two different places within the collection. Two folios are part of file 12,869 and ten of file 13,056. The division into files, however, is random, and only took place after the fire, when the collection was transferred to Istanbul. In any case, the two folios of the first category are nearly intact while the bindings of the other ten folios are heavily damaged by the fire, obscuring the first recto lines and the last verso lines. The different states of conservation clearly show that the manuscript had already been divided into several parts at the time of the fire, and without doubt even before then. The bad and incomplete condition of the manuscript probably led to its being placed in the depository for old papers, rather than in the library of the Great Mosque.

The manuscript forms a codex written on parchment folios of 24.5 cm by 12.2 cm. It was copied in an old script of a category qualified by François Déroche (1987–1989, 356–358; 1992) as 'the New 'Abbāsid style', one of many old writing styles that can be distinguished because of a set of particularities in certain characters. A significant example is the letter *alif*, which is written in the form of an inverted 's', with a hook at the left top of the vertical bar, and, when it is in a final position, it has a tip extending underneath the line. Another characteristic letter is *ṭā*, which is written with a bar inclining to the right while the top curves to the left. When it comes at the end of a word, it ends with a tiny appendix at the bottom, which slightly curves downwards.

There are many more examples that show the similarity between the handwriting in our folios and this bookish handwriting from the 'Abbāsid period. François Déroche, whom we have consulted for his expertise regarding this document, dates the manuscript between AD 850 and 900. Parchment, which on which it is written, is rarely used in the Near East after AD 900 for manuscripts other than the Qur'ān. The handwriting in the new 'Abbāsid style is well attested in the ninth century. Therefore, it must have been written shortly after the translation of the text by Ḥunayn's school before 855 AD, as it is mentioned in Ḥunayn's *Epistle*. One should therefore think of a manuscript produced in Baghdad in the close vicinity of Ḥunayn. Without the title page, it is impossible to know whether we are dealing with the translation by Ḥubayš or perhaps that of 'Isā ibn Yaḥyā, since two contemporary texts seem to have existed according to Ḥunayn (as we have seen above). At this stage, it is hard to distinguish between the stylistic differences of the various translators in Ḥunayn's school, although future research could help solve this problem.

As we have no colophon, we cannot determine how and when the text arrived at the Grand Mosque of Damascus. There are two possibilities: one earlier process would be directly related to Ḥunayn who died in 873. It is known that he went to Damascus personally to search for manuscripts, and one can imagine that he may have offered his translations there, or perhaps sent them following the close contacts which he must have formed with the members of the intellectual circles of Damascus.[17] Another possibility involves a slightly later route, related to one of the two translators of the *Commentaries*, Ḥubayš, the nephew of Ḥunayn. The biographic dictionaries give him the *nisba* al-Dimašqī, 'the Damascene', even though the exact links that connect him to Damascus are unknown.[18] As he is believed to have died at the end of the ninth century, we could simply suppose that he sent a copy of the text during his life to the city with which he apparently entertained privileged connections. Of course, much later hypotheses remain possible as well.

3 Content of the Extracts

Since title page and colophon are missing, the first problem is to determine whether our manuscript contains the same work as that which Ḥunayn mentions in his *Epistle*, namely the *Commentary on the Book 'Oath of Hippocrates'* (*Tafsīr li-kitāb 'Ahd Buqrāṭ*) by Galen. This work is also described in the famous *Catalogue* (*Fihrist*) of the Baghdad librarian Ibn al-Nadīm a century later as the *The Book 'Oath of Hippocrates' with Galen's Commentary* (*Kitāb 'Ahd Buqrāṭ bi-tafsīr Ǧālīnūs*).[19] The first indicator that they are the same is the fact that the folios of the Damascus manuscript correspond to the description which Ḥunayn gives in his *Risāla*: the Hippocratic lemmas are introduced by '*qāla Buqrāṭu* (Hippocrates said)' and Galen's commentary by '*qāla Ǧālīnūsu* (Galen said)'. We occasionally find remarks by Ḥunayn introduced by the formula '*qāla Ḥunaynun* (Ḥunayn said)'. Ḥunayn used a similar third-person style to mark his personal additions in his translation of other Galenic treatises.[20]

A second, equally important argument to determine the identity of the commentary is that some folios in the *Damascus Papers* have a very similar text to that preserved in later authors such as Ibn Abī Uṣaybiʿa and already collected, translated and discussed in Rosenthal (1956). One example will suffice to

17 Boudon-Millot (2011), 340.

18 Ibn Abī Uṣaybiʿa, *Essential Information about the Classes of Physicians*, ed. Müller (1888), vol. 1, p. 202; ed. Riḍā (n.d.), p. 276.

19 Ibn al-Nadīm, *al-Fihrist* (Beirut, Dār al-Maʿrifa, 1978), 401; ed. Flügel (1871–1872), vol. 1, p. 288; and Dodge (1970), vol. 2, p. 679 (translation).

20 For other examples, see Pietrobelli (2012), p. 107 and n. 33, listing previous literature (on the *Commentary on Hippocrates' 'Regimen in Acute Diseases'*); and Vagelpohl (2011), 253–256 and 268–288, (2014), 19 and 55–57; (2016), 66–67 (on the *Commentary on Hippocrates' 'Epidemics'*).

illustrate this point, namely a passage describing the image of Asclepius with a laurel crown on his head and an egg in his hand:[21]

جعل على رأسه إكليل متخذ من شجر الغار، لأن هذه الشجرة تذهب بالحزن. ولهذا نجد هرمس، إذا سمي المهيب، كلل بمثل هذا الإكليل. فلأن الأطبّاء ينبغي لهم أن يصرفوا عنهم الأحزان، كلل أسقليبيوس بإكليل يذهب بالحزن.

جعل على رأسه إكليل متخذ من شجر الغار لأن هذه الشجرة تذهب بالحزن. ولهذا نجد هرمس، إذا سمي المهيب، كلل بمثل هذا الإكليل فإن الأطبّاء ينبغي لهم أن يصرفوا عنهم الأحزان، كذلك كلل أسقليبيوس بإكليل يذهب بالحزن.

> He (Asclepius) wears crown made from the laurel tree on his head, because that tree removes sadness. For the same reason, when Hermes is called 'the venerable', we see that he is crowned with such as crown. Because physicians must dispel sadness, Asclepius is crowned with a crown that removes sadness.

From a methodological point of view, it is worth noting that Ibn Abī Uṣaybiʿa is extremely precise when he cites these passages.[22] This increases his trustworthiness with regard to the other, lost, passages.

Since the folios undoubtedly derive from one and the same text, their discovery represents an undeniable progress. While until now our knowledge of this commentary relied exclusively on much later citations, we now have a witness offering a continuous narrative which is directly related to the same tradition. We can now establish, for example, that the passages devoted to Hippocrates' biography are in fact part of the comment on the very last lemma. These passages include the anecdote about Hippocrates' refusal of Artaxerxes' gifts which was already known through the extracts published by Rosenthal.

Another crucial contribution of our manuscript lies in the ethical sections of the text, which where previously unknown, because compilers preferred

21 The first quotation is from the *Damascus Papers*, file 12,869, fol. 1[a]; the second is a quotation from Ibn Abī Uṣaybiʿa, already translated by Rosenthal (1956), 71. On this image, see also Strohmaier (1970).

22 For an analysis of how Ibn Abī Uṣaybiʿa quotes from his sources, see Pormann (2010); (2015).

other parts of the text for their selections.[23] If we were to place the discovered folios within the structure of the work as it emerges from the new material, it becomes clear that the two folios of file 12,869 belong to the first part of the commentary. The first folio, which discusses Asclepius, contains a more complete passage than the one preserved in Ibn Abī Usaybiʿa. It probably explains the Christianised version of the lemma: 'I swear by God, Lord of life and death and Giver of health, and I swear by Asclepius, the creator of healing and all treatments, and I swear by all the saints of God.'[24]

The second folio of this file is unrelated to the first and contains a previously unknown comment on two subsequent lemmas from the *Oath* dealing with the disciple's duties towards his master. Part of it reads: '(I swear) to regard him who has taught me this art as equal to my parents, *and to share, in partnership, my livelihood with him and to give him a share when he is in need of necessities* (ἡγήσασθαι μὲν τὸν διδάξαντά με τὴν τέχνην ταύτην ἴσα γενέτῃσιν ἐμοῖσι, καὶ βίου κοινώσασθαι, *καὶ χρεῶν χρηΐζοντι μετάδοσιν ποιήσασθαι*)', The last part of this lemma (in italics) is preserved in the manuscript:[25] 'If he requires money, I shall share and provide some of my money (وإذا احتاج إلى مال، واسيته ووصلته[26] من مالي).

The ten folios in the second file (13,056) contain the continuous commentary, lemma after lemma, of the complete second part of the Oath concerning medical ethics, the most famous part today. The text on the first preserved folio in this file begins in the middle of the comment on abortive pessaries (of which the lemma has not been preserved) and the next folios continue with lemmas and explanations until the end of the text. This part of the commentary was previously completely unknown, with the exception of a small extract in which Hippocrates refused to care for the subjects of the Persian king Artaxerxes when they suffered from the plague, because the Persians were enemies of the Greeks.[27]

---

23 Nutton (2012b), 92 previously expressed his disappointment about the lacunae in the evidence derived from later quotations: 'How much has been lost in the process of selection is far from easy to determine, but the length of the existing quotations suggests that the author devoted more space in his single book to explaining the historical and cultural background of the *Oath* than to discussing the ethical questions that exercise modern interpreters.'

24 See Strohmaier (1974), 322–323, repeated in Strohmaier (2012), 178–179 about this invocation and the presence of the pagan name Asclepius.

25 *Damascus Papers*, file 12,869, fol. 2b.

26 Ibn Abī Uṣaybiʿa read واصلته instead of وصلته.

27 See Rosenthal (1956), 77–78. This anecdote is otherwise known from the so-called 'Persian' Hippocratic Letters; see Pinault (1992), 79–93 (on 'Hippocrates and Artaxerxes'), and 115–124 (on 'The Accounts of Hippocrates and the King of Persia in the Ṣiwān and the Muḫtār'). Pinault, however, did not quote Rosenthal's translation, although the commentary must

The previous discussion shows that our commentary on the *Oath* followed a similar pattern to other Galenic commentaries. Because the manuscript is of such an early date, the ninth century, it is the earliest witness to the text of the *Oath*, apart from a small number of papyrus fragments.[28] We will not discuss the formation of the Hippocratic text here in detail, but the following preliminary remarks may be useful. The transmission of the Greek text is divided in a 'old' recension, the Marcianus gr. 269 (10th c.) and the Vaticanus gr. 276 (12th c.), and a 'new' recension, Ambrosianus gr. 134 (13th–14th c.), sometimes judged as superior to the old recension.[29] Suffice it to say that our manuscript supports Jacques Jouanna's (1996b, 262–263) conclusions. He had already emitted some doubts about how reliable the readings of Ambrosianus are compared to the two other witnesses. Take the example of the injunction against cutting—'I will not cut, and certainly not those suffering from stone (Οὐ τεμέω δὲ οὐδὲ μὴν λιθιῶντας)'—, which we shall discuss more fully below. The Ambrosianus omits this phrase and replaces it with its own: 'nor my assistants nor other assistants will I allow to participate in such an action (οὔτ' ἐμοῖσι δὲ οὔτ' ἄλλοισιν ἐκχωρήσω)'; this phrase does not relate to cutting, but to administering poison. Because the injunction not to cut is so strange, some scholars wanted to adopt the reading of the Ambrosianus. Our Arabic manuscript sides with the old recension and the Vindobonensis med.gr. 37 (Jouanna 2018, lxxxvi) against the Ambrosianus and thus confirms that the latter contains more recent innovations.

But let us now turn to the heart of the matter, namely the new information on the ethical section of the *Oath* that this manuscript brings to light for the first time. The commentary is much shorter in these sections that, for instance, the long discussion about Asclepius and to the origin of medicine, which we had already known. Nevertheless, even if the damage caused by fire renders certain passages of the manuscript unclear, these new sections contain many interesting interpretations. We will discuss some of these here, focusing on two of the most famous sections of the *Oath*, about abortion and surgery.

---

have been the principal sources of this anecdote in the Arab world. On the transmission of the Letters in the Islamic world, see Cottrell (2016): she studies London, British Library, MS Or. 12070, which associates a part of the Hippocratic Letters with two short treatises, *Law*, and *Testament*. Jouanna (1996b, 253–272) has shown that both deal with the *Oath* from a specific tradition and constitute an ethical 'triad'. Even if the Oath is absent in this Arabic manuscript, this regrouping remains suggestive.

28 *P.Oxy.* XXXI 2547, from the 4th century AD, republished by Manetti (2008).

29 Jouanna (2018, lxxii–lxxxvi) adds another manuscript neglected by the previous editors and pertaining to the new recension, the Vindobonensis med. gr. 37 (14th c.).

3.1 *Abortion*

Let us begin with the injunction against abortion, 'And likewise I will not give a woman a destructive pessary (ὁμοίως δὲ οὐδὲ γυναικὶ πεσσὸν φθόριον δώσω.)'.[30] In the manuscript, the lemma and the beginning of the commentary are absent, but what survives, even if damaged, still comprises three folios, with an addition by Ḥunayn in between two sections most likely attributable to Galen, even if a marker is missing for the first section. We will now provide a summary of the main elements of the commentary: it first discusses instances in which abortion are justified: a woman who has fallen pregnant at a very young age; an abnormally large foetus; ulcer in the womb (*fī l-raḥimi minhā waramun*);[31] situations where the lives of both mother and child are in danger; or the physician wants to avoid embryotomy, which is even more dangerous. The commentator copies the Hippocratic lemma and adds the following passage: 'I will not give abortive pessaries if someone asks me, but if I myself think I should do it, I will do it (*wa-lā uʿ*[*ṭī*] *farzaǧatan tusqitu l-ǧanīna* [*iḏā*] *ṭalabat minnī lākinnī iḏā raʾ*[*aytu*] *an afʿala ḏālika faʿaltuhū*)'.[32] According to the commentator, Hippocrates' objective was to save the mother rather than to get rid of the foetus. This passage is followed by an explicit reference to the treatise *Nature of the Child*, namely the famous passage in which a musician slave girl jumps up and down in order to expel a six-day old foetus, because her pregnancy will diminish her value.[33] The Arabic text, which is damaged here, does not speak of the value of the slave girl for her mistress, but rather of the danger imposed by her pregnancy and of the desire to remain beautiful (*tuḥibbu l-ǧamāla*).[34] Furthermore, the term 'contradiction' (*muḍādda*), is clearly readable at the end of the comment, as part of yet another reference to *Nature of the Child*.[35] The commentator clearly tolerated what we would today call a 'therapeutic abortion' in case of crucial danger of the mother's life, as can also be seen from the fact that he mentions chapter 13 of *Nature of the Child*. This

30 Whilst a lot of ink has been spilt over this passage, the most relevant article for our argument is that of Congourdeau (1997), who traced its reception in the Graeco-Roman and Arabic world.

31 File 13,056, fol. 1[a].

32 Ibid., fol. 1[b].

33 Chapter 13 (7.488–492 L.; Joly 1970, 55–56; Giorgianni 2006, p. 168, line 21–p. 174, line 2). See also Lonie (1981), 161, emphasising Galen's interest in this anecdote: 'Galen was impressed by the passage, and quotes from it four times'; and Anastassiou, Irmer (1997–2012), vol. 2.1, pp. 282–285.

34 File 13,056, fol. 2[a].

35 Ibid. fol. 3[a].

can be related to two other passages from Greek medical literature. First, Soranus (fl. ca. AD 100) speaks of a 'dispute' and shows that both supporters and opponents of abortion draw on both these Hippocratic passages to justify their opinion:[36]

> διὸ καὶ τὸν Ἱπποκράτην παραιτησάμενον τὰ φθόρια παραλαβεῖν ἐν τῷ Περὶ παιδίου φύσεως ἐκβολῆς χάριν τὸ πρὸς πυγὰς πηδᾶν. γεγένηται δὲ στάσις. οἱ μὲν γὰρ ἐκβάλλουσιν τὰ φθόρια τὴν Ἱπποκράτους προσκαλούμενοι μαρτυρίαν λέγοντος· "οὐ δώσω δὲ οὐδενὶ φθόριον", καὶ ὅτι τῆς ἰατρικῆς ἐστιν. ἴδιον τὸ τηρεῖν καὶ σῴζειν τὰ γεννώμενα ὑπὸ τῆς φύσεως. οἱ δὲ μετὰ διορισμοῦ συντάσσουσιν αὐτά, τοῦτ' ἔστιν οὐχ ὅτε διὰ μοιχείαν τις βούλεται φθεῖραι τὸ συλληφθὲν οὔτε δι' ἐπιτήδευσιν ὡραιότητος, ἀλλ' ὅτε διὰ ⟨τὸ⟩ κίνδυνον κωλῦσαι γενησόμενον ἐν ταῖς ἀποτέξεσιν, μικρᾶς τῆς μήτρας ὑπαρχούσης καὶ μὴ δυναμένης χωρῆσαι τὴν τελείωσιν, ἢ κατὰ τοῦ στομίου κονδυλώματα καὶ ῥαγάδας ἐχούσης, ἤ τινος ἐμφεροῦς περιστάσεως ἐγκειμένης. τὰ δὲ αὐτὰ λέγουσιν καὶ περὶ ἀτοκίων, οἷς καὶ ἡμεῖς συναινοῦμεν. ὅθεν ἐπεὶ τοῦ φθεῖραι τὸ κωλῦσαι γενέσθαι σύλληψιν ἀσφαλέστερον, περὶ τούτου νῦν πρῶτον ὑποδείξομεν.

> For this reason they say that Hippocrates, although prohibiting abortives, yet in his book *Nature of the Child* employs leaping with the heels to the buttocks for the sake of expulsion. But a controversy has arisen. For one party banishes abortives, citing the testimony of Hippocrates who says: 'I will give to no one an abortive'; moreover, because it is the specific task of medicine to guard and preserve what has been engendered by nature. The other party prescribes abortives, but with discrimination, that is, they do not prescribe them when a person wishes to destroy the embryo because of adultery or out of consideration for youthful beauty; but only to prevent subsequent danger in parturition if the uterus is small and not capable of accommodating the complete development, or if the uterus at its orifice has knobby swellings and fissures, or if some similar difficulty is involved. And they say the same about contraceptives as well, and we too agree with them. And since it is safer to prevent conception from taking place than to destroy the foetus, we shall first discourse upon such prevention.

36 Soranus, *Gynaecology*, 1.60 (Ilberg 1927, p. 45, lines 6–19); 1.20 (Gourevitch et al. 1988–2000, vol. 1, p. 59, lines 8–24); tr. Temkin (1991), 62–63. On this passage, also see Gourevitch (1992), 598–599.

The second passage is found in John of Alexandria (first half of the 6th century), who, in his commentary on *Nature of the Child*, also demonstrates a contradiction between this passage and the prohibition in the *Oath*:[37]

> Εἰώθασιν ἀπορεῖν ἐνταῦθα ὅτι αὐτός ἐστιν ὁ λέγων ἐν τῷ ὅρκῳ 'οὐ δώσω φθόριον'. πῶς οὖν κελεύει ἐπὶ πυγὴν πηδῆσαι τὴν γυναῖκα; καὶ πρὸς ταύτην τὴν ἀπορίαν πολλαὶ φέρονται λύσεις.
>
> It is customary to object at this point that it was [Hippocrates] himself who said in the *Oath* 'I will not give the means to induce abortion'. How is it, then, that he orders the woman to perform the buttocks leap? Numerous responses to this objection are current.

John's main aim was to save Hippocrates from the charge that he had caused an abortion. He therefore deploys four arguments against this accusation: 1) there was only semen, as the foetus had not yet formed; 2) Hippocrates merely wanted to conduct a scientific experiment for the greater good; 3) or he wanted to prevent the birth of the illegitimate child to a prostitute; and last but not least, 4) he wanted to prevent the suicide of the mother, whose pregnancy would have decreased her beauty, an intolerable situation for a courtesan.[38] Hippocrates had thus chosen to destroy not a life, but merely the semen in order to avoid losing both mother and child.

The overlap between Soranus and John on the one hand and the Arabic commentary on the other does not stop there. After quoting *Nature of the Child*, the commentator continues his discussion by distinguishing between different types of drugs, which he organises in three distinct categories: contraceptive, abortive, and expulsive. Perhaps he does so in order to defend Hippocrates here again against the charge of abortion, as he merely advised an expulsion:[39]

> ونقول بان هذا [الـ]ـقول إن الدواء المانع [من ا]لحمل غير الدواء المسقط [للـ]ـجنين والدواء المخرج له [غير]هما جميعا. وذلك .... [إن] الدواء المانع من الحبل [هو] الذي إذا تنوّل منع المر[أ]ه من الحمل. وأما [المسقط] للجنين فالذي إذا أد[ني يفسد] الطفل. وأما المخر[ج] فالذي يخرج الجنين با[لدواء] وبالطفرة فالذي أ[دني من] الجارية الفتية إنما [كان] مخرجا لا مسقطا.

37 John of Alexander, *Commentary on Hippocrates' 'Nature of the Child'* 18 (Bell et al. 1997, p. 146, lines 16–19 [text]; p. 147, lines 15–17 [translation].)

38 Ibid. (Bell et al. 1997, p. 146, lines 19–32 [text]; p. 147, lines 17–33 [translation].)

39 File 13,056, fol. 2^{a-b}.

> Regarding this we assert that the medicine that prevents pregnancy (contraceptive) is different from the abortive medicine, and that the medicine that makes [the foetus] come out (expulsive) is different from the both of the other medicines. For (…). The contraceptive medicine is the medicine that, when taken, prevents the woman from getting pregnant. The abortive medicine is the medicine that when administered destroys the child. The expulsive medicine brings out the foetus by medicine and jumping. And the courtisan used the expulsive medicine and not the abortive one.

This tripartite classification into contraceptive (*māniʿ mina l-ḥamli*, ἀτόκιον), abortive (*musqiṭ*, φθόριον), and expulsive (*muḫriǧ*, ἐκβόλιον) is also found in Soranus just before the passage quoted above:[40]

> Εἰ φθορίοις καὶ ἀτοκίοις χρηστέον καὶ πῶς.
>
> Ἀτόκιον δὲ φθορίου διαφέρει, τὸ μὲν γὰρ οὐκ ἐᾷ γενέσθαι σύλληψιν, τὸ δὲ φθείρει τὸ συλληφθέν· εἴπωμεν οὖν ἄλλο ‘φθόριον’ καὶ ἄλλο ‘ἀτόκιον’. τὸ δὲ ‘ἐκβόλιον’ οἱ μὲν συνωνυμεῖν τῷ φθορίῳ λέγουσιν, οἱ δὲ διαφέρειν τῷ μὴ ἐν φαρμάκοις νοεῖσθαι, κατασεισμοῖς δὲ καὶ πηδήμασιν ….

> Whether One Ought to Make Use of Abortives and Contraceptives and How?
>
> A contraceptive differs from an abortive, for the first does not let conception take place, while the latter destroys what has been conceived. Let us, therefore, call the one ‘abortive (*phthórion*)’ and the other ‘contraceptive (*atókion*)’. And an ‘expulsive (*ekbólion*)’ some people say is synonymous with an abortive; others, however, say that there is a difference because an expulsive does not mean drugs but shaking and leaping ….

In the Arabic translation we can easily identify the three Greek terms φθόριον, ἀτόκιον and ἐκβόλιον, which proves again that the source of the Arabic must have been Greek. These seem to be the only two texts to adopt this tripartite classification.[41] If the Arabic commentary goes back to Galen in one way

40 Soranus, *Gynaecology*, 1.60 (Ilberg 1927, p. 45, lines 1–6); 1.20 (Gourevitch et al. 1988–2000, vol. 1, p. 59, lines 1–7); tr. Temkin (1991), 62.

41 The passage in Aetius of Amida 16.17 combines abortive and expulsive agents and thus reduces the three categories to two: φθόριον: Ἀτόκιον δὲ φθορίου διαφέρει· τὸ μὲν γὰρ ἀτόκιον οὐκ ἐᾷ γίγνεσθαι σύλληψιν, τὸ δὲ φθόριον φθείρει τὸ συλληφθὲν καὶ ἐκβάλλει (Zervos 1901, p. 18, lines 1–3).

or another, this similarity would be even more remarkable, since Galen never mentions Soranus' *Gynaecology* in his extant works.[42]

3.2 *Bladder Stone Operation and Surgery*

The second example demonstrating the importance of the newly discovered manuscript relates apparent prohibition of surgery 'I will not cut, and certainly not those suffering from stone, but I will cede [this] to men [who are] practitioners of this activity (Οὐ τεμέω δὲ οὐδὲ μὴν λιθιῶντας, ἐκχωρήσω δὲ ἐργάτῃσιν ἀνδράσι πρήξιος τῆσδε.)'. The lemma in our manuscript understands this passage to be a prohibition of bladder stone operations: 'I will no cut patients suffering from stones in their bladder, but I will leave this to those whose profession this operation is ([*wa*]*-lā ašuqqu ayḍān ʿan man fī maṯānatihī* [*ḥiǧā*]*ratun lākin atruku fiʿla ḏālika ilā* [*man*] *kānat ḥirfatuhū hāḏā l-ʿamala*)'.[43] Even on this narrower interpretation, this phrase has been controversial, because bladder stone operations were often performed by the versatile Greek physicians of the day.[44] The commentator first lists past criticisms against Hippocrates, who is accused of abandoning his patients to their fate, in what must be an allusion to other commentaries on the *Oath* which have not survived:[45]

وقد لام بعض الناس الشيخ بقراط [في] هذا القول فقالوا إنه لم يصب [في] منعها بيمين من الشق عن الحجارة وهي علة ذات خطر يحتاج فيها إلى معونة الطبيب.

> Some people have criticised the master Hippocrates about this lemma, saying that he was wrong to forbid in an oath to cut out bladder stones, although this is a very dangerous disease which requires the help of a physician.

But to support Hippocrates and justify the prohibition, the author adds innovative and sophisticated arguments:[46]

---

42 Gourevitch (2009), 256: 'Galen's interest in the past history of therapeutics seems to be limited to works of pharmacology and cosmetics. We have, for instance, established that Galen did not know [Soranus'] *Gynaecology*—or at least he did not mention it. (La recherche du passé thérapeutique entreprise par Galien semble strictement limitée à des ouvrages de pure pharmacologie, ou, à la rigueur, de cosmétologie. Nous avons constaté par exemple que Galien ne connaissait pas le *Traité des maladies des femmes*, ou du moins n'en faisait pas état.)'

43 File 13,056, fol. 4[a].

44 See Leven (2018), Witt (2018).

45 File 13,056, fol. 4[a].

46 Ibid., fol. 4[b].

> أبقراط لم يمنع من الشـ[ـق عن] الحجارة، لكن من شق من لا حجارة في مثانته.
>
> Hippocrates did not forbid cutting bladder stones, but cutting those who do not have stones in their bladder.

The commentator thus denounces unscrupulous physicians who exploit the fact that many bladder diseases have similar symptoms and convince their patients that they suffer from bladder stones, even when they do not; they then operate for no other reason than to make money. Even if the bladder stone is imaginary, the operation is not, and the charlatan will go so far as to bring a small stone resembling an extracted stone to make the patient believe that the operation has been successful.[47] It is therefore out of caution and concern for the physician's reputation that Hippocrates advised against this operation. Because there were just too many fraudulent cases, he recommended to leave it to specialists, namely surgeons.

A little further, the commentator also criticises the false physicians who do not enter homes except to corrupt their inhabitants, in contrast to the ideal physician embodied by Hippocrates and those who respect the Oath:[48]

> [و]ذلك أنّا نجد قوما ينتحلون صناعة الطب ويدخلون [إ]لى منازل الناس فيفسدون [في؟] بعض الأوقات العبيد على مواليهم وفي بعضها الأبناء على آبائهم و [...] أفسدوا أيضا النساء على ا[لرجال؟] إلا أن هذه الأشياء لا [...] أحدا ممن قبل إيمان [...]
>
> There are, however, those who claim [to master] the art of medicine and enter the houses of people to corrupt slaves by pitting them against their masters, and sons against their fathers [...] they also corrupt women, pitting them against [their husbands]. However, these things [...] anyone who has taken the *Oath*.

---

47 Interestingly, Abū Bakr al-Rāzī (d. c. 925) later denounced this trick used by charlatans in his Book for al-Manṣūr (*al-Kitāb al-Manṣūrī*) 7.27; Savage-Smith (1996, 937) cites this passage: 'Sometimes they remove stones from the bladder and replace them with others which they proceed to extract. Frequently, they do not even check to see if there are stones in the bladder. Instead, they have the audacity to cut it open recklessly and insert a finger in the incision. If they find a stone, they take it out, but if not, they place one there to take out.' We know from other extracts that al-Rāzī must have read this commentary, and this passage is therefore probably directly influenced by it.

48 File 13,056, fol 6[a–b].

Using the Hippocratic ideal to denounce charlatans who abuse their position is a familiar theme in the medical ethics of Galen. Here, a fake bladder stone is secretly introduced and then extracted. We find a very similar pattern in Galen's treatise *Diseases That Are Hard to Cure*; although it is lost in Greek, we have some Arabic fragments. In one of them Galen inveighs against a charlatan who made a patient believe that he had extracted a worm from his tooth, although he had actually had brought it in a little bottle.[49]

4 Was Galen the Author?

These similarities between the commentary and Galen's other works raise again the question, already briefly broached at the beginning of the article, whether the commentary on the *Oath* actually is an Arabic translation of a work by Galen. Space does not permit to discuss this issue exhaustively, so that we merely highlight some points that show the similarities between the two. The commentator twice denounces charlatans and contrasts them with the figure of Hippocrates. He also emphasises that physicians should treat slaves and free men equally, without any concern for money.[50] These themes are well known leitmotifs of Hippocratic ethics, as revived by Galen. We already knew that the commentator quoted from the *Prognostic* and was familiar with the Hippocratic *Letters*;[51] the new passages show that he was also conversant with the *Nature on the Child*, and in particular with chapter 13, from which Galen himself often quoted.[52]

A different kind of reference, not medical but poetic, can be retrieved from a passage considerably damaged by the fire. It speaks of a person called Fūlūksānī in Arabic:

49 See Pormann (2005), 196 (according to al-Qifṭī and Ibn Abī Uṣaybiʿa): 'The man was saying to them: "I am one of the inhabitants of Aleppo. I have encountered Galen, and he taught me all his sciences. This is a remedy that helps against worms in the teeth." This wicked man had [previously] prepared a ball made out of tar and cotton. He placed it onto amber and fumigated the mouth of the patient who believed that he suffered from worms in his teeth. The patient had to close his eyes. Once he had closed them, this man slipped a worm into his mouth, which he had at hand in a box. Then he extracted it from the mouth of the patient suffering from tooth[ache]. After he had done this, the fools threw the things they had to him [i.e., gave him their money].'; see also Boudon-Millot (2003a).

50 See Jouanna (1996), 234–235 about Hippocrates' disdaining money and treating the poor.

51 Rosenthal (1956), 70, quoting the beginning of the *Prognostic*.

52 See above note 33.

تكون فولوكساني المذكورة في الشعر يقال إنها لما بلغت الموت [...] أ]ن يكون شكلها في [...]
الذي يسقط فيه [...] لا حسنا كما قال اور[يبد]س في قصيدته.

... Fūlūksānī, who was mentioned in poetry, is said to have reach death ... her shape was ... into which falls ... no beauty, as Euripides said in his poem.

This Fūlūksānī mentioned by Euripides is Polyxena, the youngest daughter of Priam and Hecuba. In his eponymous play *Hecuba*, Euripides writes about Polyxena as she is about to be sacrificed on the tomb of Achilles:[53]

ἡ δὲ καὶ θνῄσκουσ' ὅμως
πολλὴν πρόνοιαν εἶχεν εὐσχήμων πεσεῖν,
κρύπτουσ' ἃ κρύπτειν ὄμματ' ἀρσένων χρεών.

but she, even in death,
took good heed to fall with grace,
hiding from the gaze of men what must be hidden.

This quotation depicts Polyxena as 'having a good shape (εὐσχήμων)' even in death, and therefore probably relates to the injunction of modesty in the *Oath*. Galen uses this same passage in his *Commentary on Hippocrates' 'Prognostic'*, but this time in a comment on the word πρόνοια in the sense of 'foresight', which has an unusual and technical meaning in the *Prognostic*.[54] This passage, however, has been cited repeatedly in medical Greek literature, and the similarity between the commentary on the *Oath* and Galen may therefore go back to a common source which was later reused within the school of Alexandria.[55]

We will conclude with a last possible understanding, this time from within the Galenic corpus. The comment on lithiasis mentioned above ends with a surprising affirmation of the inferiority of the surgeon with respect to the physician:[56]

53 Verses 568–569, translated by Coleridge (1938).

54 Galen, *Commentary on Hippocrates' 'Prognostic'* 1.4 (18b.7.16–8.2 K.; Heeg 1915, p. 201, lines 6–9).

55 This passage is also cited by Stephen of Alexandria in his *Commentary on Hippocrates' 'Prognostics'* (Duffy 1983, p. 38, lines 16–19), and in *Theriac to Piso*, part of the Galenic corpus although not by Galen himself. We thank Véronique Boudon-Millot for making us aware of this last citation; see now her edition, Boudon-Millot (2016), ch. 8.12, pp. 38–39, and note 1 on pp. 185–186.

56 File 13,056, fol. 5[a].

وقد نجد [بـ]ـقراط في هذا القول [يشـ]ـرّف الأطباء ويقدّمهم [على] أصحاب الجراحة ويجعل [مر]تبة عمل الجراحة بعقب مرتبة العلاج بالتدبير.

> We see that in this lemma Hippocrates here wishes to make physicians more noble and superior to surgeons; he makes the rank of surgery come after that of treatment by regimen.

We find an echo of this passage in Galen's treatise *How to Recognise the Best Physician*.[57] Galen there says the following about surgery and regimen:[58]

> I say that you should consider a physician learned and wise, trained and skilful, if he can cure with drugs diseases which surgeons treat by making incisions (...). You should praise a physician's knowledge of drugs if he can cure all these diseases with drugs without resorting to incision, unless compelling necessity calls for such treatment. (...) Praise also their knowledge of drugs if they cure elephantiasis or disperse stones formed in the bladder and the kidney or prevent the formation of stones in the joints or disperse those which are already formed. (...) A skilful physician can cure all these illnesses by drugs together with diet.

In this way, Galen insists that a good physician can cure with drugs and diet what a surgeon cures by operating. He specifically mentions bladder stones, thus creating an implicit hierarchy between the physician and the surgeon and their respective medical practices. All these elements constitute indications in favour of an attribution to Galen, but none of them is conclusive, and the complete absence of any reference to the *Oath* in Galen's other medical works remains problematic.

Another argument against Galen's authorship is length. Galen normally gives very long-winded explanations in his other commentaries. The author of this commentary on the *Oath* could possibly draw on a common source of

---

57 See Nutton (1990), especially p. 240 on the question of whether it is really by Galen. This Galenic treatise *How to Recognise the Best Physician* like the commentary on the *Oath* is never mentioned in the extant Greek works by Galen nor in bio-bibliographical sources in the Graeco-Roman world, whereas we find numerous quotations of both in medieval Arabic sources. Ḥunayn in particular list the treatise in his *Epistle* (no. 112) and does not express any doubt that it is by Galen; moreover, Ḥunayn does not list this treatise among the books not mentioned by Galen in *My Own Books* nor among the books falsely attributed to him (see Iskandar 1990, 13, 27–30).

58 Iskandar (1988), 117–118.

medical scholarship, no doubt related to the Alexandrian school of medicine. Be that as it may, his medical and literary knowledge is extensive, as Nutton already noted.[59] It would perhaps be even more interesting for the reception history of Hippocrates, if the author of this commentary were a physician other than Galen.

The question remains open and can perhaps be answered once we have edited, translated and analysed all the extant new fragments, as we hope to do. This unexpected discovery within the documentary-like *Damascus Papers* is only one of a line of recent discoveries that have given us quite a few hitherto unknown treatises by Galen. One could mention *Avoiding Grief*, discovered in Thessaloniki by A. Pietrobelli and published by J. Jouanna and V. Boudon-Millot in 2010.[60] However fragmentary and damaged by the fire, this new witness from the ninth century AD, one of the oldest known Arabic medical manuscripts, represents the missing link in the transmission history of the *Oath* in the East, between Ḥunayn's *Epistle* and later quotations by Arabic bio-bibliographical authors. Above all—whoever the author may be—this manuscript has restored the ethical part of a commentary on one of the most famous Hippocratic treatises, of which until recently no remnants were thought to have survived. The commentary rediscovered among the *Damascus Papers*, 60 years after F. Rosenthal's article, illustrates again the richness of the Oriental collections and the future discoveries that are still to come.

59 Nutton (2012b), 99–100: 'one may conclude that the tradition of Hippocratic scholarship represented here even in fragmentary form, was broader and more extensive than Galen leads us to believe. Galen became a less isolated figure than might have been supposed. The author is a man of considerable erudition, able to draw on a variety of traditions and to quote poetry, as well as being interested in things beyond the Greek world. If he is not Galen, then we have yet another doctor with intellectual claims to our attention.'

60 See Manetti (2012), Nutton (2016), and Singer (2018a and b); and Petit (2018) more generally.

CHAPTER 6

Beyond and behind the Commentary: Galen on Hippocrates on Elements

Peter N. Singer

> The present discussion is not designed for one used to discourses of human nature which go beyond what is relevant to medicine.
>
> HIPPOCRATES, *Nature of Man* 1 (6.32 L.; Jouanna 2002, p. 164, lines 3–5)

•••

> Hippocrates, our guide in all that is good
>
> GALEN, *Prognosis* 1 (14.602 K.; Nutton 1979, p. 70, lines 16–17)

Galen is a voluminous and important commentator on Hippocratic texts; and certain Hippocratic texts—or certain interpretations of them—are of central theoretical importance to him in the formulation and presentation of his own views.*

These facts are well known; and there is a considerable volume of recent scholarship on Galen's scholarly and interpretive work on Hippocrates. The fact—or the risk—that we read 'Hippocrates' through Galen's eyes has also been an important finding of modern scholarship.[1]

* I am grateful to Peter E. Pormann and the conference organizers for the invitation to participate in the Colloque Hippocratique at Manchester in 2015, and for their hospitality during the event; and I am indebted to the other participants, most especially to Sabrina Grimaudo, Jim Hankinson, David Leith, Daniela Manetti, Amneris Roselli, Ralph Rosen and Roland Wittwer, for their instructive feedback and discussion. This paper was written during research funded by the Wellcome Trust and the Alexander von Humboldt Foundation, to both of which institutions I extend my sincere gratitude.

1 An essential introduction to Galen's Hippocratic scholarship is Manetti and Roselli (1994); amongst extensive recent work, on Galen's scholarship in general and his scholarship on Hippocrates in particular, see also especially: Manuli (1984), Lloyd (1993), Mansfeld (1994), Vegetti

© PETER N. SINGER, 2021 | DOI:10.1163/9789004470200_008

Building on that body of recent work, and on that perception, the present paper aims to point out four specific aspects, or results, of Galen's very particular engagement with Hippocrates. First, on the basis of a range of Galenic texts and remarks, I aim to show that for Galen Hippocratic commentary and exposition of his own views are enmeshed more closely, and in a more complicated way, than has sometimes been realized. Secondly, I point to the central importance of a particular Hippocratic text, *Nature of Man*, and a particular intepretation of that text, within the structure of Galen's own argumentation on element theory. Thirdly, I suggest that behind this Galenic argumentation we may discern a fundamentally different position, in relation to the value and status of element theory for medicine—an anti-theoretical, or theoretically minimalist, position which Galen's rhetoric does its best to obscure, but which *also* claims the authority of the same Hippocratic text. Fourthly, I suggest that Galen's particular interpretation of Hippocratic element theory casts a long shadow on subsequent interpretation of Hippocrates—a shadow, indeed, from which we have not entirely emerged. The conclusions will thus represent a contribution both to the interpretation of Galen and the nature of his influence, on the one hand, and to the understanding of the history of commentary on Hippocrates, on the other.

1 Commentary and Non-commentary

In the proem to his commentary on *Fractures*, Galen makes an apparently obvious and common-sense distinction: between the accurate elucidation of a previous author's text—the task of a commentary—and the demonstration of true and refutation of false doctrines, or defence of the author, on the other.[2] In a similar vein, in his commentary on the Hippocratic *Prognostic*, he makes reference to other works as the correct place to learn the full theory of prognosis: here, by contrast, he is simply explaining the *léxis* of Hippocrates.[3]

But how clear-cut is this distinction for Galen, in theory or in practice? In the very same passage of the *Fractures* commentary, in fact, he proceeds to justify a

(1999), Von Staden (2009), Manetti (2012), Boudon-Millot (2015). On Galen's 'appropriation' of Hippocrates, see especially Smith (1979); also Temkin (1932), Lloyd (1988), Singer (1996). Specifically on Galen's use of *Nature of Man* in relation to element theory, see Jouanna (2000), as well as the introduction and notes to his edition of the text; also Tassinari (1997), Todd (2015), Hankinson (2015), (forthcoming), and his contribution to the present proceedings.

2 18b.318 K.

3 3.6 (18b.229–236 K.; Heeg 1915, 328–331).

certain level of non-exegetic activity, even for the exegete; nor, indeed, can one deny that the *Prognostic* commentary does, itself, spend a considerable time setting forth Galen's own views and defending Hippocrates from attacks (see further note 19 below).

Of course, we may doubt the plausibility of the distinction between exegesis and exposition—insofar as it relates to Hippocrates—from the outset. Galen's professed admiration for and self-alignment with the master is bound to have certain consequences for his exegesis. He is reluctant to attribute views wildly divergent from his own to Hippocrates; conversely, he seeks in that author's texts views which are identical to his own, albeit less fully articulated. Such an approach inevitably affects his view as to which texts can be regarded as authentically Hippocratic; Galen's undoubtedly sophisticated historical scholarship is vitiated—or at least strongly guided in its direction—by a prior view of the kind of doctrines the 'divine' Hippocrates can be thought to have held. Moreover, the style or *léxis* of a particular passage—arguably a still more subjective and fluid criterion—may also be brought forward in arguments for or (especially) against authenticity; and in the context of such arguments in relation to problem passages Galen will give his own evaluative judgements as to what Hippocrates can and cannot plausibly be taken to have written.[4]

Indeed, in relation to authenticity, Galen applies a sliding scale, in accordance with the reliability or unreliability of the view expressed.[5] Thus, the text of *Nature of Man* itself is divided into sections which are 'in accordance with the Hippocratic art' (the first two parts, which are therefore considered authentic), inconsistent with observed fact and with what 'Hippocrates' says elsewhere (the next section, dealt with in book 2 of Galen's commentary, including the anatomical material—therefore inauthentic); very close to the right level (the last part, also known as *Regimen in Health*—therefore by the pupil Polybus).[6]

4 The situation is, in fact, more complex than the present brief sketch can convey. See Börno and Coughlin (2020), who both give a rich account of Galen's use of one particular stylistic term, *kakozēlía*, to deny authenticity to 'Hippocratic' passages and point out the potential conflict in the criteria Galen himself claims to use in his quest of the authentically Hippocratic: these include not just linguistic style (*léxis*) but also antquity of the manuscripts consulted (a criterion which in theory trumps that of the 'implausibility' of a reading). See further Hankinson, in this volume.

5 The very fact that the term for 'authentic' admits of grammatical degrees is revealing; see for example the superlative form γνησιωτάτοις at *Commentary on Hippocrates' 'Nature of Man'* 1 (15.14 K.; Mewaldt 1914, p. 9, line 24).

6 *Commentary on Hippocrates' 'Nature of Man'* 1 (15.9–12 K.; Mewaldt 1914, p. 7, line 15–p. 8, line 29); 2 (15.108–109 K.; Mewaldt 1914, p. 57, lines 4–21); cf. also *Commentary on Hippocrates' 'Nature of Man'* 1.44 (15. 102–107 K.; Mewaldt 1914, p. 53, line 15–p. 56, line 6), a lengthy discussion associating the concepts of correct method and Hippocratic authenticity. A sim-

Works too difficult to incorporate in a Galenic discourse are not only rejected as inauthentic (as for example with the passages of *Nature of Man* just discussed) but, in some cases, rather overlooked, passed over in near-silence.[7]

The very nature of the literary enterprise, of course, which justifies extremely lengthy exegesis of words or phrases which are in themselves sketchy, notional, even cryptic, allows the commentator to interpret creatively, or at least optimistically. One thinks here particularly of Galen's belief in the high level of Hippocratic anatomical science or, in another context, of the pages-long exposition of Galen's own views of the importance of the psychological in patient pathology, occasioned by a single word, *gnṓmē*, in book 6 of the *Epidemics*.[8]

On the other hand, Galen almost completely ignores certain texts which appear to offer him support in certain of his central arguments. *Sacred Disease* and *Breaths*, for example, are pretty much the only Hippocratic texts which offer something like a brain-centred view of rational activity; and *Ancient Medicine* offers something close to a Galenic view of regimen.[9] It seems likely here that certain other intrinsic features of these texts make him anxious to ignore them—in the cases cited, the phlegm-based humoral theory of *The Sacred Disease* and the anti-theoretical stance of *Ancient Medicine*. So, here again, a rejection on historical grounds is intimately connected with an antipathy to intellectual content.

---

ilar sliding scale applies to the authenticity of the books of the *Epidemics* according to Galen: books 1 and 3 are completely authentic, books 2 and 6 compilations based on authentic material by Hippocrates' son Thessalus, books 4, 5 and 7 forgeries. For a summary of the relevant Galenic passages and literature see Vagelpohl (2014), 12–14, with notes. Cf. the somewhat different perspective of Hankinson in this volume, emphasizing the overall coherence and the argued nature of Galen's position, in relation to *Nature of Man* in particular.

7 I do not mean to enter here into any discussion of modern attempts to identify—or even to find more or less plausible candidates for—the authentically Hippocratic within the Corpus. There is of course a vast literature in this area. Alongside the classic Edelstein (1967), see especially Lloyd (1991) and Craik (2015) for appropriately cautious accounts; Smith (1979) on the historical construction of 'Hippocrates'; and van der Eijk (2015), problematizing the very use of the term 'Hippocratic' as a demarcator within the corpus of classical medical writing.

8 *Epidemics* 6.23 (5.352.8–9 L.), commented by Galen in his *Commentary on Hippocrates' 'Epidemics' 6* 8 (Wenkebach and Pfaff 1956, 485–487).

9 Galen wants to attribute his Platonic tripartite psychology, with the rational in the brain, to Hippocrates, and can only most tenuously detect it in the texts on which he does rely: on this point see Singer (1996), Vegetti (1999); on *Ancient Medicine* and Galenic regimen, see Grimaudo (2008), as well as her chapter in this volume.

Let us turn then to Galen's 'commentaries', and consider their relationship with the non-commentary treatises. A substantial part of this commentary work seems to belong to a rather late period in his output, and perhaps relatedly to an increasingly leisured focus on more purely scholarly endeavour, after the writing of his main works of anatomy, physiology and medicine.[10] Let us however consider some problems in maintaining the distinct nature of the commentary genre.

If we turn to the text which will be our central focus in the next phase of this paper, *Elements According to Hippocrates*, this is clearly very far from 'commentary' in any usual sense of the word. It cites verbatim, or even refers to, only a very small part of the text upon which it is 'commenting'; and it is centrally concerned to lay out Galen's own views and refute those of his opponents (and not just in their interpretation of Hippocrates). It is, moreover, a text to which Galen himself refers in a number of other places in his oeuvre as that in which the correct theory of the elements has been demonstrated.[11]

Yet Galen explicitly refers to *Elements* as an *exhḗgēsis* of the Hippocratic text *Nature of Man*. More than that, he claims elsewhere that it was precisely its adequacy in this role that made him refrain from writing 'another' commentary: he does not like to do the same thing twice. The reason that he finally *does* decide to write a line-by-line commentary is apparently to be attributed to certain features of the text's argumentative presentation, rather than to any inadequate coverage of the text 'commented': it takes too much for granted, because of the particular level of knowledge of the intended recipient.[12] Conversely, the *Commentary on Hippocrates' 'Nature of Man'*, which *is* a line-by-line commentary and undoubtedly falls within that genre, is an argumentative work which goes far beyond the exegesis of Hippocrates. It is, in fact, a work which—even more so than *Elements*—attempts an exposition of Galen's own detailed understanding of the fundamental composition of the world, and of the notions of element, principle, quality and matter—an exposition which

10 On the chronology see e.g. Jouanna (2000), as well as the discussion of Hankinson (forthcoming); but see also further below for more detailed considerations on the chronological progression of his commentary work, on Galen's own account.

11 *Mixtures* 1.1 (1.509 K.; Helmreich 1904, p. 1, lines 5–7); cf. *Preservation of Health* 1.4–5 (6.13 K.; Koch 1923, p. 8, lines 10–15).

12 *Commentary on Hippocrates' 'Nature of Man'* 1 (15.1–2 K.; Mewaldt 1914, p. 3, lines 1–19); *Doctrines of Hippocrates and Plato* 8.2 (5.663–664 K.; De Lacy 1978, p. 492, lines 11–21). The latter passage goes on to say that that former *exhḗgēsis* was not done *kath' hekástēn léxin* ('word by word'), as most writers of *exhēgḗseis* do, but 'of those statements that give continuity to the doctrine (*synechóntōn tò dógma*), along with their proper demonstrations' (ibid. 5.664–665 K.; De Lacy 1978, p. 492, lines 25–30).

involves technical arguments and terminology that go far beyond anything in any Hippocratic text, drawing in particular heavily on Aristotle.[13]

With this notion in mind—that a work like *Elements* is, in a sense a commentary, an *exhḗgēsis*, as much as the later, line-by-line *exhēgḗseis* which come under that heading in Galen's work on his own books—let us turn now to that very text, *My Own Books*, and consider the discussion of his own commentary work there:[14]

> I did not have the expectation that my works giving exegesis of Hippocrates' writings would reach a wide audience, any more than any other of those works which I gave to friends. For to begin with I had occasionally written[15] notes on them for my own personal training, as I did in each part of the science of medicine, preparing them for myself—notes which contain all the things stated by Hippocrates in accordance with the art of medicine, [things which] have both a clear and a fully elaborated exposition. For I wrote specifically on *Critical Days according to the Opinion of Hippocrates*, specifically on *Crises*, specifically on *Difficulty in Breathing*, and on all the other matters; I also produced the *Method of Healing* in fourteen books, [consisting of] all matters to do with healing and, in addition to that, what is in accord with his opinion …

Now, there are several oddities, as well as textual difficulties, presented by this important passage of self-analysis of Galen's oeuvre. I pass over these here (but see note 15). What is true, on *any* reading, is that Galen goes on to refer to some of his own central works of clinical theory and practice as, in a sense, works on Hippocrates. He refers explicitly to his own work *Critical Days*, as *Critical Days according to Hippocrates*.[16]

13 *Commentary on Hippocrates' 'Nature of Man'* 1 (15.5–9 K.; Mewaldt 1914, p. 5, line 10–p. 7, line 14), with its dedicated discussion of the precise definition of *stoicheîon*, and of related concepts.

14 *On My Own Books* 9 [6] (19.33–34 K.; Boudon-Millot 2007, p. 159, line 10–p. 160, line 1).

15 This passage and its problems, both textual and interpretive, are considered much more fully by Singer (2018b: 101–107). While the translation here follows the text of Boudon-Millot ('ἐμαυτὸν γυμνάζων'), other possible readings of this particular phrase are: 'I had never even written notes on them for my own … (οὐδ' ἐμαυτὸν γυμνάζων)' (Singer) and 'I had occasionally written notes on them, not for distribution, but for my own … (οὐδὲν πρὸς ἔκδοσιν ἀλλ' ἐμαυτὸν γυμνάζων)' (Müller).

16 And, indeed, the dual status of these works, *Crises* and *Critical Days* in particular, as *both* central to his own medical practice *and* authentic accounts of Hippocrates, is strongly asserted also in Galen's central work of self-publicization, *Prognosis*. There he remarks, as a coda to an account of his own spectacularly successful diagnoses and cures: 'I recounted

What Galen is in fact doing here is characterizing several of his own major clinical and diagnostic writings as works which so fully expounded the views of Hippocrates that it seemed redundant at this stage also to write line-by-line commentaries. What he was doing was, in a sense, Hippocratic exegesis; but he was doing it thematically—according to each branch (*kath' hékaston méros*) of the medical science (*theōría*), and treating each subject specifically (*idíāi*[17])—not text by text. In a very striking sense, then, Galen is here eliding the distinction between commentary and treatise.

In concluding this summary of Galen's own account of his commentary work, it seems important to deal briefly with another distinction, which is raised in the continuation of this same passage of *My Own Books*. Important, because the distinction has been misunderstood or at least interpreted simplistically in previous scholarship; briefly, because it is less directly relevant to the commentary/non-commentary distinction which is our main focus here.[18] I refer to the apparent division of his own commentaries into two categories: earlier, 'private' works, or ones for a more restricted audience, and later ones 'for general distribution', which also engage more directly with views of rival commentators.

One might doubt the validity of such a straightforward distinction on intrinsic grounds; and indeed, as Heinrich von Staden has pointed out, the differences theoretically implied by Galen's developmental account often seem not to be borne out in practice.[19] But in any case the distinction, in the form that it

this ... along with the fact that I had just recently written ... *Critical Days* and ... *Crises*, in which I showed that the science by which one may foreknow what will happen in infirmities has been written down by Hippocrates' (ch. 12; 14.664 K.; Nutton 1979, p. 132, lines 27–31).

17 N.b. the translation in the authoritative edition of Boudon-Millot (2007) misses the sense here, understanding a reference to the nature of the audience (or non-audience): 'à l' usage privé'. But the meaning of *ídios* as 'specific', in the sense of subject-matter, is standard in such Galenic contexts, and clearly borne out by the context here.

18 I have discussed the issue, and the Galenic notion of *ékdosis*, more fully in Singer (2018b); the present account essentially summarizes that one.

19 For example, the *Prognostic* commentary, supposedly in the former category, is quite polemical in its account of erroneous interpretations, e.g. in relation to Herophilus (1.4; 18b.12–20 K.; Heeg 1915, p. 203, line 19–p. 207, line 24); the errors of other commentators are in fact given as the reason for the request to Galen to write the commentary in the first place (3.6; 18b.230–231 K.; Heeg 1915, p. 328, lines 13–22). This same passage again elides the distinction between commentary and non-commentary texts by stating that some matters have been dealt with thoroughly in one place and some in the other: repetition (even between commentaries and non-commentaries) is to be avoided. One may also doubt how significant the difference is between the 'two groups' in terms of their scholarly precision and level of references to other commentators. The commentary on *Epidemics* 1,

has been understood by scholars, is not, in fact, supported by a close reading, both of the passage in question from *My Own Books*[20] and of his much fuller account of the different phases of his commentary work, in his *Commentary on Hippocrates' 'Epidemics'* 3. In the former text, it is a later *attitude* on Galen's part to the fact of 'wider distribution', not a new *reality* of distribution, which (he claims) determines his new way of proceeding: that is the sense of the phrase πρὸς κοινὴν ἔκδοσιν ἀποβλέπων.[21] In the latter,[22] it emerges that, far from any such simple dichotomy, there is, in fact, a *seven*-phase development in his compositional procedure and intent. Here, then, is no straightforward distinction between 'private' and 'public'. Indeed, while acknowledging the need to respond to a wider debate, Galen claims that, in *each* of these seven phases, his commentaries are always written in response to requests which come almost entirely from those in his intimate circle (*hetaîroi*). And, even in the above passage from *My Own Books*, the wider class of people who receive the works in the 'general distribution' is contrasted with the actual intended addressees: the latter are explicitly referred to by the phrase 'the actual recipients alone (ἐκείνων μόνων τῶν λαβόντων)'. Consciousness of—indeed engagement with—a wider audience and debates is not, for Galen, in any way inconsistent with the claim that his *intended* audience comprises specific individuals or a close group of followers.

2 Hippocrates and Galen's Element Theory in *Elements according to Hippocrates*

I turn to the main part of the paper, which is centred on the argument in relation to Hippocrates in *Elements According to Hippocrates* and which will

from the 'first' group, mentions a specific reading by Capito (2.57; 17a.154 K.; Wenkebach 1934, p. 78, lines 21–24; Vagelpohl 2014, p. 276); certainly, the commentary on *Epidemics* 2, from the 'second' group, has a few more such references, but the difference does not seem dramatic. Similarly, the commentary on *Nature of Man*, supposedly in the later phase, has only one reference to a specific reading by Capito in book 1, and no such reference (though there are two citations of readings by Dioscorides and two mentions of Sabinus) in book 2; see Von Staden (2009), suggesting that 'the truth might be less straightforward' (135) than Galen's own account of his intentions and imagined readerships suggests.

20 *My Own Books* 9 [6] (19.34–35 K.; Boudon-Millot 2007, p. 160, lines 1–21).

21 And this is completely consistent with what he says about *ékdosis* at the beginning of *My Own Books*: he does not initiate it distribution himself, with *any* of his works, but responds to the fact that it takes place.

22 2, preface (17a.576–584 K.; Wenkebach 1936, 60–66); again, see the fuller discussion of the passage in Singer (2018b), esp. 110–111.

jointly address the second and third of my main points: the importance of Hippocrates in the structure of Galen's argumentation on the elements, and the possibility of discerning rival contemporary views through the lens of that argumentation. In what will necessarily be a simplified account of a highly intricate text, my attempt will be to point to certain key moves in the argument and investigate what they tell us about Galen's intellectual motivations, his use of Hippocratic textual authority, and his engagement with the use of it by his rivals.

The first important leg in Galen's argument (ch. 1; 1.413–415 K.; De Lacy 1996, 56–58) is that a distinction must be made between things which are smallest, or primary, in our perception and those which are so in reality, or in nature, and a consequent assertion of the limitations of an individual's sense perception to discover the latter. It follows, then, that we need a theoretical 'method' by which to identify these entities. This, Galen says, is the 'method taught by Hippocrates' (ch. 2; 1.415 K.; De Lacy 1996, p. 58, lines 6–7); one might characterize it, in theoretical terms, as an enquiry which has as its basis the observed phenomena of the physical, especially the biological, world, but which uses theoretical or logical processes of argument to reason from these phenomena to the underlying truth. Hippocrates 'disdains the simplest and primary in relation to sensation'; that is to say, the scientific-medical enquiry must proceed beyond that point.

Galen might appear here to be simply offering some fairly uncontentious opening remarks; on closer inspection of the intellectual background, however, this turns out to be very far from the case.[23] Such a distinction between 'perceptible least parts' and 'least parts in truth and nature' seems to reflect the verbal formulation of medical practitioners who are not (at least in the medical context) interested in that latter, more theoretical, category. The followers of Erasistratus restrict themselves to discussion of the 'proximate' first elements, that is to say the homoeomerous parts (in particular artery, vein, *neûron*).[24]

23 David Leith (2015) has explored and analysed this intellectual background.

24 See *Method of Healing* 2.5 (10.107 K.), where Galen characterizes Erasistratus as departing from the kind of 'ultimate study of nature (ἄκρας φυσιολογίας)' associated with philosophers, and regarding it as sufficient rather to treat artery, vein and nerve as 'proximate principles and as it were elements (ἀρχὰς προσεχεῖς καὶ οἷον στοιχεῖα).' The passage is cited by Leith (2015, 465–466), who, surely correctly, contests Frede's view that what is referred to in this passage is an invisible but theoretically posited network (*triplokía*): the point is precisely that in this enquiry one is *not* considering such non-evident entities. The *Anonymous of London* further claims, however, that Erasistratus advanced beyond what is proper to medical science to arteries, veins and nerves which are 'posited by theory (λόγῳ θεωρητά)' (21.26; Manetti 2011, 46); but, as Leith (2015, p. 469, note 12) argues, this

Apparently with a similar methodological thrust, Herophilus is supposed to have said, also of the homoeomerous parts: 'let these be primary, even if they are not [in fact] primary'.[25] The precise implications of Erasistratus' and Herophilus' theoretical commitments here continue to be debated. But two things seem clear: that such statements represent a reluctance to rely on a certain kind of theoretical abstraction (at least in the medical context), in strong contrast to Galen's theoretical confidence; and that this debate over what, for medical purposes, should be taken as 'elements' forms a relevant background to Galen's polemic here.

I shall argue that a similar refusal to engage in discussion of fundamental element theory on the part of Athenaeus or his followers lies at the root of Galen's criticism of them; if so, the opening remarks above are in fact already laying the groundwork for the development—and for the polemical dimension—of his central methodology. And Galen's presentation of this methodology involves a simultaneous invocation, right at the outset, of Hippocrates as methodological guide. The appeal to Hippocrates in Galen's account of his element theory is well known, and has been usefully explored in recent work.[26] The process, within the present text, is well summarized by a phrase of David Leith's: 'designed to transplant Hippocratic terminology into an Aristotelian *analytical framework* of element theories'.[27]

This invocation of Hippocrates, at the very beginning of Galen's theoretical argument, points to the inextricable relationship of the insistence on a certain interpretation of the Hippocratic text and the insistence on a certain view of element theory. As we shall see, his opponents' failure to get it right about Hippocrates is at the heart of their failure to get it right about the elements. Or, to look at it in socio-intellectual terms: there are rival physicians in second-

---

specific statement is probably to be taken as a misunderstanding of Erasistratus' position on the part of the author. The very formulation, however, 'πόρρω τοῦ ἰατρικοῦ κανόνος (away from the remit of medicine)' (21.24–25; Manetti 2011, 46), is significant for our identification of an anti-theoretical strand in the medical tradition. Further Galenic texts on the Erasistratean view are: *Natural Faculties* 2.9 (2.125–129 K.; Helmreich, 1893, 192–195) and *Commentary on Hippocrates' 'Nature of Man'* 1, preface (15.6–9 K.; Mewaldt 1914, 5–7).

25 τὸν Ἡρόφιλον εἰπόντα κατὰ λέξιν οὕτως· 'ἔστω ταῦτα εἶναι πρῶτα, εἰ καὶ μή ἐστι πρῶτα' (*Method of Healing* 2.5; 10.107 K.; Von Staden 1989, T50b); there is a similar formulation also at *Anonymous of London* 21.18–23 (Manetti 2011, 45–46).

26 See Leith (2014), showing the complex ways in which Galen aims to incorporate the Hippocratic text in a discourse on the elements which has much closer links to Aristotelian thought; also Kupreeva (2014); and Hankinson (2015), as well as his contribution to the present volume.

27 Leith (2014), 232 (the specific reference there is to Galen's particular use of the phrase 'one in form and power').

century Graeco-Roman society, who, every bit as much as Galen, believe that their methodological approach to the constituents of the body is justified by their reading of *Nature of Man*. It is these individuals whom Galen—using the twin weapons of scholarship and theoretical argument—is at pains to quash.

We proceed now to a central move in Galen's 'Hippocratic' argument against rival theories, and (ultimately) in favour of his own, four-quality theory: the consideration that if the fundamental component of all things in nature were one, there could be no pain (De Lacy 1996, 62–68). This is broadened to include not just pain but sense-perception in general.[28] Galen here bases himself on an argument which is indeed vital to the first part of *Nature of Man*. There, it is directed against opponents (real or imaginary) who take the fundamental component in human beings to be a single humour, e.g. phlegm or blood. In the Galenic context, the target is rather atomism of various kinds—specifically, that of Epicurus and Democritus, as well as the related *ónkos* theory of Asclepiades. The sense in which these theorists are taken to espouse the view that 'all is one' is that their atoms (or *ónkoi*) are all qualitatively identical.

This move—that of subverting an argument against some form of monism to serve as an argument against atomism—is striking.[29] The sense in which the argument against monism works equally as a refutation of atomism is that atoms are taken to be 'one in form and capacity'. That is to say: there is, on this atomic theory, no distinction of properties between different atoms; there are only differences in the ways in which these qualitatively identical entities are 'put together', their composition.[30]

The 'Hippocratic' argument that if all were one there could be no pain nor sense-perception is elucidated as follows: 'if the elements are themselves neither sentient nor liable to change, then the product of their composition cannot be sentient' (De Lacy 1996, 64).

We might describe this as an argument against the notion of emergent properties, or supervenience; or, more precisely, against one particular form

28 Sense-perception is not directly discussed in the Hippocratic text, but is taken by Galen as the general term under which the experience of pain is subsumed; the move is discussed by Kupreeva (2014).

29 See Leith (2014), 217, pointing out that Galen here goes so far as apparently to deny that the Hippocratic argument is directed against monism at all.

30 The question arises, how fairly or accurately Galen represents ancient atomic theory. Certainly (as Kupreeva 2014 points out) Epicurus has different sizes and shapes of atom; to the extent that these different sizes and shapes at the micro-level may be taken to account for qualitative differences at the macro-level, that will undermine Galen's anti-atomist argument. But it is noteworthy that Galen subsumes a number of different thinkers under this anti-atomist polemic.

of emergentism or supervenience, namely that whereby emergent properties may come about through composition—that is, the arrangement and relationship with each other of the elements—alone. Galen's own theory, whereby two elements may combine with each other to produce a third substance which is qualitatively different from either of them, could also be characterized as an 'emergent-properties' view: the property of the third substance did not exist in either of the elements. What is crucial for Galen, however, is that this fundamental change, or new property, can only arise through those elements being *themselves* fundamentally altered in the process of the combination; such change could not come about simply through a particular *combination* of unaltered elements.

Galen's argument proceeds, by elimination of each of the other possible pairings of these two terms (sentient and liable to change; sentient but not liable to change; non-sentient but liable to change; non-sentient and not liable to change), to the conclusion that elements must be non-sentient but liable to change. The essential argument can, I think, be summarized as follows.[31] There are sentient beings. Let us suppose that the world, and these sentient beings in particular, are composed of a single type of element. That type of element, as we know, is not itself sentient.[32] Unless, then, that element itself undergoes change in the process of composition, what is composed from it cannot be sentient either. Thus, our original supposition fails. As an argument against atomism it is sound, provided that both (a) the atoms are indeed a single type of element, that is, they are qualitatively indistinguishable, and (b) the particular form of emergentism already mentioned has been ruled out, namely that whereby fresh properties may arise merely from the *organization and relationship between each other* of (unchanging) elemental bodies—their 'composition'—rather than from a fundamental change within the elemental bodies themselves.

It seems to me that we have to take (b) as simply Galen's strong intellectual intuition: it is not further supported by argument (and indeed would be denied, for example, by modern physics: differences in the mere *arrangement* of microscopic particles do account for qualitative or perceptible differences at the macroscopic level). As for (a), we note the fact that Galen's argument is

31 Cf. the rather intense logical analysis of Kupreeva (2014). While not disagreeing with her analysis in any fundamental, I suggest that Galen is in fact presenting a somewhat over-elaborate statement of a fairly straightforward argument.

32 As far as I can see, Galen takes this proposition—that elements are not sentient—as obvious and universally agreed.

specific to the context of ancient atomism (if indeed he is interpreting these correctly; see n. 30 above). His position will not have any purchase—or at least, will require considerable further argument—against an atomic theory which envisages distinct properties for different atoms; what is essentially an attack on the explanatory power of monism will be fundamentally undermined if the atomic theory in question includes a multitude of essentially distinct entities.

So, by the end of chapter 2 Galen takes himself to have refuted monism, and in the process atomic theory as he understands it. Galen proceeds, then (from De Lacy 1996, 72), to adumbrate his own views on the *kind* of mixture of elements which is required to explain change and emergent properties. Still, by the time we reach De Lacy (1996), 80, the propositions that Galen can take himself to have demonstrated are only (a) that the fundamental elements are more than one in number; and (b) that they are not *apathê*, that is, unaffected, non-liable to change.

We now arrive (from De Lacy 1996, 82 onwards) at a discussion of the opening of Hippocrates' *Nature of Man*, which turns into a detailed textual analysis of certain words and phrases. We may be tempted to think of this as something of a digression. Actually, as we shall see, it is of crucial strategic importance in his argument. The establishment of this text as authority for his own view is rhetorically important precisely because there is a radically opposed group which may equally hope to take it as authority for theirs.

Let us look at the crucial—and very well known—passage of the Hippocratic text:[33]

> The present discussion is not designed for one used to discourses of human nature which go beyond what is relevant to medicine. For I state that the human being is absolutely not [or, is not entirely] made of either air, fire, water or earth, nor of any other thing which is not manifestly present [or, is not manifestly the one thing] in the human being.

Central to Galen's interpretation of this passage is an insistence that Hippocrates is *not* here attacking the notion that the human body is composed of elements which cannot be observed as such within it, but *is* attacking the notion that it is composed of any *one* such element. The interpretation is, at least, contentious, and (as we shall see below) Galen adopts at least two controversial readings of individual words or phrases in order to support it. At the

33 *Nature of Man* 1, 6.32 L.; Jouanna (2002) p. 164, lines 3–7.

same time, it must be said that Galen's interpretation has found modern as well as ancient proponents.[34]

It is clear from the very opening remark that the text is attacking at least *some* form of abstract theorization about the components of the human body. The claim that the, or at least a, main target of the attack is monism, is undeniable; but the claim that this is the *only* target seems flatly incompatible with that opening remark.[35] What is the sense of 'beyond what is relevant to medicine' if there is not a reference to some category of theoretical entity, or some mode of theoretical discussion, which the author does reject?

There are two crucial Galenic views here, both of which he attributes to Hippocrates and to this text: one, that the hot, the cold, the wet and the dry are the ultimate explanatory principles in the composition of the human body; two, that these explanatory principles are inextricably connected with their related bodies or elements as observed in the world outside the human body—fire, air, water and earth.

For convenience I shall henceforth refer to the first set of entities (hot, cold, wet, dry) as the 'element-qualities' and to the second (fire, air, water, earth) as 'element-bodies'. (Galen himself sometimes uses 'element (*stoicheîon*)', in relation to both, although he clarifies that properly speaking the latter set—the ultimate items into which bodies are *physically* divisible—are elements, while the former—the end points of our *conceptual* division—are principles, *archaí*.)[36]

Of these two crucial Galenic views, then, as I shall now argue, the second definitely, and the first possibly, were rejected by certain other element theorists of Galen's time—and were rejected by them not just as accounts of the truth, but as interpretations of Hippocrates. I will argue, further (in the fourth and final part of this paper), that the Galenic interpretation constitutes a strong misreading of this Hippocratic text in the interests of supporting his own theory; and that this interpretation has been and remains influential in the way

34 See Hankinson (2015), note 18, as well as his contribution to the present volume.

35 Cf. Jouanna's comment in his edition on *Nature of Man*, acknowledging the difficulty of the opening remark but essentially following Galen's line: 'cette polémique, *malgré les premières indications de l'auteur*, ne vise pas tous les philosophes en bloc, comme c' est le cas dans l'Ancienne médecine, mais simplement ceux qui soutiennent que la nature humaine est constituée d'un élément unique' (Jouanna, 2002, 39, my italics; cf. 226–227). The situation is discussed also by Hankinson in the present volume, who points out that Galen is indeed aware of the problem. See also below.

36 *Commentary on Hippocrates' 'Nature of Man'* 1.3 (15.30 K.; Mewaldt 1914, p. 17, line 30–p. 18, line 5).

that we read *Nature of Man*. That last question, however, is separate from that to which we now turn concerning *ancient* conflicts over the interpretation of Hippocrates.

Let us consider the further progress of the argument in *Elements according to Hippocrates*. After the attack upon atomism via monism (De Lacy 1996, 86–88), Galen proceeds to a different form of argument, still tied to his interpretation of the Hippocratic text:[37]

> It would be terribly illogical if all four [element-bodies] were to be rejected on the grounds that no one of them appears unadulterated in the body; by the same reasoning, surely, one would then reject the proposition that the so-called *tetrapharmakos* is composed of wax, resin, pitch and tallow, since no one of these appears in it whole and complete.

Hippocrates is not rejecting element theory; and, more generally, it is illogical to base such rejection on the grounds that no element is visible in unadulterated form:[38]

> Nor, certainly, should one reject the proposition that the bodies of animals consist of a mixture of the four elements, on the grounds that here too none of these is unadulterated or complete; nor should one for this reason concede that the cosmos consists of the four, but take animals out of the realm of coming-to-be from these, as though they had arrived from somewhere else and had not come about within the cosmos.

We thus have (1) an argument against a particular kind of ground for rejecting the four-element theory and (2) an argument against the notion that one might accept four-element theory at the cosmic level but reject it at the human level. Both arguments may be persuasive, given certain prior commitments; but one may note, first, that an argument against a particular ground of rejection is not the same as an argument for acceptance; secondly, that the force of the second argument depends precisely on a prior acceptance of the cosmic-level element theory.

We saw that by the middle of chapter 3 (De Lacy 1996, 80), Galen takes himself to have proved both the falsity of atomic theory and the necessity of posit-

---

37 *Elements according to Hippocrates* 5 (1.452 K.; De Lacy 1996, p. 96, lines, 7–12).

38 *Elements according to Hippocrates* 5 (1.452–453 K.; De Lacy 1996, p. 96, lines 17–21).

ing more than one fundamental element, but does not take himself to have shown the precise number of the elements. Is there anything more demonstrative here? A key moment, in the transition from the destructive arguments against monism and against a misunderstanding of the distinction between prime matter and elements to the constructive arguments on Galen's own theory, seems to be the following:[39]

> let it suffice for you, when you see this part that is cold, dry and thick, to be reminded of earth, and this one which is rarefied, wet and fluid, to arrive at the conception of water. Great heat in an animal body, meanwhile, should remind you of fire; and the nature of breath, without which no animal can be put together, should remind you particularly of air …

The argument works by making a conceptual leap on the basis of our empirical observations. But it is quite a leap—one which essentially forges a link between the element-quality theory and the element-body theory without argument. The ground has been laid for this leap—it has been rendered more plausible—by the macrocosm–microcosm, or cosmic–biological, parallel, which has been the subject of the last couple of pages. Yet all that was introduced merely as support for the proposition: 'you should not accept four elements in the cosmos and then reject them in biology', that is to say it had the status of a hypothetical or conditional argument. The acceptance of those four elements in the cosmos (the element-body theory) is not itself argued for at this point. All that we have here beyond that is the intuitive move that 'great heat should remind you of fire', and so on.

Now this, perhaps, can be made rather more solid. The underlying proposition here is that any perceptible quality encountered can only be understood, is only explicable, in terms of an extreme version of that quality existing somewhere—or at least potentially existing somewhere—in the universe. That extreme version of the quality provides the explanation, by its 'coming into' matter and interaction with other such elements which are explicable in the same way, of the actual instantiation of hotness, coldness, and so on. But this causal relationship between theoretially posited extreme versions of qualities and their instantiations in the world must, as far as I can see, be taken as somehow axiomatic or obvious for Galen. Such a view is not self-evident; and it was, perhaps, precisely this which was among the propositions disputed by the rival doctors against whom Galen polemicizes.

---

39 *Elements according to Hippocrates* 5 (1.454 K.; De Lacy 1996, p. 98, lines 13–17).

The following passage of argument (chapter 5, De Lacy 1996, 98–100) is again addressed at those who might accept the four-element theory in a cosmic context but deny its use in biology: one needs fire and air to explain the growth of seeds to plants and of animals, *too.*

We move, then, to an attack on a follower of Athenaeus of Attalia. This is interesting from a number of points of view. One is that Athenaeus and his followers appear also in *Mixtures*, Galen's other major work relating to fundamental bodily composition. There they are a target, but one, it seems, which, while getting certain fundamental things wrong, represents the closest near-contemporaries to Galen's own views. Again, we note in this passage the way in which criticism of theory and of Hippocratic interpretation go hand in hand: Athenaeus has 'betrayed the ancient account', Galen says says (1.460 K.; De Lacy 1996, p. 104, lines 14–17); a little earlier, also in the context of his attack on Athenaeus, he stated: 'I know of no one who treated accurately of the art of medicine, nor who worked out and completed the methods passed down to us by the [ancients]' (1.457–458 K.; De Lacy 1996, 102, lines 10–12). 'Ancient' in this context must be understood as referring essentially to Hippocrates. Indeed, in the following course of the argument Galen shows himself very much aware of a more widespread phenomenon of disagreement with his interpretation of 'Hippocratic' element theory on the part of 'those who call themselves Hippocratean' (1.478 K.; De Lacy 1996, p. 124, line 12). But the most interesting point is precisely the core of his disagreement here with Athenaeus on the nature of elements; and it is here we see most clearly the rhetorical importance to Galen of his own interpretation of Hippocrates.

It is, of course, perilous and ultimately impossible to reconstruct an author's views from another's criticisms.[40] What is clear is that Athenaeus' follower is trying to advance a theory of the components of the body *without* advancing a broader, or cosmic, element theory, or at least without equating the two. It seems to me at least highly plausible that what is at stake here—and obscured by Galen's presentation of it—is a fundamentally different epistemological approach. The follower of Athenaeus, I suggest, wishes to preserve a theoret-

40 See again Leith (2015). A full overview of Athenaeus will emerge from Coughlin (forthcoming); but see already Coughlin (2018), suggesting a close simliarity between Athenaeus and Galen especially in the area of their use of medical–philosophical authority. That similarity, which is of obvious relevance for our present argument, may, he argues, extend indeed to a direct influence from Athenaeus upon Galen. Explicit evidence that Athenaeus does, indeed, take himself to be following Hippocratic authority is provided by a passage from the (still unpublished) Arabic version of Galen's commentary on the Hippocratic *Airs, Waters, Places*, cited and discussed as T1 by Coughlin and Lewis (2020), 209–210; see that chapter also for further analysis of Athenaeus' element theory.

ical minimalism which is diametrically opposed to Galen's confident assertions in the field of abstract physics. This, it seems, is how we are to make sense of Galen's claim that his opponent held that 'the elements are evident and not in need of demonstration' (De Lacy 1996, 102, lines 4–5): what is meant by 'elements' here is empirically perceptible qualities which admit of no doubt and involve no theoretical postulates. That is to say, one observes the hotness, coldness, and so on, of a body empirically; to do so involves no physical theory, or theory of the elements of which that body is composed. In this context, the Athenaean reluctance to commit oneself to an element theory that mentions earth, air, fire and water would make perfect sense. Galen ridicules what he takes to be conceptual or logical inconsistencies, including the statement that the hot, the cold, the dry and the wet are the elements 'both of bodies and of the whole art of medicine'. But again, such a statement, nonsensical though it be within Galen's conceptual scheme, would be perfectly understandable if what was meant by 'element' in this rival theory were, rather, a purely empirical concept involving no theory of composition. The meaning would be simply that the doctor's empirical experience of hot, cold, and so on, provides the basis on which he proceeds in clinical examination of and prescription for the patient.[41]

Now, it is possible that Athenaeus and his followers are not, in fact, as theoretically minimalist as the above account suggests. It may be that they do accept a theory of composition of the human body in something like the Galenic sense—that is, as consisting ultimately of hot, cold, wet and dry.[42] What seems absolutely clear, however, is that the Athenaean approach rejected the very view that is so crucial to Galen in his interpretation of the opening chapter of *Nature of Man*: that the element-quality theory inevitably entails the element-body theory. And if, as I have suggested, the mention of 'distortion of the ancients' is an implied reference to Hippocratic interpretation, it seems that

41 A fascinating parallel is provided by a passing, dismissive remark made by Galen at *Preservation of Health* 3.13 (6.228 K.; Koch 1923, p. 100, line 33–p. 101, line 1), where he mentions—with outrage at its frivolity—the saying attributed to Quintus, that 'regarding hot, cold, dry and wet, these are words for types of bath'. It seems to me not implausible to see behind this attack a situation in which Quintus was advocating just such a non-theoretical use of the terms 'hot', 'cold', and so on, as that which I am here attributing to Athenaeus.

42 Further evidence for Athenaeus' views in this area is assembled by Leith and Coughlin (see note 40 above). There is indeed a considerable oddity in Galen's account of the disciple of Athenaeus in our present text, namely that there is no mention whatever—in relation to a thinker elsewhere characterized as 'pneumatist', indeed as the founder of the pneumatist school—of *pneûma*. This point of course reminds us further of the partial and fragmentary nature of our sources in such cases; but it also perhaps invites still further caution as to the reliability of Galen as witness in this particular argumentative context.

the Athenaeans rejected that entailment while also claiming—just as much as Galen does—Hippocratic authority for their view.

As we shall see in the last part of the paper, Galen's attribution to Hippocrates of the element-body theory is in fact the most tendentious of his claims in relation to *Nature of Man*; so, evidence for a rival contemporary interpretation is indeed of interest. Here are contemporary medical theorists—and apparently ones who enjoyed some influence—explicitly rejecting the view of Hippocrates which Galen is at such pains to support: namely, that he holds the cosmic element-body theory.

Galen's attack on the follower of Athenaeus relies on two key moves: (1) any view of the elements as hot, cold, wet and dry depends on the notion of those elements as being at the *extreme* of those qualities, so that Athenaeus and his followers have no account to give of what these are without going, at least theoretically, *beyond* actual human or animal bodies; (2) such a notion of elements being at the extremes of their respective qualities will inevitably lead to their identification with fire, earth, air and water (i.e., element-quality theory entails element-body theory). Now, its seems unclear, on Galen's evidence, that his opponents do in fact subscribe to (1); nor, as far as I can see, does he explicitly say that they do. He merely asserts that no element theory makes sense without that bit of theory.

There is a further bit of theory, too, to which Galen says Athenaeus should be committed: (3) an element (*stoicheîon*) arises from a principle (*archḗ*) coming into quality-less matter. But there seems no reason to suppose that Athenaeus will feel himself committed to (3), either, if he does not accept (1). The only justification Galen gives for his contention that Athenaeus *should* be committed to (3), it seems, is that it is 'agreed by all the philosophers whom Athenaeus wishes to follow' (chapter 6; De Lacy 1996, p. 114, lines 15–16).[43]

As for proposition (2), one may or may not find it persuasive in itself—or, what is more to the point, one may or may not suppose it to have been persuasive within Galen's socio-intellectual milieu. I would suggest that the very way in which this connection is introduced may point to the fact that Galen is

43 The identity of these 'philosophers' is of course of interest. Athenaeus is traditionally thought to have been fundamentally influenced by Stoic philosophy; 'the Stoics' might, then, be thought to be the obvious reference. Yet the phrase is a surprisingly vague one if Galen intends to be so specific: he could easily have mentioned the Stoics or Chrysippus, as he often does. True, if Athenaeus did take himself to follow an orthodox Stoic view, he should indeed accept the notion of a quality combining with quality-less matter as a part of his element theory. It should be noted here that Kupreeva (2014) suggests a quite different interpretation of Galen's attack on Athenaeus, whereby what lies behind Athenaeus' (for Galen) problematic characterisation of the elements is not a rejection

aware of a lack of clear argument available to him to bolster it. Here, too, then, we observe the vital importance of Hippocrates—as read by Galen, that is—as providing support for an otherwise wobbly leg of his argument.

In the above, I have asserted a stronger and a weaker claim in relation to Athenaeus: the weaker, I think uncontroversial, one is that he denied (at least as far as human bodies are concerned) the entailment of the element-body theory by the element-quality theory; the stronger one is that he was exercised to remain at a level of theoretical minimalism, committing himself only, in the medical context, to statements about what is empirically evident.

Both possibilities, but especially the latter, are worth considering in the light of the evidence already touched upon in relation to Erasistratus and Herophilus. It is possible to see these important medical authors as wishing to avoid a certain kind of universalizing theory based on entities which are not clearly visible in the human body—and thus as representing an intellectual trend pulling in a fundamentally different direction from Galen's.

It is perhaps unclear, on the basis of our sources, whether such theoretical reticence is based on a complete rejection of fundamental bodies or qualities as primary elements, or rather on the view that such entities may be primary in some abstract sense, but are nonetheless not those with which medicine should be primarily concerned. Moreover, the answer may not be exactly the same for the three authors mentioned. The precise 'physical theory' of these authors is, in a sense, beside the point; it is at least arguable that modern analysis which attempts to hold them to a particular physical element theory risks playing exactly the same distortive game that Galen does, that is, to categorize them in terms of a particular kind of speculative natural-philosophical discourse which they either reject or regard as irrelevant to medicine.

My claim, then, is that there was a significant contemporary rival strand to the Galenic medical approach to 'elements', a rival strand which drew on a significantly distinct view of Hippocrates, and of the Hippocratic *Nature of Man* in particular. This claim may seem to be in need of further support. Such support, I suggest, is provided by a text already touched upon above, namely the *Anonymous of London*.

of abstract theoretical commitments, but, precisely, a positive commitment to specifically Stoic ones, in particular the notion that qualities are bodies, and the distinct role of pneuma. Without space to engage with that interpretation in detail here, I suggest that these commitments are difficult to extract from what Galen says about Athenaeus (either here or in *Mixtures*), and the identity of 'all the philosophers whom Athenaeus wishes to follow' with Stoics at least uncertain.

3 The Anonymous of London: Further Challenges to Galen's Hippocrates?

In-depth analysis of this extremely difficult text and its doxographical implications would, of course, be far beyond my scope here.[44] One aspect of the text, namely the light it sheds on the epistemological or methodological views of Herophilus and Erasistratus, has already been considered (see notes 24 and 25 above). What is relevant to us now is what the anonymous author tells us about Hippocratic doxography—that is, specifically, about views current in a period not long before Galen's own as to what (if anything) was Hippocrates' 'element theory'.

We are thus now concerned with the work's 'doxographic' section (4.18–21.9), which in some way reflects Aristotelian views[45] on a range of earlier medical and philosophical authors. This section, whose central focus is these authors' accounts of disease causation, divides them into two fundamental categories: those who attribute diseases to 'residues arising from food' and those who attribute them to the elements (4.26–29; Manetti 2011, 8). The first point to note is that 'Hippocrates' is placed in the former group. When we reach the summarization of Hippocrates' views, however (5.35–7.40), this already complex and layered text presents us with an extra layer of complexity: the author breaks off to make a distinction between Hippocrates' account of disease causation 'according to Aristotle' and what Hippocrates actually says himself. He thus presents us with two alternative accounts of Hippocrates and his fundamental medical theory. But there is one more complexity still, for our purposes: firmly within the second part of the division—that of 'element' as opposed to 'residue' theorists—we arrive at the figure of Polybus (19.1–18); but the Polybus here meant is (by scholarly consensus) the author of *Nature of Man*. It should be mentioned, finally, before we attempt to elucidate this situation, that at the precise moment when the author introduces Hippocrates' own views—immediately after the words 'αὐτὸς Ἱπποκράτης λέγει (Hippocrates himself says)' (13.44; Manetti 2011, 13)—the text becomes, for several lines,

44 The difficulties are essentially two in kind: textual, due to the extremely lacunose nature of the papyrus, on the one hand, and (though by no means unrelated) interpretive, due to the complexities or elusive nature or the work's structure and intent. The essential overview is Manetti (1999); for particular aspects see also Manetti (1996) and Leith (2015).

45 This Aristotleian material was previously associated with a lost medical doxography by Meno, a pupil of Aristotle, which is mentioned by Galen, or thought to have reached its author through some other indirect transmission; Manetti (1999) argues that it in fact derives from the author's own reading of Aristotle.

extremely lacunose; one cannot here—nor, indeed, in the case of the later entry on 'Polybus', also seriously vitiated—aspire to reconstruct the summary with precision.

But let us consider the relevance of the material here to our argument. First, in the Aristotelian account of Hippocrates (5.35–6.43), the latter is credited with a view which focuses on the role of breath or air (*phŷsa* or *pneûma*) in disease causation.[46] One 'humour'—or at least the physical entity—is thus dominant, against the four-humour theory of *Nature of Man*; as we have seen, the broader aetiological context according to this doxography is that of 'residues from food': the harmful *phŷsai* arise from problems in the digestion of food. This Aristotelian account of Hippocrates is then superseded by the author's own. In spite of the textual problems already mentioned, some things become clear. First, at least some of the entities normally known as 'humours'—referred to by the author as 'ὑγρά (fluids)'—play an important role: bile and phlegm certainly, and blood possibly, are prominent in the causal account. Secondly, heating and cooling seem to have a role, though certainly there is no mention (in the recoverable lines) of 'the hot', 'the cold', and so on. Thirdly, there is a binary attribution of diseases to either air (πνεῦμα/ἀήρ) or diet/lifestyle (διαιτήματα), which seems clearly to recall chapter 9 of *Nature of Man*.

Finally, we have the (Aristotelian) entry on Polybus. As already observed, scholars have agreed that the text here summarized is a part of *Nature of Man*. Definitely present are the terms 'cold' and 'hot', also 'phlegm' and 'black [presumably bile]', as well as various terms for bodies and mixtures. Manetti's reconstruction of the text, largely following that of Diels, sees here a two-level composition, the second one—that of the four humours or fluids—arising on the basis of the first—that of the hot, cold, wet and dry. We are thus presented with a piece of text which not only functions as a summary of the doctrine of *Nature of Man*, but also does so in a way which would suit Galen: the element-qualities are explicitly identified. One should, perhaps, adduce a note of scholarly caution. While the reconstruction seems highly plausible, it is also true that it was carried out, from the beginning, with input from chapter 4 of *Nature of Man*: the prior assumption of the relevance of this text—and arguably even a particular interpretation of this text—have conditioned the reconstruction, from Diels onward.[47]

---

46 Attempts to identify the 'Hippocrates' here meant, in terms of extant texts (especially *Breaths*, possibly *Sacred Disease*) have occupied a considerable amount of scholarly literature, surveyed by Manetti (1999), 103, note 20. On the broader matter of attempts to identify plausible candidates for the historical Hippocrates, see note 7 above.

47 Both Diels and Manetti include an extensive quotation from *Nature of Man* in their appar-

We have, then, three doxographical accounts of relevance to contemporary views of Hippocrates and Hippocratic element theory. To take the last first: the facts that in Aristotelian circles Polybus was considered the author of *Nature of Man*, and that this text was interpreted as expounding element theory, are, as far as they go, fine from Galen's point of view. On the first fact, Galen himself says that Polybus departed 'not at all' from Hippocrates in his doctrines,[48] so in a sense that distinction is unimportant to him (though clearly he would prefer to refer to this central work in his construction of the Hippocratic as by 'Hippocrates'); on the second, we might take this to show that the view of Hippocrates as an element-quality theorist was current in Peripatetic circles; we might even speculate that Galen was influenced by such an interpretation. (Although, be it said, we see no hint, even here, of an interpretation which attributes to the text an *element-body* theory.)

The fact that Peripatetic doxography identified Hippocrates as a distinct figure from Polybus, however, and more especially the fact that the central point in the distinction was that the former was, explicitly, a 'residue' and not an 'element' theorist, are of course of considerable interest for our purposes. But there is more: we have, as noted above, an apparent reference to chapter 9 of *Nature of Man* in this summary. So, not just the Aristotelian picture of Polybus, but also the Anonymous' own picture of Hippocrates, draw upon our same 'foundation text', albeit in a different way. As Manetti shows, this latter picture both focuses on different chapters of our text and places it alongside other texts, in particular *Diseases* 1.[49] Through this different positioning of the *Nature of Man*, and through the highlighting of different passages and aspects of it—the emphasis on humours or fluids, the more prominent causal role of heating and cooling, as opposed to the other quality pair, the focus on the innate and permanent character of humours in the human body—we gain a completely different picture of the text and its intellectual world-view from Galen's construction of it.

As Manetti suggests, such a reading—less concerned with debates with or against philosophers—was probably quite plausible in the imperial medical milieu. (She even adduces another papyrus, P. Strasb. gr. inv. 27, of the second century AD, which similarly cites the two texts, *Nature of Man* and *Diseases* 1,

atus at this point, as justification for the details of the reconstruction. It should be added that there is a substantial quotation from *Nature of Man* (chapter 11) at Aristotle, *History of Animals* 3, 512b12–513a7, with Polybus mentioned as the author of the text there quoted. The fact that *Nature of Man* was attributed to Polybus in the Aristotelian tradition thus seems fairly well established.

48 *Commentary on Hippocrates' 'Nature of Man'* 1 preface (15.12 K.; Mewaldt 1914, p. 8, lines 25–46).

49 Manetti (1996), 300–303.

together.[50]) If so, it would have constituted a challenge to Galen's 'Aristotelian' account of the text in terms of element-qualities and element-bodies.

Finally—although, as we have remarked, the overall structure and connections between parts of *Anonymous of London* remain problematic—we should recall the passages already noted on the epistemological approach of Herophilus and Erasistratus (notes 24 and 25 above), which come in the final, 'physiological' section. There is, as David Leith has explored, a connection between the homoeomerous parts, which the author presents as central to an analytical account in this last section, and the residues or 'fluids' (we could also say 'humours') which are presented, in contradistinction to 'elements', as underlying the accounts of previous authors in the first part of the doxographical section. The less theoretical, or less philosophically speculative, self-restriction to talk of fluids or humours may thus be seen as linked to a particular empirically based approach in research and in clinical medicine—and one which, at least arguably, is seen by our author as 'Hippocratic'.

4 Galen's Hippocrates and Our Hippocrates

Let us return to the thorny, foundational Hippocratic text, *Nature of Man*, which is the bone of contention between these rival interpretations. In what follows, I consider what justification there is for Galen's reading of it as justifying *either* his element-quality *or* his element-body theory. In the process, I hope it will emerge that the rival theorist whom he attacks in *Elements* may, at the very least, be on as strong ground as he is, in terms of their Hippocratic interpretation. The significance of this, if correct, is twofold: first, it adds to the likelihood that there existed in Galen's time an interpretation substantially contradictory to his own; secondly, it may affect our own view of the position of *Nature of Man* in relation to other Hippocratic texts. In particular, the dichotomy between the 'natural philosophy' of this text and the anti-*hypothesis* position of another key 'Hippocratic' text, *Ancient Medicine*, might tend to disappear.[51]

Let us state it rather baldly at the outset: the Hippocratic text nowhere states that the fundamental elements are the hot, the cold, the wet, the dry (element-

50 Manetti (1996), 304, asserting that 'both the Anonymous and the Strasburg papyrus allow us to discern the meagre remnants of an alternative Hippocratism to that represented by Galen' (my translation).

51 The dichotomy is in a sense asserted by Galen by his very ignoring of the latter text; and it continues to be asserted in modern scholarship. For a particularly helpful discussion of the (anti-)theoretical stance of *Ancient Medicine*, see Hankinson (1992).

quality theory), still less that they are fire, air, earth and water (element-body theory). The former position can be found at best by extrapolation from hints in the text; the latter is simply absent.[52] First, on the element-quality theory. There are in fact only two passages in the text (a and c below) which mention the qualities as abstract entities, using the singular neuter article *tò*: '*the* hot', and so on. In addition to these two, one must take into account one (b below) in which the verbal forms appear in an apparently fundamental explanatory context; and one (d below) where they appear in the plural. Let us consider each of these passages.

(a) chapter 2; Jouanna (2002), p. 166, line 12–p. 168, line 3; 6.34–36 L.: the argument here is that doctors who propound a monist theory—namely that of blood or bile—then claim that this single substance changes its form and capacity *under the compulsion of the hot and the cold*. This rival view, however, the author proceeds immediately to deny: thus, at this appearance, 'element-qualities' are being mentioned only within an account of a theory which is rejected.

(b) chapter 2; Jouanna (2002), p, 168, lines 6–8; 6.36 L.: 'there are many [*a plurality of*] things in the body, which, when heated, cooled, dried and wetted contrary to the natural, give rise to diseases; so that there are many forms of diseases, and more than one cure'. Again, the central point here is the refutation of the thesis that there is only *one* substance (e.g. blood) in the body. Clearly, heating, cooling, and so on, are of explanatory importance; but—unless we start from the prior assumption that the element-quality theory is present in this text—there is no reason why we should take this as an exhaustive list of causes, let alone as part of a theory of *components* of the body.

(c) chapter 3; Jouanna (2002), p. 170, lines 11–14; 6.38 L.: the thesis here is that generation cannot take place without a balance of 'the hot, the cold, the wet, the dry'. Further, the text goes on to say that each of these will go back to its origin in nature at death—wet to wet and so on (Jouanna 2002, p. 172, lines 5–8; 6.38 L.). There is here, undoubtedly, a very cursory foray into the cosmological, although such speculation is not later followed up or explained in detail, and one must emphasize, here again, that the main thrust of the argument here is

52 Although some of what I argue here is comparatively uncontroversial, at other points I depart significantly from what appears a modern consensus. Hankinson (2015, 440), for example, agrees that 'Galen clearly goes too far in supposing that Hippocrates really intended us to infer that he espoused the four element theory in Galen's own preferred form'; however, I am here arguing against his further claim that Hippocrates 'does imply more than is usually supposed' (ibid. 440–441), as well as with his remark (ibid., 424) that Galen is 'correct that the author attacks *only* monistic theories which invoke them [*sc.*, earth, water, air, fire]' (my italics). See also Hankinson in this volume.

polemical, as part of a refutation of one-component theories, not as advancing his own theory in detail. We may add that it is not completely obvious, from this very brief account, that the phrases 'each of the things brought together in the process of generation (ἕκαστον τῶν συμβαλλομένων ἐς τὴν γένεσιν)' (Jouanna 2002, p. 172, line 4) and '[its] nature is composed from all these items mentioned, and ends in the manner (*or*, in the items) mentioned (συνίσταταί τε γὰρ αὐτῶν ἡ φύσις ἀπὸ τούτων τῶν εἰρημένων πάντων, καὶ τελευτᾷ κατὰ τὰ εἰρημένα)' (Jouanna 2002, p, 172, lines 10–11) are referring straightforwardly and univocally to those four, considered as an exhaustive account of the ingredients.

This last passage is the *only* one in which 'the hot, the cold, the wet and the dry' are mentioned as abstract entities by this author in a theory that he is actually proposing, as opposed to rejecting; moreover, the positive theory in question, as enunciated here, is a causal one: the specific context is that of generation and decay. Even if we take it that the hot, the cold, the wet and the dry are central to a causal account of how bodies come about (and what happens to them at death), that does not entail that they are the fundamental elements *of the living body*, or the key conceptual items that should be referred to in its description. These 'qualities' are still not here clearly presented as components.

Which, indeed, leads us to the most obvious and serious problem for the notion of this text as offering an element-quality theory of bodily composition, namely that, in chapter 4, its author proceeds immediately to give his positive account of what he *does* take the components to be: phlegm, blood, yellow bile and black bile.

Those few words in chapter 3, then, are the only explicit justification one can find for the notion that this author subscribes to the theory that everything in the natural world, human beings in particular, is ultimately composed four element qualities. One may add the evidence of chapter 7, with its account of the influence of the seasons. But, while this account, and the correlations it suggests, may seem broadly consistent with Galen's views, it is never clearly suggested that the analysis in terms of humours is reducible to one in terms of element-qualities. It is the humours, *not* element-qualities, that are the explanatory items with which one works when giving accounts of health and disease in the human body.

Before proceeding further, we should consider a further point, which represents, as it were, the other side of the same coin. For the Galenic problem, in relation to *Nature of Man*, has two aspects: one, which we have been considering, is that of the presence or absence of (Galenic) element theory in Hippocrates; the other is that of the presence or absence of (Hippocratic) humoral theory in Galen. And the mismatch in this latter context is at least as striking as in the former.

One might indeed argue that Galen has been even more spectacularly successful in persuading us that he is a follower of Hippocrates in the four-humour theory than he has in persuading us that Hippocrates shares Galenic element theory—and that the former claim is even more strikingly tendentious. The situtation, however, is slightly different in the two cases. Galen's statements in the former area are much less direct than in the latter; in fact, he studiously avoids openly stating that he has adopted the four-humour theory of *Nature of Man*, relying on somewhat oblique formulations, and implying rather than asserting his adoption of the theory, by suggesting the mutual interdependence of the humour theory and the element theory.

So, Galen wishes to *suggest* that he has adopted the four-humour theory; but the way that he does this is by evasive allusion, and by avoidance of close analysis of the specifics of that theory—analysis which would bring into the open the clear contradiction between his own understanding of *chymós* and the Hippocratic one. To summarize: for Galen, the four humours are key causes and indicators of health and disease, but are not the fundamental *components* of the body; indeed, with the exception of blood, the humours are considered mainly (following Aristotle) as residues, *perittṓmata*, rather than as building-blocks or levels in biological composition. Thus the scholarly view, fairly commonly stated, that the humours are key components in the formation of the body, constituting a level above elements but below uniform or homoeomerous parts, seems to represent at best an over-reading of some of the evidence and at worst a considerable distortion; and the view—much more widely stated, beyond academic circles—of Galen as essentially a four-humour, rather than a four-element, theorist is simply wrong.[53] One may, however, be tempted to say

53 See the introduction to Singer and van der Eijk (2018), especially p. 29 and p. 32, note 126. In general terms, it must be said that the role played by phlegm, yellow bile and black bile play in Galen's system (prominently, for instance, in *Preservation of Health* or in *Mixtures*, with which one may compare many instances in the pharmacological work) is almost always as residues, the excess of which will have negative implications for health, and the level of which may be increased or reduced by certain foods, activities or drugs. For a good theoretical summary see *Natural Faculties* 2.8; 2.117 K.; Helmreich (1893), p. 186, lines 14–19, asserting that blood is produced from nutrition through good balance of the internal heat, the other humours through its poor balance; and compare also Galen's summary of his own views in *My Own Opinions* (12), where he regards it as at least a possibility that blood alone is our 'proper' fluid, while the others arise only as necessary consequences. It must be pointed out, further, that the suggested hierarchical sequence elements—humours—homoeomerous parts would run into considerable theoretical difficulties, since for Galen as for Aristotle blood itself is, in fact, a homoeomerous part. On the specific question, whether Galen does *on occasion* suggest a fundamental role for the humours in the structural formation of the body, see *Commentary on Hippocrates' 'Nature of Man'* 1 (15.59–97 K.;

that the historical and ongoing confusion—given Galen's own commitment to his self-presentation as an ardent proponent of *Nature of Man*, which *does* propound such a theory—is not entirely surprising.

One should also in this context consider the conception of *chymós* in Galen's *Simples*, where the term refers to the fundamental flavours or properties of substances, especially plant substances, in the natural world.

Here, then, we have *chymoí* assuming a much more central importance; but, by the same token, this is a model of *chymoí* quite different from, and much more broadly conceived than, the four of *Nature of Man*: there are many relevant such *chymoí* in the natural world. One might object that this is simply a different, homonymous use of the term; and that indeed Galen himself specifies such a distinct usage in that work, saying that he will use the term *chymós* for 'tasteable property (*dýnamis geustḗ*)', preferring the alternative form *chylós* to refer to actual substances or fluids. But this objection cannot stand, for two reasons. The first is that this would simply displace the apparent problem from *chymós* to *chylós*: if *chylós* is the term for fluid or humour in *Simples*, then *chyloí* are understood in a much broader sense than the four *chyloí* of *Nature of Man*. Secondly, Galen *does* seem to want to suggest that *chymoí*, understood in precisely this sense of fundamental *dynámeis geustaí*, can be mapped onto the *chymoí* of the Hippocratic text. This is made clear by a mention of Praxagoras, who is said to have proposed a set of ten *chymoí*. Now, *chymoí* here must surely be understood in the sense of the larger set of 'tasteable properties' which Galen discusses in *Simples*.[54] Yet Galen wishes to relate *precisely this theory* of the *chymoí* to the Hippocratic one: his claim is that Praxagoras, in proposing ten *chymoí* (not counting blood!) is 'not departing from Hippocrates, but dividing those originally stated by Hippocrates into *genera* and *species*'.[55] Galen's making this claim, of course, is dependent precisely on his

Mewaldt 1914, 32–51, commenting on *Nature of Man* 1.19–40) and *Doctrines of Hippocrates and Plato* 8.3 (5.672 K.; De Lacy 1978, p. 498, lines 23–34). While these passages may seem superficially to support such a view, it is in fact clear throughout (a) that the fundamental level of analysis, to which Galen always wishes to return, is that of the *elements*, and (b) that—consistently with his view in *Semen* and elsewhere—it is *blood* which is the key physical component in embyronic formation. (The sense in which, in the above passage of *Doctrines of Hippocrates and Plato* and at *Commentary on Hippocrates' 'Nature of Man'* 1, 15.94 K.; Mewaldt 1914, p. 50, lines 13–15, blood is 'composed from the four humours', seems to be simply that it never appears in completely pure form, having always a small admixture of the others.)

54 This seems clear from our other evidence regarding Praxagoras on the humours (see Lewis 2017, 194, also arguing that Galen has distorted Praxagoras' view).

55 *Natural Faculties* 2.9 (2.141 K.; Helmreich 1893, p. 203, lines 19–22).

not laying out either Hippocrates' or Praxagoras' theory in any detail at this point; again we have allusiveness and elusiveness as the major tools in Galen's project of presenting himself as broadly subscribing to Hippocratic humoral theory.

But let us return to the other question, that of the dubious presence of element theory in *Nature of Man*. Given the absence—at least explicitly—of Galen's theoretical scheme from the Hippocratic text, it seems striking how successful Galen has been in persuading us to read the text as he would have it. While the presence of the element-bodies—to which I shall return shortly—is a different matter, Galen's reading of this text as subscribing to the theory of element-qualities (both within the human body and in the world around it) seems uncontentious in modern scholarship. Two examples—from two of the most prominent scholars of ancient medicine of recent years—may stand for many.

First, consider this passage from ch. 7, dealing with the changes due to the seasons:

> (d) The year as a whole partakes of all [things, those] which are hot, cold, dry and wet. Within the world, nothing could subsist for any time without all [the things] that are in it: if one were removed, all would disappear (for it is by the same necessity that all have come together and are nourished by each other). So, too, if any of these [things] which have come together were removed from the human being, it would not be able to live.

As already remarked, the terms here are in the plural, not the singular neuter forms normally translatable as 'the hot, the cold', and so on. Yet consider the translation in the authoritative French edition: '… l'année participe pendant toute sa durée à tous les éléments, le chaud, le froid, le sec et l'humide …' (Jouanna, 2002, 185–187). Here, the term 'éléments' has interpretively—and Galenically—been supplied. Or consider another highly authoritative and influential summary, from the introduction to the standard English-language anthology of Hippocratic texts:[56]

> … the synthesis he [*sc., the author of Nature of Man*] proposes is, in certain respects, more elaborate and comprehensive than any extant earlier system …. The basic constituent substances, in terms of which all phys-

56 Lloyd (1978), 26.

> ical bodies are to be analysed, are the hot, the cold, the dry and the wet. … each of the humours is associated with one of the four seasons … and with two of the primary opposites, hot, cold, dry and wet.

Again, although legitimate as an interpretation of the text, this summary is just that—an interpretation, and one which follows the Galenic line. So much, then, for the element-qualities, and their shady presence in *Nature of Man*.

When we turn to fire, earth, air and water—the identification of which in this text is, we have seen, a central part of Galen's argument—he is on much shakier ground yet. As possible candidates for the fundamental elements, they are mentioned only in the first chapter.[57] In that introductory passage, the author is certainly not openly saying that air, earth, fire and water are the components of the body. He at first appears—at least—to be openly denying that theory. On Galen's reading, he is rather denying that any *one* such element is the *single* component; even on that reading, however, the denial that one element-body is the single component is not the same as the assertion that a particular four element-bodies *are* the components. And such an assertion, quite simply, the text never makes.

As already observed, the rhetorical thrust, at least, of that first sentence seems hostile to any such theory. But let us consider Galen's reading of that sentence:

> Ὅστις μὲν οὖν εἴωθεν ἀκούειν λεγόντων ἀμφὶ τῆς φύσιος τῆς ἀνθρωπίνης προσωτέρω ἢ ὅσον αὐτῆς εἰς ἰητρικὴν ἀφήκει, τούτῳ μὲν οὖν οὐκ ἐπιτήδειος ὅδε ὁ λόγος ἀκούειν· οὔτε γὰρ *τὸ πάμπαν* ἠέρα λέγω τὸν ἄνθρωπον εἶναι, οὔτε πῦρ, οὔτε ὕδωρ, οὔτε γῆν, οὔτε ἄλλο οὐδὲν ὅ τι μὴ φανερόν ἐστιν *ἐνεὸν* ἐν τῷ ἀνθρώπῳ·

I have highlighted in italics the two cases, first, where Galen adopts a contentious interpretation of a phrase, and secondly, where he proposes an alternative reading.

The following translations represent (1) the Galenic and (2) the non-Galenic version:

> (1) For I state that the human being is *not* [*made*] *entirely* [*of*] either air, fire, water or earth, nor [of] anything else which is *not manifestly the one thing* in the human being

57 There is only one further mention, of two of them (fire and water), in a possibly relevant context, but the argument there has no apparent implication for an element-body theory (chapter 5; Jouanna 2002, 176, lines 3–9; 6.42 L.).

(2) For I state that the human being is *absolutely not* [*made of*] either air, fire, water or earth, nor [of] any other thing which is *not manifestly present* in the human being.

We might, further, add an alternative version of the first part of the non-Galenic alternative:

(2a) For I state that the human being is *not, in its entirety,* [*made of*] either air …

According to versions (2) and (2a) of the first part, the Hippocratic text is denying, respectively, the notion of element-bodies as components of the human body altogether, and that of element-bodies as their sole components. Either interpretation is fatal to Galen's view. Now, it should be said that Galen is on stronger ground with his reading here than with the second pair of variants, which we will consider shortly. The translation of *tò pámpan* with the negative, as 'not entirely' is certainly possible, and arguably more grammatically likely than the alternative ('absolutely not').

What makes the alternative 2/2a seem more plausible, however, is precisely the argument that follows, which seems to state as the reason for rejecting this proposition the fact that *none* of these things is manifest in the human body. The non-manifest nature of *any* of these elements (earth, air, fire, water—and it is suggested there could be more of this sort) at least *seems* very clearly to be an argument against accepting them as elements altogether, not an argument against accepting only one of them.

And it is in awareness of precisely this problem that Galen emends the text. He reads 'ἓν ἐὸν (being one)' or 'being a single thing' for 'ἐνεὸν (being present)'.[58] The position that the Hippocratic text rejects, then, is not element theory but monistic element theory, and the argument from what is 'not manifestly present' in the body becomes an argument from what is 'not manifestly a single thing' in the body. If we made entirely of water, then (the argument thus construed goes), this water would be clearly manifest, as it would be the only thing in us.

As an argumentative structure imagined to be persuasive against monism, without simultaneously attacking element theory in general, this seems implausible; and Galen's emendation here seems forced ('spécieux' is Jouanna's word for it). Stylistically speaking, while the phrase μὴ φανερόν ἐστιν ἐνεὸν seems

58 As pointed out to me by Roland Wittwer, this change does not, in terms of ancient palaeography, strictly speaking constitute an emendation: written Greek of the Hippocratic

a fairly natural, idiomatic way of saying 'not obviously present', the alternative, μὴ φανερόν ἐστιν ἓν ἐὸν ('not obviously being one thing'), seems somewhat unnatural.[59]

From a rejection of Galen's reading it does not immediately follow that the rest of his argument is vitiated. But it does follow that there remains something to explain, which Galen has thus by-passed, namely: why does the author bring forward the non-manifest nature of element-bodies as an objection, if not to cast doubt on element-bodies in quite general terms? Galen is undoubtedly right in his claim that the author has as a target various forms of monism: in the remaining part of the chapter he specifically attacks forms of element-body monism, before moving in the next chapter to combat humoral monism. My claim is that he is wrong in his contention that element-body monism is the *only* target: at the very outset, the text also attacks the hypothesization of abstract elements altogether. What is admittedly confusing is the speed with which the text moves from that first target to the second (cf. note 35 above); yet, however confusing, that does seem to be what the author does. There is, in this rhetorical preamble to the text, a slide from the broader attack to the narrower. On my interpretation, then, the various forms of element-body monism are not the primary target, but introduced as a particularly absurd manifestation of element theory—and indeed also as pointing out the total failure of unanimity *between* element theorists.

Even if one does take it, however, that the author subscribes to an element-quality theory (and still more if one takes it that he subscribes to an element-body theory!) one must at the very least admit that such theories are in no way central to the work's main theoretical thrust. The theoretical models which *are* thus central are that of the four humours on the one hand, and that of treatment by opposites on the other. Both, moreover, involve entities or phenomena which are, the author may argue, directly observable; they do not rely on abstractions or hypotheses. That term, of course, is deliberately chosen: on a plausible interpretation of *Nature of Man*—and, more importantly, on one which was plausibly adopted by Galen's contemporaries—the text may in fact

---

period would—in the absence of both aspiration marks and spaces between words—have no means whatever of distinguishing between the two options. The *verbal* and *logical* difference remains, however, in spite of the ambiguity inherent in the written form; and so the following remarks as to the plausibility of one or other reading remain equally applicable, even if one should perhaps prefer the terminology of 'interpretation' to that of 'emendation'.

59 The point is admittedly debatable: as already mentioned (note 34 above), Hankinson has defended the Galenic reading; see below p. 154.

be rather close in its methodological outlook to the theoretically minimalist *Ancient Medicine*, which has often been thought to oppose its position, and which explicity attacks 'hypotheses'.

5 Conclusion

There were, amongst Galen's medical predecessors and contemporaries, very significant methodological or epistemological differences in the approach to element theory. These lie essentially in the reluctance of certain other medical thinkers either (a) to be drawn into discussions of fundamental element theory in medical contexts, on the grounds of its irrelevance to medical practice, or, more strongly (b) to commit themselves to an element-body theory or element-quality theory at all. I suggest that Athenaeus, or his school or followers as represented in *Elements*, was anti-theoretical or theoretically minimalist; that such theoretical minimalism, motivated by a desire to confine oneself to discussion of what is empirically evident and relevant to medical practice, reflected a significant strand in ancient medical thinking which Galen felt the need to oppose; and that it is *both* such theoretical minimalism *and* the (arguably justified) appeal to *Nature of Man* in support of it which Galen perceives as such a large threat.

Galen, I suggest, has not just been brilliantly successful in persuading doctors and scholars from late antiquity to the present day to read Hippocrates as his kind of element theorist; he has in the process also succeeded in obscuring an alternative medical approach to both element theory and Hippocratic interpretation. The text of *Nature of Man* represents the battleground on which rival element theories and rival epistemologies, in various polemical and exegetical contexts, have been and continue to be fought.

CHAPTER 7

Galen the Hippocratic: Textual Analysis and the Practice of Commentary

R.J. Hankinson

Galen reveres the ancients as much as he reviles the moderns; and supreme among the great men of the past is Hippocrates, his model, so he tells us, in physics and philosophy as much as in physiology and medicine. But Galen was aware that there was a 'Hippocratic Question': which of the many works in circulation under his name was actually the work of the Master? and which of the rest, if not genuine, none the less reproduced his doctrines more or less faithfully? Of course, Galen's answers to these questions are not disinterested; indeed, he is attempting to create a canon of the true Hippocrates as much on the basis of his own views as to what he takes to be the truth as on the basis of pure textual criticism. But for all that, he does not eschew the latter, and is relentlessly critical of earlier exegetes, in particular Dioscorides, Artemidorus Capito, and Sabinus. In this paper I examine the complex manner in which he goes about undertaking this task, in particular in regard to his commentary on *Nature of Man*, where this drive to canonize (and equally to stigmatize) is at its most obvious.

1 In the Footsteps of the Master

In Galen's view, Hippocrates was the founder, and the greatest exponent, of a properly philosophical medicine, one based on accurate physiological knowledge:[1]

> [Hippocrates] thought that one should have a precise understanding of the nature of the body, saying that this was the origin (or principle: *archḗ*) of the whole theory of medicine.

1 *The Best Doctor is also a Philosopher* 1.54 K.; Müller (1891), p. 1, lines 11–13; Boudon-Millot (2007), p. 284, line 13–p. 285, line 2. For texts of Galen, at their first appearance, I cite their full title in English, followed by a citation in Kühn (1819–1831), where possible, followed

© R.J. HANKINSON, 2021 | DOI:10.1163/9789004470200_009

Moreover, such knowledge required an understanding of fundamental physics:[2]

> Hippocrates already understood this even before Aristotle; since, prior to any other doctor or philosopher of whom we know, he undertook to demonstrate that there are four qualities in total which act upon one another, as a result of which everything which is subject to generation and destruction is generated and destroyed. Moreover it was Hippocrates before anyone else who realized that these were wholly mixed with one another through and through; and one can in his writings find the beginnings at least of the demonstrations which Aristotle was later to undertake.

Elsewhere he writes:[3]

> The doctrine that all bodies … are composed of hot, cold, wet and dry is common to virtually all the most reputable doctors ('Diocles, Mnesitheus, Dieuches and Athenaeus') as well as to the best philosophers ('Chrysippus and Aristotle') … but I call them 'Elements according to Hippocrates' because I think it proper to credit him who first propounded and demonstrated them.

Elements according to Hippocrates is the title of an early treatise[4] in which Galen seeks to show that Hippocrates not only deployed the four qualities, but indeed argued (albeit enthymematically, as the quotation from *Natural Powers* above suggests), for their existence and primacy. Indeed, he did not stop there. At the end of the first book of his *Commentary on Hippocrates' 'Nature of Man'* he writes:[5]

> Those things which are common to all things and which are simple and genuinely primary are properly called 'elements'. And Hippocrates

by detailed references to later and better texts (where available), as here. For Galen's self-presentation in this text, see Boudon-Millot (2009).

2 *Natural Faculties* 2.5 K.; Helmreich (1893), p. 103, line 25–p. 104, line 11; also available with English translation in Brock (1929).

3 *Method of Healing* 10.462–463 K.

4 Edited with English translation and commentary in De Lacy (1996).

5 15.103 K.; Mewaldt (1914), p. 54, lines 5–9; cf. *Elements according to Hippocrates* 1.476–477 K.; De Lacy (1996), p. 122, lines 4–14; and *Doctrines of Hippocrates and Plato* 5.676 K.; De Lacy (1978), p. 502, lines 14–25.

> named these things after the qualities, hot and cold, wet and dry, and not things intermediate between their extremes, but the extremes themselves, namely fire and earth, water and air.

Elsewhere I have examined the extent to which Galen's fathering of traditional Greek element- and quality-theory on Hippocrates may be justified,[6] and I shall not re-plough that field here. But central to this contention is his claim that at least the first part of this text is the purest of echt Hippocrates:[7]

> The first part of it [sc. *Nature of Man* 1–8; on the divisions of the text, see further below] constitutes as it were the foundation-stone of the whole of the Hippocratic art. This why I said that I was astonished by those people who would make it seem alien to Hippocrates' thought. The majority of those familiar with the Hippocratic art number it among the genuine works, and suppose it to be the work of the great Hippocrates himself. Some, however, think it by Polybus, who was both his pupil and the man charged with passing on his teaching to new pupils, and who clearly departed in no way at all from Hippocrates' doctrine in any of his books.

Galen is firmly in what he at least claims (with what justification is quite unclear) to be the majority camp. But even if it were by Polybus[8] (as for example is maintained in *Menon's Medical Writings*),[9] that would not sully its claims to ideological purity. Indeed, one might well wonder why, given that this is the case, he is so concerned to vindicate genuine Hippocratic authorship for it. After all, as he himself says, what matters is whether what it says is true, not who wrote it.[10]

---

6 In an earlier contribution to this series: Hankinson (2015); see also Hankinson (2008a, 2009, 2017).

7 15.11–12 K.; Mewaldt (1914), p. 8, lines 19–26.

8 Polybus of Cos, one of Hippocrates' major students, was probably also his son-in-law, although this tradition relies on only one isolated reference in Galen (*Difficulties in Breathing* 7.960 K.; see Jouanna 1999, 20, 27, 48, 51). Galen regularly mentions him as an especially-favoured acolyte: see for instance, *Best Doctor is Also a Philosopher* 1.58 K.; Müller (1891), p. 5, lines 12–14; Boudon-Millot (2007), p. 289, lines 2–4. On Polybus's putative authorship, see Jouanna (1999), 56–57; and 61–62, 284–285, 309.

9 *Iatrikà Menṓneia* 19, 1–18; Manetti (2010), 40–41; *Menon's Medical Writings* are mentioned approvingly by Galen in his *Commentary on Hippocrates' 'Nature of Man'* (15.25–26 K.; Mewaldt 1914, p. 15, line 26–p. 16, line 4) in the context of establishing that no one *prior* to Hippocrates had adopted a full-blown four-humour physiological theory; see Manetti (2010).

10 15.106 K.; Mewaldt (1914), p. 55, lines 26–28.

The answer may well be largely emotional. *Nature of Man* is 'the foundation-stone of the whole of the Hippocratic art'; and it would be agreeable if the foundation were in fact laid by the founder. Galen's concern to discern the authentic Hippocratic grain from the spurious chaff is in large part driven by his own doctrinal commitments. Equally, his refusal to accept as Hippocratic, or even Polybean, parts of the text which he takes to be manifestly absurd and incompetent, in spite of the testimony of other, earlier sources, is clearly also at least partially ideological in character. This is most obvious in the case of the bizarre and schematic account of the structure of the blood-vessels in chapter 11 (Jouanna 2002, 192, line 15–196, line 15). Galen devotes a long and particularly splenetic passage of commentary to lambasting its absurdity,[11] thinking it manifestly unworthy even of Polybus (to whom Aristotle confidently ascribed it).[12] Galen's scorn is spectacular: he refers four times to the fabricator of this sorry account as 'our modern Prometheus'—and says that no one remotely acquainted with the facts of anatomy, as Polybus clearly was, could have accepted it for a moment.[13] It is significant that Galen, who knew Aristotle's biology well and quotes extensively from it on numerous occasions, is as silent about this ascription as he is about *Menon's Medical Writings*' attributing the four-humour physiology to Polybus.

2 The Structure and Provenance of 'Nature of Man'

In Galen's time *Nature of Man* was already substantially in the form in which we now have it. The only exception is that the spurious chapter 24 of our manuscripts, and which in fact reproduces the first chapter of *Affections*, was evidently missing from his text. What appeared as the final chapter in his text, the equally spurious chapter 23 in ours, he clearly recognizes as an intrusion.[14] The final section of the work (chapters 16–22), which he treats as an independ-

11 15.130–148 K.; Mewaldt (1914), p. 67, line 14–p. 77, line 13.

12 Aristotle, *History of Animals* 3.3 (512b12–513a7).

13 Thus it is in sharp contrast with the largely accurate account of *Epidemics* 2.4.1; Galen comments on it at *Hippocrates' 'Epidemics'* 2 (Vagelpohl 2016, 617, line 4–679, line 6).

14 15.222–223 K.; Mewaldt (1914), p. 113, lines 1–16; it is clearly borrowed from *Diseases* 2.12, although Galen does not acknowledge this. Jouanna (2002, 309–310; cf. 23) plausibly suggests that the curious state of the end of the treatise preserves the remains of two distinct orderings of the collection. In one of them, what we now know as the second part of *Diseases* 2 was the immediate successor of our text. In the other, our text was followed by *Affections*. At some later date the two tail-pieces became amalgamated, and joined to the text proper.

ent treatise and labels *Regimen in Health*,[15] he attributes provisionally (and thus largely approvingly) to Polybus:[16]

> While the *Nature of Man* is in every way sound, and the material added in between the two books is in every way unsound,[17] *Regimen in Health* is for the most part sound, depending as it always does on the Hippocratic element-theory, although one might certainly find fault with it in a few particulars. It may be ascribed to Polybus, as many have believed.

In spite of that tart judgement, however, his earlier position is somewhat more nuanced. Here is a lengthy passage from the Proem:[18]

> One might well be astonished at those who think that the book *Nature of Man* is not one of the genuine books of Hippocrates, but rather, as they are accustomed to call them, spurious; but they have been deceived by the elaborations and interpolations in it, of which I will give a fuller account in this very work. For now it suffices to repeat what was said in my work on *The Genuine and Spurious Texts of Hippocrates*,[19] where I wrote as follows:
>
> 'The first part of this book, part "A" [chs. 1–8], extends for 240 lines and shows that animals' bodies come to be from hot, cold, dry and wet, as well as expounding the nature of the humours. What follows is complicated. The first part of it distinguishes the so-called sporadic diseases from epidemics and plagues, and gives a general account of the particular treatment of each kind [chs 9–10]. The part after this discusses the anatomy of the blood-vessels [ch. 11], after which there is a complicated exposition concerning diseases [chs 12–15]. Next there is an account of healthy regimen .... It is clear, then, that the book as a whole is cobbled together and composed from many sources, and extends as a whole to not far short of 600 lines.'[20]

---

15 An appellation which survives into modern editions, although it has no manuscript support, and is rejected by Jouanna (2002, 19–22), who adopts a Unitarian approach to the whole of *Nature of Man* as we have it; see further note 21 below.

16 15.174–175 K.; Mewaldt (1914), p. 89, lines 1–14; the quotation is taken from 15.175 K.; Mewaldt (1914), p. 88, lines 10–14.

17 This is an exaggeration: even in Galen's jaundiced view, some of this 'additional material' is perfectly sound; see also the next quotation.

18 15.9–11 K.; Mewaldt (1914), p. 7, line 19–p. 8, line 18.

19 Now lost.

20 Mewaldt prints all the remainder of this passage as part of the quotation from the lost work; but this seems to be an error.

> The first discourse, which deals with the elements and humours, is completely in accord with the Hippocratic art, as indeed is the second, which distinguishes between sporadic and epidemic diseases. The part dealing with the anatomy of the blood-vessels is clearly added on, and wholly inferior; for it is both inconsistent with the evident facts, and also conflicts with what is said in the second book of the *Epidemics*. Of what follows, some is interpolated, about which there will be more precise information when we elucidate the book for you, while some parts are reputable, and express the truth concisely, and are in accordance with the Hippocratic art, as also are the parts concerned with regimen in health.

In his view, then, things are complicated.[21] For the sake of clarity, let us follow Galen in labelling our chapters 1–8 as Part 1; our chapters 9–15, in spite of their various provenance and reliability, as Part 2; and chapters 16–22 (*Regimen in Health*) as Part 3. Galen's commentary itself divides into three books corresponding to these parts. Nothing more is known about the lost text Galen quotes from here. But the title of another lost text, *That Hippocrates Evidently Adopts the Same Doctrine in His Other Writings as He Does in 'Nature of Man'*,[22] clearly indicates Galen's exegetical priorities, as well as the extent to which the case was both controversial and controverted in his own time. There was as little agreement about such matters in his own day as there is now; but he does not let that stand in his way:[23]

> So, as I said, pretty much every other doctor … was convinced that the book *Nature of Man* [i.e. Part 1] is by Hippocrates. And Plato was well aware of it too: for he wrote, in the *Phaedrus*, the passage I transcribed

21 Modern scholars too are divided on the issue of whether the whole of it (that is all of Parts 1–3, with the exception of the misplaced additions of chapters 23 and 24) forms a unity. Jouanna (2002, 22–38) offers a very clear and comprehensive overview of the issue, opting in the end for the view that all of it was written by the same author, and as a unified text. This may well be right, although what we and Galen know as *Regimen in Health* does at least represent a detour into new and different subject-matter. See also note 15 above.

22 Galen referred twice to this work in his *Commentary on Hippocrates' 'Nature of Man'*. He first described it (15.15 K.; Mewaldt 1914, p. 10, lines 9–12) as not yet written, while in the coda to Book 1 (15.106–107 K.; Mewaldt 1914, p. 55, line 26–p. 56, line 6), where he deals in general with the authenticity of chapters 1–8, he says that it has already been composed. Galen also lists it in *My Own Books* (19.36 K.; 9.12, Boudon-Millot 2007, p. 161, 18–20); and refers to it in *The Soul's Dependence on the Body* 4.799 K.; Müller (1891), p. 58, lines 11–14.

23 *Commentary on Hippocrates' 'Nature of Man'* 15.12–13 K.; Mewaldt (1914), p. 8, line 29–p. 9, line 10.

> a short while ago,[24] which begins (270c–d): 'So do you think it possible to understand the nature of the soul in a proper manner without understanding the nature of the whole? If one should believe Hippocrates the Asclepiad, not even the body can be understood other than by this method.' Those who talk random nonsense should pay attention to this passage and consider which of Hippocrates' books concerns the method praised by Plato. For it will be clear that in not a single one of them apart from the one which is our current subject, namely *Nature of Man*, does Hippocrates investigate first whether the human body is simple or multiform and then each of the other things which Plato enumerated.

This passage, from his other great intellectual hero, is understandably a favourite of Galen's, and he quotes it elsewhere, always claiming that it refers unequivocally to *Nature of Man*.[25] Others, both in antiquity and more recently, have been less sanguine about the attribution.[26] But Galen's commitment to the Hippocratic centrality of Part 1 is unwavering; and his commentary is in large part concerned to vindicate the genuine parts of the texts, and to demonstrate their doctrinal unimpeachability. In what follows I examine how he seeks to do this.

3 Establishing the Text and the Refutation of Monism

Galen believes that Part 1 of *Nature of Man*, the part to which the title properly attaches, both presents and defends a version of what I have elsewhere labelled[27] 'the standard model' of Greek physics. That is, a theory of the four fundamental elements, earth, water, air, and fire, which in turn embody the even more basic four qualities of hot, cold, wet, and dry. This means, of course, that he must reject the standard interpretation of the opening chapter which sees it as precisely denying that theory:[28]

---

24 15.4–5 K.; Mewaldt (1914), p. 4, lines 21–26, and later at 15.103–104 K.; Mewaldt (1914), p. 54, lines 13–25. Unsurprisingly, Galen liked it, mentioning it also at *Method of Healing* 10.13–14 K. and *Composition of Drugs according to Kind* 13.594 K.

25 See the previous note.

26 Littré thought it must refer to *Ancient Medicine*; others (e.g., Hutchinson 1988) have pressed the candidacy of *Regimen*; Jouanna (1999), 58–59 offers a brief and suitably sceptical resumé of views on the issue.

27 Hankinson (2008a, 2015); Galen's version of the theory is fundamentally Aristotelian.

28 *Nature of Man* 1.1, Jouanna (2002), p. 164, lines 3–7.

> Whoever is in the habit of listening to those who talk about human nature in terms further removed from those which pertain to medicine will not find this discourse congenial to him. For I say that man is neither wholly (*pámpan*) air, nor fire, nor water, nor earth, nor anything else which is not evidently the one thing[29] in man, but rather leave them to those who wish to say such things.

This passage is, Galen acknowledges, hard to interpret; and 'a more superficial impression', he says, might indeed suggest that its target is four-element theory. But on closer examination, one should realize that in fact what Hippocrates objects to is the thought that man (or indeed any animal) is basically composed of only one of them.[30] The target is monism, rather than element-theory as such. For the latter construal, the word '*pámpan*', which I translate as 'wholly', and which Galen takes as modifying the substantives (air, etc.), has to be construed with the main verb ('I make no such claim': see note 29). Even so, so far[31]

> One might think either of the [interpretations] to be true; but in what is said in the next passage, it is clear that it is the second which the writer upholds. But if you really apply your mind to it, even in this passage, where he says 'for I say that man is neither wholly air', he is not saying that there is no air in us at all, and no fire or water or earth either, but only that [the body] is not this 'wholly', this expression signifying 'not entirely', not 'not at all'.

So Galen certainly has an axe to grind, and he proceeds to grind it at some length throughout the rest of his commentary on Part 1. But for all that, his

29 Reading '*hèn eòn*' rather than '*eneòn*', as favoured by some manuscripts and most modern editors and commentators, including Jouanna (2002, 229–230); the latter yields the sense 'I make no such claim that man is air … nor anything else which is not evidently contained within man'. I defend Galen's reading of the text here in Hankinson (2015), note 18; Galen defends it in his *Commentary on Hippocrates' 'Nature of Man'* 15.20 K.; Mewaldt (1914), p. 12, line 26–13, line 9. Perhaps the biggest stumbling block to Galen's reading is the phrase 'in terms further removed from those which pertain to medicine' of the next passage. Galen glosses it as meaning that such monistic accounts are incompatible with medical *truth*, since they imply that pain is impossible (see *Nature of Man* 2.3, Jouanna 2002, p. 168, lines 4–6; 15.35–37 K.; Mewaldt (1914), p. 20, line 25–p. 21, line 24). Galen defends this rather strained construal at greater length at *Elements according to Hippocrates* 1.451–457 K.; De Lacy (1996), p. 96, line 1–p. 100, line 24.

30 15.17–18 K.; Mewaldt (1914), p. 11, line 15–p. 12, line 2.

31 15.18–19 K.; Mewaldt (1914), p. 12, lines 2–9.

position is neither perverse nor unargued. Indeed, both here and elsewhere he shows himself to be a sensitive and serious textual critic.

4 The Shortcomings of the Earlier Exegetes

The very sentence that he has just been interpreting was the subject of a dispute between Galen and one of his predecessors, whose excessive radicalism comes in for criticism elsewhere as well:[32]

> Artemidorus (who was also called Capito) produced an edition of Hippocrates' works which was not only highly regarded by the emperor Hadrian, but is even now taken reasonably seriously by many people; and his colleague Dioscorides produced one as well. They made many emendations, altering the old readings which were the only ones the earlier exegetes of Hippocrates' works had known. Along with many others, Capito also emended the very passage we are now concerned with, writing it as follows: 'For I say that man is neither wholly air, nor fire, nor water'. For since he had not found any book written by an ancient author which said that earth alone was the element, nor anything reported by the Peripatetic authors who most diligently collected information concerning this particular type of research, to the effect that anyone had adopted this view, he recklessly altered the reading [i.e., by suppressing 'nor earth'].

Artemidorus Capito flourished around AD 120. His edition of, and emendations to, Hippocratic texts are mentioned by Galen on numerous occasions in his commentaries.[33] He is also often associated, as here, by Galen with Dioscorides (who is not to be confused with the important writer on pharmacology of the same name), for example at *Commentary on Hippocrates' 'Epidemics' 6*, 17a.795 K.; Wenkebach (1956), 4, lines 15–17 Wenkebach, where Galen also accuses them of making rash emendations.[34] They are both further censured

32 15.21–22 K.; Mewaldt (1914), p. 13, line 19–p. 14, line 4.

33 See, for instance, *Commentary on Hippocrates' 'Epidemics' 6*, 17b. 75, 97–98, 154, 310 K.; Wenkebach (1956), p. 164, lines 19–22; p. 176, lines 13–26; p. 208, lines 15–16; p. 320, lines 11–13.

34 See also 17b. 30–31, 104 K.; Wenkebach (1956), p. 139, lines 19–23; p. 180, lines 8–16. Disocorides is mentioned on his own at 17a. 888, 909, 914 K.; Wenkebach (1956), p. 55, lines 17–19; p. 66, lines 19–20; p. 69, lines 18–19; 17b. 32, 35, 72, 75, 123, 193, 194 K.; Wenkebach (1956), p. 140, lines 19–23; p. 142, lines 8–13; p. 163, lines 4–6; p. 164, lines 16–18; p. 190, lines 24–27; p. 232, lines 20–21; p. 233, lines 14–17. In his *Hippocratic Glossary* 19. 64 K., Galen takes him

for trying to re-write *Epidemics* in a 'Coan' dialect to make it more 'authentic';[35] Galen evidently considered that they were both far too ready to make unnecessary alterations to texts, as in Galen's view (and surely rightly) is the case here. As he goes on to point out, the mere fact that no example of an earthy monism survives does not show none ever existed.[36] Books get lost and destroyed for all sorts of reasons,[37] and there may have been people who held such a doctrine, but who never bothered to write it down. Hippocrates mentions all sorts of mistaken views even though it is impossible actually to impute any of them to anybody.[38] Indeed, as Galen might have said, but does not (at least directly—he perhaps hints at it), the reference to earth might simply have been there for the sake of completeness.

Galen has one further criticism:[39]

> Capito was certainly wrong, then, recklessly to emend the old reading without even going on to say how it was possible that the original scribe had mistakenly written one thing instead of the other.

In other words, any textual emendation needs to be buttressed by a palaeographical explanation of how the supposed error that is being corrected could have come about in the first place. And while it might indeed be easy enough to come up with something in this case (an 'unintelligent correction' to bring the number of elements up to the canonical four, for instance), Capito apparently did not do so.[40]

---

to task for pointlessly glossing words which are perfectly familiar, and hence require no elucidation. For Artemidorus, see also 17b. 30–31, 104 K.; Wenkebach (1956), p. 139, lines 19–23; p. 180, lines 8–16.

35 *Commentary on Hippocrates' 'Epidemics' 6*, Wenkebach (1956), p. 483, lines 24–30.

36 Aristotle, in his general treatment of material monism (*Metaphysics* 1.8, 988b22–989a19), explicitly says that no *physikós* championed the claim of earth to be the single element: 989a5–12. He also reports (*On the Soul* 1.2, 405b8–11) that 'no one has claimed that the soul is earth'.

37 In addition to the fact that unworthy books are unlikely to get copied, all sorts of things can prevent transmission, including the envious malignity of those desiring to conceal the reputable views of earlier writers; and that's before you get to natural disasters (to which he refers at 15.23–24 K.; Mewaldt (1914), p. 14, line 25–p. 15, line 10). Tellingly, Galen mentions fires and earthquakes destroying sanctuaries as one such cause—he had lost his own library as well as a valuable collection of medical supplies in the disastrous fire at the temple of Peace in 192; see *Avoiding Distress* 2–37 = Boudon-Millot/Jouanna (2010), p. 2, line 11–p. 13, line 2.

38 15.22–24 K.; Mewaldt (1914), p. 14, line 4–p. 15, line 10.

39 15.24–25 K.; Mewaldt (1914), p. 15, lines 11–13.

40 In this context, it is worth stressing that Galen's understanding of the text of *Nature of*

5 The Errors of Sabinus

Galen, then, espouses a fairly sophisticated and rigorous approach to the business of textual establishment, as well as a preference for a conservative cautiousness of approach when it comes to making changes for which there is no manuscript support. This goes just as much for additions as it does for seclusions, as the immediately subsequent passage shows:[41]

> But equally wrongly some of the exegetes misrepresented Xenophanes, as for example Sabinus did, when he wrote the following words: 'For I say that man is neither wholly air, *as Anaximenes did*, ⟨nor fire, *as Heraclitus did*,⟩[42] nor water, *as Thales did*, nor earth, *as Xenophanes did somewhere*';[43] for nowhere can Xenophanes be found making any such statement.[44] Moreover, it is clear from his own words that Sabinus is falsifying here, rather than simply making a mistake out of ignorance; otherwise he would also have mentioned by name the book in which he [sc. Xenophanes] expounded these things. But as it is, he wrote: 'nor earth, *as Xenophanes did somewhere*'.

Sabinus was a 'Hippocratic' physician of the first or second century AD. He is mentioned by Galen as a commentator on Hippocrates at *The Order of My Own Books* 19.57 K.; Boudon-Millot (2007), p. 98, line 13; and he wrote expanded paraphrases of several Hippocratic texts,[45] which indeed this brief extract exemplifies, the italicized phrases being the expansions. He also dealt with textual issues, which will become relevant later. Galen is fairly respectful of the general quality of his work, although he takes issue with many of his particular suggestions,[46] as he does here. The error is not one of textual establishment,

---

Man 1.1 (Jouanna 2002, 164, lines 3–7 quoted above) involves no orthographical variant: the received texts would have been without breathings or word-spacing, and so *hèn eòn* and *eneòn* would both have appeared as *ENEON*; see note 29 above.

41 15.25 K.; Mewaldt (1914), p. 15, lines 13–21.

42 This is an editorial addition to our manuscripts of Galen made by Mewaldt; but it may not be necessary.

43 My italics indicate Sabinus's exegetical editions.

44 Xenophanes appears to have made both water and earth basic: fragments 21B29, 33 DK; he also supposed that we lived on the upper surface of an infinite column of earth (21 B 28 DK), but this is not a claim about elements, much less a monistic one; see note 37 above.

45 *Epidemics* 2, 3, and 6; and *Aphorisms* in addition to *Nature of Man*; see the next note.

46 See the article by Jacques Jouanna, who discusses a number of passages which mention Sabinus from Galen's *Commentary on Hippocrates' 'Epidemics'* 3. Galen, however, also mentions him (along with Rufus of Ephesus) as someone whom it is particularly surprising,

but rather of commentary; and it involves a mistaken expansion, rather than an unjustified excision. Sabinus' mistake is thus the opposite of Capito's, and in more than one way—but it is no less egregious for all that. Just as we should not delete a claim just because we can find no one to attribute it to, equally we should not invent an attribution to justify the claim. Both of Galen's objections, then, equally exemplify his general conservatism of editorial approach.

Galen also mentions Sabinus in connection with two passages from Part 2 of our text, which he considers to be a messy hodge-podge of material culled from various sources, none of it directly ascribable to Hippocrates, but some at least consistent with what he (and of course the correct opinion) would have said. The first passage is the (very brief) chapter 13:[47]

> Those diseases which occur rapidly (*ex olígou*) and those whose occasions (*propháseis*) are well known, are the ones whose course can most reliably be predicted. For the cure should be constructed by opposing the cause of the disease, since in this way what it is producing the disease in the body will be removed.

Galen begins by noting that this seems to conflict with the doctrine of *Aphorisms* 2.19: 'in the case of acute diseases, it is not entirely safe to predict either recovery or death'.[48] In general, Galen thinks that *Aphorisms* is unimpeachably Hippocratic,[49] and Galen comments approvingly on this one at *Commentary On Hippocrates' 'Aphorisms'* 17b.490–492 K.: the outcomes of acute diseases are indeed harder to predict; they are, comparatively at any rate, short-lived; and they can involve rapid exacerbations. Sabinus points to the apparent contradiction, and infers that this cannot be genuinely Hippocratic. But he misunderstands the text here, which refers not to short-lived, violent, acute diseases, but rather to diseases that arise very soon after their evident occasions. It is both the obviousness of the antecedent cause, and brevity of the interval between that cause and the onset of the disease, which renders prediction easier, not the nature of the disease itself. Thus, when the force of *ex olígou* is properly under-

---

in view of his 'genuine familiarity with the works of Hippocrates' to discover making an elementary error of omission (*Commentary on Hippocrates' 'Epidemics'* 6, 17a. 849 K.; Wenkebach (1956), p. 32, lines 3–10); this renders Galen's hostility towards him here all the more remarkable.

47 Jouanna (2002), p. 200, lines 13–16.

48 This aphorism is one of Galen's favourites; he also quotes it in his *Commentary on Hippocrates' 'Nature of Man'*, 15.20 K.; Mewaldt (1914), p. 12, lines 16–17.

49 *Commentary on Hippocrates' 'Epidemics'* 3, 17a.577–579 K.; Wenkebach (1934), p. 60, line 15–p. 62, line 14.

stood, there is no conflict between this passage and Hippocratic orthodoxy. Sabinus is reduced to babbling, as he so frequently is, as a result of misunderstanding.[50] This chapter, then, is one of those parts of the middle section which, in the words of the proem quoted above, 'are reputable, and express the truth concisely'.

Galen returns to Sabinus at the end of the commentary on the middle section, in relation to chapter 15. This chapter lays out an account of the periodicities of recurrent fevers, their causes and their relative durations,[51] one which Galen himself thinks is mistaken in more than one particular. Sabinus, among others, it turns out, agrees with him. But even so, Galen's attitude is both angry and condescending:[52]

> Many of the commentators, including Sabinus, seem to be suffering from something similar to the man who was ill with dropsy, but who thought that the doctor Phylotimus ought to treat him for a whitlow:[53] … either he did not see that that whole of him was ill, or else he did not think he needed treatment at all. In the same way, one should think that the commentators are either mentally blind, or that they suppose that, while mild complaints require some treatment, the serious ones do not need any remedy at all. It is as if they have been awoken from a deep slumber; they perceive how this passage conflicts with Hippocrates in asserting that quotidian fever is less long-lasting than tertian, while Hippocrates clearly said, both in the first book of the *Epidemics*[54] and in the *Aphor-*

50 *Commentary on Hippocrates' 'Nature of Man'*, 15.161–162 K.; Mewaldt (1914), p. 82, line 17–p. 83, line 6; for Sabinus' irrelevant babbling, see *Commentary on Hippocrates' 'Epidemics'* 3, 17a. 516–517, 521, 547–548 K.; Wenkebach (1934), p. 22, lines 20–24; p. 25, lines 2–9; p. 40, lines 7–19. He is also accused of lack of clarity, and of being 'an exegete who is himself in need of another exegete': 17a. 595 K.; Wenkebach (1934), p. 72, lines 12–18.

51 *Nature of Man* 15.1–5; Jouanna (2002), p. 202, line 10–p. 204, line 21.

52 15.167–169 K.; Mewaldt (1914), p. 85, line 18–p. 86, line 5.

53 *Parōnychía*, a painful suppuration under the nail, mentioned at *Epidemics* 2.6.27, where treatment with black oak-gall in honey is recommended: see *Galen's Commentary on Hippocrates' 'Epidemics'* 2 (Vagelpohl, 2016, p. 927, line 17–p. 928, line 14). Plutarch gives two slightly different versions of this story at *On Hearing* 43b, and *How to Tell a Flatterer from a Friend* 73b (fr. 26 Steckerl).

54 *Epidemics* 1.24–26 (2. 670.16–680.11 L.; Jones 1923, 180–184) treats of the different types of periodic fever at some length: 'the most acute, severe, difficult and fatal are continuous; the safest and easiest and longest of them all is the quartan … nocturnal fever is not very fatal, but is long-lasting. The diurnal is longer still, and in some cases turns to consumption. The septan is long, but not fatal. The nonan is even longer, but not fatal. The proper tertian comes quickly to a crisis, and is not fatal' (1.24; 2. 672.3–674.11 L.; Jones 1923, 182). Cf.

> *isms*,[55] that the tertian is resolved most quickly of all. And so they say that this book is not Hippocratic, since what is said here is both manifestly false as well differing from what Hippocrates wrote elsewhere. But if it is only here that they recognize that the man responsible for these interpolated passages says things that are both false and in conflict with Hippocrates, then they do indeed resemble the man who notices the whitlow, but fails to observe that his whole body is in terrible shape.

This is peculiar in more ways than one. As we have just seen, in his *Commentary On Hippocrates' 'Nature of Man'*, Galen rebukes Sabinus for condemning a passage that was in fact doctrinally sound. Yet here he is accused, along with the unnamed 'other commentators', with uncritically accepting all of the previous material, and not seeing how hopelessly bad it (or at least most of it, after chapter 10) was. Things are not helped by the fact that we have no other evidence as to what Sabinus thought about any of the individual passages apart from what Galen says here. It is hard, though, to imagine that he, writing in the Imperial era, could have had much truck with the long-exploded, jejune vascular anatomy of chapter 11, which so arouses Galen's ire. But whatever we are to make of that, Galen finds fault with him here for noting what is (apparently) a relatively minor, if none the less genuine, departure from the true doctrines of the Master, and failing to see the enormity of the other errors elsewhere in the text.

But for all that, Sabinus et al. are correct, at least in stigmatizing the doctrine in question as un-Hippocratic. Indeed, nowhere else in the corpus is it suggested that the tertian lasts longer than the quotidian. But even so, Galen seeks to minimize the culpability of the mistake on the part of the author of the passage, and at the same time to emphasize the extent of the delinquency of Sabinus and his associates. Supposing that quotidians last longer than tertians, the author certainly betrays his unfamiliarity with the medical facts, but his is an understandable error, made as a result of a plausible piece of reasoning, one deriving ultimately in fact from Plato in the *Timaeus* (86a). The different periodicities (and severities of onset and resolution) of the different recurrent fevers are due to their differing elemental bases: fire in the case of the continu-

---

Epidemics 1.6 (2. 620.6–10 L.; Jones 1923, 156), where the author writes that the tertians prevalent (in Thasos) were all resolved in seven periods (i.e. fourteen days), which is shorter than the other types of epidemic fever.

55 Mewaldt (1914) cites *Aphorisms* 4.59 (4. 522.15 L.; Jones 1923, 150); but this only says that tertians do not last longer than fourteen days.

ous, air for the quotidian, water for the tertian and finally earth for the quartan; the more sluggish the element, the more difficult it is to dislodge.[56] Indeed our author's view is more plausible than that of Plato,[57] since it allows that all fever is a result of heat, and assigns the differentiae of fevers to the different intensities of the heat, and other factors.

In other words, from the standpoint of medical theory, the error is a relatively venial one. Galen will no doubt also have been inclined to leniency here by the fact that our author holds black bile responsible for quartans;[58] and indeed largely for similar reasons he is also inclined to overlook Plato's rather more serious mistake.[59] For all that, Sabinus and his ilk make a meal out of this; and compound their mistake by ascribing the text, absurdly, to Polybus:[60]

> One might also wonder how Sabinus and the majority of commentators (who invariably praised all these supplementary additions, saying that this is 'wonderfully said' by the man, or that 'angelically', or the other 'divinely') can now immediately forget all of that, and because of a single discrepancy no longer think that this is a work of Hippocrates, but ascribe it instead to Polybus, as if they have not read the *Aphorisms* and the first book of the *Epidemics*, though Polybus himself had read them. As a pupil of Hippocrates, he must have frequently heard him discuss the differences of fevers, and have often read his writings, as well as having observed for himself in the case of patients that the tertian quickly reaches a crisis, while the quotidian takes longer. For Polybus was certainly not one of those pontificators of Alexandria, who have never seen anyone actually

56 15.169–170 K.; Mewaldt (1914), p. 86, lines 5–24; see also Galen's *Doctrines of Hippocrates and Plato*, 5.696–699 K.; De Lacy (1978), p. 526, line 26–p. 528, line 35, where he accuses Plato of two errors. First, that of 'explaining the causes of periodic fevers in terms of the common elements of all bodies, rather than those of blooded animals', since it is better in these cases to point to things which are actually observable, rather than to their theoretical bases (5.697–698 K.; De Lacy 1978, p. 528, lines 11–15). Secondly, and more seriously, 'he did not even come close to the real cause of quotidian and tertian fevers' (5.698 K.; De Lacy 1978, p. 598, lines 15–16); in the former, 'an excess of phlegm-like humour, which is wet and cold, is clearly evident; and in tertians an excess of yellow bile, which is extremely hot and dry' (5.698 K.; De Lacy 1978, p. 598, lines 16–18). Thus Plato should have associated tertians with fire and quotidians with water, if he was going to go down the elemental route, while quartans would then be associated with black bile and earth (5.698 K.; De Lacy 1978, p. 598, lines, 19–21).

57 15.170–171 K.; Mewaldt (1914), p. 86, line 25–p. 87, line 14.

58 *Nature of Man* 15.5; Jouanna (2002), p. 204, lines 8–21.

59 *Doctrines of Hippocrates and Plato*, 5.696 K.; De Lacy (1978), p. 526, lines 28–31.

60 15.171–172 K.; Mewaldt (1914), p. 87, line 7–p. 88, line 4.

> sick, but spend their time in conjectures, saying nothing sound, nor any of the things which those who actually practise observe to be plainly evident in their patients.

This passage brings to the foreground another regular source of Galen's contempt for the failures of others: their total inexperience of practical medicine. It is a charge he regularly raises against 'so-called' physicians, calling them 'word-doctors (*logiatroí*)',[61] who are like people who seek to pilot ships by following handbooks.[62] It is central to Galen's own self-presentation that he manages to marry intellectual rigour and honesty, and scholarship that ranges both deep and wide, with the sort of extensive practical experience without which no one can be an effective doctor or judge of medical opinion.

6 Linguistic Considerations: *oúrēma* and *sýnochos*

There are reasons other than doctrinal inadequacy for rejecting the inadequate farrago of error that constitutes our chapter 15, however. The language itself is clearly, in Galen's view, un-Hippocratic:[63]

> It is quite clear that neither Hippocrates nor Polybus would have said 'urinations (*ourḗmata*)', since they could have said 'those whose urines (*oûra*) are bloody'; for while Hippocrates frequently wrote 'urine', in no passage did he ever say 'urination'. And many other things in these appended writings clearly indicate that they are the work neither of Hippocrates nor of Polybus.

The word *oúrēma* is indeed rare; in fact it occurs nowhere else in the corpus (see Jouanna, 2002, 292). Galen was extremely proud of his philological knowledge, and wrote widely on matters of vocabulary and usage, both in specific texts now

61 For instance in his *Commentary on Hippocrates' 'Epidemics'* 3, 17a.574 K.; Wenkebach (1934), p. 59, lines 3–4, where he writes 'for this is what many people who see them behaving disgracefully in actual practice call them'.

62 *Composition of Drugs according to Genera* 13.604–605 K.: people who derive their anatomical knowledge solely from books are like 'the proverbial helmsman who steers by the book'; the proverb is a favourite of Galen's: *My Own Books* 19.33 K.; Boudon-Millot (2007), p. 158, lines 24–26; *The Powers of Simple Drugs* 11.796–797 K.; *Composition of Drugs according to Places* 12.894 K.; *Powers of Foodstuffs* 6.480 K.; Wilkins (2013), p. 24, lines 2–6; see Wilkins note ad loc.

63 15.164 K.; Mewaldt (1914), p. 83, line 27–p. 84, line 2.

lost (see *My Own Books* 19.48 K.; Boudon-Millot 2007, 173, lines 5–15), as well as throughout his Hippocratic commentaries, and his writings on food and drugs (see Manetti 2009). Whether his insistence here is correct depends on controversial questions of dating, and even more intractable ones concerning what if anything may be ascribed to the historical Hippocrates. But Galen's own evidence is perhaps the best we have got; and while he was certainly capable of making serious errors of ascription which also involve mistakes of dating (the most egregious case, perhaps, being his insistence that *Nutriment* is a genuine Hippocratic text),[64] his opinions should not be merely dismissed. In addition to being proud of his own philological skills, Galen was also concerned with the proper way of expressing oneself in technical prose in such a way as to ensure maximum precision and comprehensibility.[65] Sometimes this involves making clear precise shades of meaning; sometimes it is rather more simply a matter of translating local terminology into a more widely accepted and understood vernacular (this occurs particularly in the pharmacological treatises, in which Galen recalls his own extensive travels in search of herbs and other medicaments: Manetti 2009, 171–173). Galen wrote a number of works on linguistic issues, including the surviving *Hippocratic Glossary* (19.62–157 K.), which is probably genuine.[66]

But at all events, Galen discerns no particular shade of meaning in the use of *oúrēma* as opposed to *oûron*; and indeed it is hard to see what any distinction might amount to. This seems to be no more than a not particularly elegant case of *variatio*. Even so, Galen thinks that it is certain that the term is late, or at any rate later than Hippocrates and his immediate circle.

The same is true in the case of the term *sunochos*, as applied to non-remitting fever:[67]

> The term 'continuant' (*sýnochos*) is also a proof of the fact that the man who appended these things is more recent. For nowhere did Hippocrates, or indeed any other of the ancients, call a continuous fever 'continuant', just as they never called urine *oúrēma*; rather these are terms of the more recent doctors, who were ignorant of the ancient form of expression.

---

64 He wrote a (lost) commentary on it (*My Own Books* 19.35 K.; Boudon-Millot 2007, p. 160, line 24), and quotes approvingly, if selectively, from it in numerous places.

65 For Galen's attitudes towards, and studies in, language, see Morison (2008); von Staden (2009); Manetti (2009); Manetti and Roselli (1994).

66 *My Own Books* 19.37 K.; Boudon-Millot (2007), p. 162, lines 2–3; for Galen's list of his own linguistic works, see ibid. 19.48 K.; Boudon-Millot (2007), p. 173, lines 5–15.

67 15.172 K.; Mewaldt (1914), p. 88, lines 7–12.

Again, Galen is right; '*sýnochos*', does not occur anywhere else in the Hippocratic Corpus. Jouanna (2002, 294) notes this fact, but also remarks that there are other cases of words which do appear sparingly in the Corpus, and which only re-appear much later (the term '*sýnochos*' was revived by the Pneumatists in the first century BC). This is not, then, a proof of the hypothesis of later authorship; but it is certainly evidence in favour of the view.

Elsewhere, in the course of an interesting discussion of the classification of fevers,[68] Galen writes that 'more recent doctors' use the term for wholly unremitting continuous fever, reserving the more common '*synechḗs*' (which does appear regularly in the Hippocratic corpus) for continuous fevers of varying intensity;[69] and later he repeats the point.[70] In his *Method of Healing* (10.599–604 K.), Galen remarks on the inappropriateness of the name 'ephemeral' being applied to a certain type of unremitting fever, since it may well last longer than a day, and says that such fevers should more properly be called '*sýnochoi*'. Later developments in diagnosis and classification, then, allow, and perhaps call, for a greater precision in terminology; but no such distinctions are in play here. What we apparently have is a simple variant in naming, without any hint of any particular motivation for it. That suggests that this passage is written by an individual prone to deploy an unusual diction. And that in turn suggests that he is an outlier, at least linguistically and hence possibly chronologically, even if not necessarily doctrinally, which further serves to distance this text (or rather in Galen's view, this particular part of it) from classical Hippocratic medicine.

7 Conclusions

This brief, and necessarily incomplete, discussion of Galen's approaches to textual and authorial establishment in his *Commentary on Hippocrates' 'Nature of Man'* may allow us finally to draw some tentative conclusions. First of all, there is no point in trying to deny, or even to minimize, the fact that Galen is far from being an independent and disinterested seeker after the pure and literal truth. He is motivated above all by the desire to establish that Part 1 of the text (which he thinks of as being the foundation-stone of all that is right and good in medical physiology) is unimpeachably the genuine product of his great med-

68 *Commentary on Hippocrates' 'Epidemics'* 1, 17a.219–224 K.; Wenkebach (1934), p. 111, line 5–p. 113, line 11.

69 Ibid. 17a. 220 K.; Wenkebach (1934), p. 111, lines 13–18.

70 *Commentary on Hippocrates' 'Epidemics'* 6, 17a.890 K.; Wenkebach (1934), p. 56, line 22–p. 57, line 1.

ical exemplar, Hippocrates. This drive to secure its position as echt Hippocrates is thus fundamentally driven by doctrine. Here is the only place in the Hippocratic corpus as it was available to him (and indeed as it is to us) in which the complete and as he saw it true and demonstrable doctrine of the four humours was preserved in its correct form. Indeed, so he thinks, Hippocrates not only here commends the doctrine—he also seeks to establish it on a firm demonstrative basis, even if he does not spell out the proofs in their full and lucid generality, since he need make no concession to the intellectual weaknesses of a later, more degenerate age.

Equally, Galen's own commitment to the reducibility of four-humour physiology to the fundamental physics of the four qualities, by way of the traditional Greek elements—earth, air, fire and water—that are supposed pre-eminently to embody them, leads him improbably to discern an equivalent commitment to the postulation of the four elements, as well as the four basic causal qualities, in the text of *Nature of Man*. And that, in turn, leads him to construe the object of Hippocrates' attack in the opening chapters as being material monism, rather than four-element theory as such, a construal which in turn prompts particular readings, and interpretations, of the text. Finally, the constraints of doctrinal orthodoxy, as well as the irresistibility of the ascription of the basic text to Hippocrates himself, force Galen to suppose that the treatise as a whole as he had it, that is, all of Parts 1–3, is a pastiche, a pastiche of material culled from different and sometimes markedly inferior sources. And they also force him to ignore evidence ascribing not only the four-humour theory of Part 1, but also the despised vascular anatomy of chapter 11 of Part 2, to the estimable Polybus, evidence derived from texts that he not only knew but in general respected and admired.

All of these views may be mistaken—although I have hinted above, and argued elsewhere, that at any rate some of them may be defended[71]—and some of them certainly are. But for all that, Galen's selective and impassioned defence of the Hippocratic authenticity of Part 1 of the text, and the un-Hippocratic mediocrity of much of the rest of it, is not simply a product of his ideologically-blinkered party allegiance. As I hope to have shown, he deploys not merely great ingenuity and argumentative skill in combatting the follies, as he sees them, of his commentatorial opponents. He also displays considerable acuteness, as well as genuine learning, in identifying linguistic peculiarities and inconcinnities. His criticisms of his opponents are typically sharp, and sometimes characteristically caustic and intemperate. But for all that, they are not

71 See Hankinson (2015).

mere partisan vituperation. Galen's Hippocrates is, to be sure, the misbegotten product of an over-zealous ideological commitment, and as such a chimaera. It is nonetheless not, paradoxical as it may seem, a purely baseless fabrication. For it rests also on serious, and seriously-deployed, textual and linguistic criticism. The case that is made is special pleading, of course, and ultimately unconvincing special pleading at that. But it is no mere casuistry.

CHAPTER 8

Galen's Hippocratic 'Commentary' on *The Capacities of the Soul Depend on the Mixtures of the Body*

Ralph M. Rosen

One of the central questions of Galen's treatise *The Capacities of the Soul Depend on the Mixtures of the Body* (Latin title abbreviated as *Quod Animi Mores* or *QAM*) is to what extent the bodily mixtures of the hot, cold, wet and dry—which, in his view, affect so profoundly the functioning of the soul—are themselves affected by external forces.[1] The short answer for *QAM* is that external factors may certainly affect the body's mixtures, and any change in a person's behaviour should be conceptualized as a direct consequence of these mixtures. Only indirectly, then, should we think of the soul's changed behaviour as a consequence of the external force. Too much wine (i.e., an external influence), to use one of Galen's favourite examples, changes a person's behaviour because it changes the body's mixtures, which in turn affects the soul, and then a person's behaviour.[2] This formulation, of course, only works if we assume that the soul is in some sense 'material', that the mixtures of the body's elements (which *are* material) will in fact interact in a physical way with a physical 'something' within the body that drives a per-

1 Singer (2013), 339: 'are there any factors apart from mixtures which are causally relevant? Two points should be considered here: whether mixtures are the only *bodily* factors in play; and whether there are also relevant *non-bodily* factors'.

2 As, e.g., *QAM* Müller (1891), p. 41, lines 1–6 (4.778–779 K.): 'For it is certainly true that wine, if drunk in moderation, will have a very great effect on digestion, distribution, blood-production and nutrition, while also making our souls gentler, and braver, too—which is, of course, by means of the mixture in the body, which is itself brought about by means of the humours. (ὄντως γάρ, εἰ συμμέτρως ποθείη, καὶ πέψει καὶ ἀναδόσει καὶ αἱματώσει καὶ θρέψει μεγάλα συντελεῖ μετὰ τοῦ καὶ τὴν ψυχὴν ἡμῶν ἡμερωτέραν ⟨θ'⟩ ἅμα καὶ θαρσαλεωτέραν ἐργάζεσθαι διὰ μέσης δηλονότι τῆς κατὰ τὸ σῶμα κράσεως, ἥντινα πάλιν [αὐτὴν] ἐργάζεται διὰ μέσων τῶν χυμῶν.)' (Singer 2013, 384; all subsequent translations of *QAM* from Singer). See also, *QAM* Müller (1891), 70–71 (4.811–812 K.), another passage on the damaging effects of wine on the soul, in which Galen concludes that it is 'through the medium of mixture that these activities of the soul are damaged when we drink wine (διὰ μέσης τῆς κράσεως αἱ εἰρημέναι τῆς ψυχῆς ἐνέργειαι φαίνονται βλαπτόμεναι πινόντων ἡμῶν τὸν οἶνον)' (Müller 1891, p. 71, lines 11–13).

© RALPH M. ROSEN, 2021 | DOI:10.1163/9789004470200_010

son's behaviour. There is considerable ambiguity in *QAM* about Galen's precise position on the matter: his approach is undeniably 'materialist' in the *broadest* sense, but he was aware of the logical complexities that arise in trying to think through all the factors that drive the soul to make an individual act as it does.

Examples that were material and involved the body directly, such as wine, are slightly less problematic: there is a liquid one can point to and taste, and then ingest; one can visualize how it would affect the body's mixtures fairly easily, tracing it through the digestive organs and into the humoral systems. So if the soul is also material, or even if the mixtures are somehow held to 'be' the soul—akin perhaps, as Singer (341) suggests, to the Aristotelian notion of the soul as '*eîdos* of the body'—the mechanism by which wine effects one's behaviour is, at least, not hard to imagine. Above all, one can observe what appears to be cause and effect: too much wine will change a person's behaviour fairly predictably.

More complicated for Galen, however, are questions about innate character as a function of the soul's *phýsis*, by which he meant its *dynámeis*, or 'capacities' as a function of the body's mixtures.[3] Galen believed that the mixtures people are born with account for their basic character, but that external environmental influences—from climate and geography to education and acculturation—can influence these mixtures to shape that character for better or worse. Galen's overall rhetorical strategy of arguing against contemporaries (here 'various Platonists', 'Aristotelians' and some 'Stoics') by invoking the authority of the great classical troika of Plato, Hippocrates and Aristotle, will be familiar enough. Even though Plato's and Aristotle's positions on the nature of the soul, and the soul's relationship with the body, are not always consonant with Galen's fundamentally physicalist approach, he nevertheless works hard in the *QAM* to align them with his own thinking, partly to enhance his polemic against his opponents, and partly, as it seems, to help him work through the complexities of the issues themselves.

The Hippocratic *Airs, Waters, Places* (*AWP*) plays a prominent role in this agenda in *QAM*, and Galen quotes liberally from it to support his argument about the influence of the environment on the soul. As we shall see, the frequency of his citation from *AWP*, and its systematic presentation, are striking and, as I will argue, suggest that Galen was also conceptualizing his quotations as if they were lemmas on which his discussion in *QAM* could serve as a form of exegetical commentary.

3 See Singer (2013), 375–376.

The quotations from Hippocrates are placed strategically in the last part of the treatise after Galen has worked through the views of Plato and Aristotle, with a brief introduction signaling Hippocrates' special status (Müller 1891, 57; 4.797 K.):

> ὧν καὶ παρεθέμην ἄν τινας ῥήσεις, εἰ μήτε μακρολογίας ἔμελλον ἀποίσεσθαι δόξαν ἀναλίσκειν τε τὸν χρόνον μάτην ἐξὸν ἐπὶ τὸν πάντων ἰατρῶν τε καὶ φιλοσόφων πρῶτον εὑρόντα τὴν θεωρίαν ταύτην ἀφικέσθαι μάρτυρα, τὸν θεῖον Ἱπποκράτην.

> I would juxtapose some quotations from that work [Aristotle's *History of Animals*] here too, if it were not that I would then get a reputation for longwindedness, as well as wasting time to no purpose, when we have available to us the witness of the man who discovered this study first of all doctors and philosophers—the divine Hippocrates.

The blunt instrument of Authority is especially evident in Galen's deployment of Aristotle as he prepares for his Hippocratic showcase at the end, which is intended to demonstrate that both authors agree with him that the 'capacities of the soul depend on the mixtures of the body'. In *QAM* 7 (4.791–794 K.; Müller 1891, p. 51, line 12–p. 54, line 13) Galen cites passages from *Parts of Animals* 2 which are supposed to show how the nature of an animal's blood (or in non-blooded animals such as insects, the liquid analogous to blood) accounts for various aspects of their nature—such as levels of intelligence, boldness, or timidity. Galen rounds out this section by quoting *Parts of Animals* 650b14–651a12 as proof for his own position:[4]

> ταῦτα προειπὼν ὁ Ἀριστοτέλης ἐφεξῆς αὐτοῖς συνάπτει ταῦτα· 'πολλῶν δ' ἐστὶν αἰτία ἡ τοῦ αἵματος φύσις καὶ κατὰ τὸ ἦθος τοῖς ζῴοις καὶ κατὰ τὴν αἴσθησιν, εὐλόγως· ὕλη γάρ ἐστι παντὸς τοῦ σώματος· ἡ γὰρ τροφὴ ὕλη, τὸ δ' αἷμα ἐσχάτη τροφή. πολλὴν οὖν ποιεῖ διαφορὰν θερμὸν ὂν καὶ ψυχρὸν καὶ λεπτὸν καὶ παχὺ καὶ καθαρὸν καὶ θολερόν.'

> After this preamble, Aristotle proceeds to add the following: 'The nature of the blood is the cause of many things in animals both in relation to character, and in relation to perception, reasonably enough: for it is the

4 *QAM* 4.794 K.; Müller (1891), 54.

> matter of the whole body; for nourishment is matter, and blood is the ultimate nourishment. And so it makes a great difference whether it is hot, cold, fine, thick, pure or cloudy'.

From the effects of mixtures on character, Galen then moves to physiognomics, citing Aristotle again as his authority, with quotations from the *History of Animals* (1), that mixtures can influence not only character but even physical form.

This section is, in fact, somewhat distracting from his main thesis, and the argument becomes rather blatantly circular: from Aristotle's assertions about how mixtures affect the appearance of the body, Galen cites passages to illustrate the reverse, namely, that there are many physiognomical characteristics which 'give indication of the mixture directly, without any intermediary; so it is with colour and hair, and also with activities of the parts'.[5] His last quotation from *History of Animals* (492a34–492b3), concerning the size and shape of human ears, threatens to take us entirely off-topic from mixtures: 'moderate ones are a sign of the best character, the large and prominent ones of stupidity and talkativeness.'[6] But Galen's associative train of thought then takes us to 'the divine Hippocrates', and it is here, in chapter 8 (Müller 1891, p. 57, line 14; 4.798 K.), as a complement to his appeal to Aristotle's authority on mixtures and character that Galen introduces the testimony of the Hippocratic *Airs, Waters, Places*.

This is a strategy that may be tried and true for Galen,[7] but which seems to take us even farther afield. This extended section on *AWP*, is, at least on first reading, really no more helpful for Galen's argument than Aristotle on physiognomics. Lloyd (1988, 26) noted that Galen's citations from Aristotle do little to *argue for* a thesis that character traits 'depend on/follow' the *mixtures* of the body. He also pointed out that Galen more generally ignores Aristotle's most important discussions of the moral capacities of the soul in the *Nicomachean* and *Eudemian Ethics*, which are concerned with moral acculturation and individual choice rather than questions of how the soul interacts with the material body. Similarly Lloyd noted how tendentious the next section invoking the

5 4.795–796 K.; Müller (1891), p. 55, lines 7–11: ἔνια δὲ τῶν φυσιογνωμονικῶν ἄντικρύς τε καὶ δι' οὐδενὸς μέσου τὴν κρᾶσιν ἐνδείκνυται. τοιαῦτα δ' ἐστὶ κατὰ τὰς χρόας καὶ τρίχας, ἔτι δὲ τὰς φωνὰς καὶ τὰς ἐνεργείας τῶν μορίων.

6 4.797 K.; Müller (1891), p. 57, lines 3–5: τὰ δὲ μέσα βελτίστου ἤθους σημεῖον, τὰ δὲ μεγάλα καὶ ἐπανεστηκότα μωρολογίας καὶ ἀδολεσχίας.

7 See Strohmaier (2004), 2 on Galen's engagement with the 'time-consuming job of commenting upon the corpus of a very old and in some respects even obsolete author'.

Hippocratic *AWP* is, particularly in its selective citation of the work and the omission of parts that would be difficult to square with his own basic thesis about influence of mixtures on the soul (e.g., Lloyd 1988, 30–32). As Lloyd pointed out, it is not clear from this section of *QAM*, for example, how Galen would account for the Hippocratic assertion—which he omits from his discussion—that the character of Asians was influenced by their *political* system (although by the end of *QAM*, he does seem more open to such external, non-physical influences on the capacities of the soul).

Lloyd explained Galen's tendentious deployment and selective citation of *AWP* as a function of a rhetorical strategy designed to persuade the reader that a doctor's intervention in the constitution of one's bodily mixtures can have positive effects on one's moral and psychological life. From a purely practical point of view, the treatise shows the reader how Galen can 'help you to acquire the best possible physical *krâsis*, which in turn will contribute both to moral excellence and to your intellectual capacities.' (Lloyd 1988, 39). Certainly, the ability to offer his readers at least the impression that the greatest thinkers of the past corroborate his own views is more important than the fact that they may not always actually say what he wants them to say.[8]

Lloyd's conclusion[9] is reasonable and probable enough on one level, but I would like to suggest here that there are additional forces at work in Galen's engagement with *AWP* in *QAM*, if only because the misalignment between the two works seems so glaring. As a supplement to Lloyd's discussion, then, I would propose that we read the section on *AWP* in *QAM* as itself a form of *commentary*, or perhaps, a 'proto-commentary' on the Hippocratic treatise.[10] By this I mean that at the same time as Galen adduces these passages as corroboration of his own argument in the treatise, he is also *interpreting* the Hippocratic passages, as one would who is actively engaged in an exegetical project on a target text. If pressed on the question of the legitimacy of his parallels from *AWP* for his argument in *QAM*, Galen would have defended these Hippocratic passages by arguing that any inconsistency with his own ideas was only apparent, namely, that Hippocrates was saying things in *AWP* which could in fact be

8 See also Strohmaier (2004), 2–3.

9 Also endorsed by Singer (2013), cf. p. 336, n. 4; p. 344, n. 27; and pp. 345, 355.

10 I use the term 'proto-commentary' to suggest that the markedly exegetical format of this section of *QAM*, with its systematic focus on *AWP*, anticipates the later formal commentary Galen came eventually to write on *AWP*. We cannot, of course, say whether Galen was consciously anticipating the later commentary on *AWP* while writing QAM, although it seems not unlikely. See Craik in this volume, and note her use of the term 'quasi-commentary', pp. 24–27.

seen as logically foundational for his views about the interaction of mixtures and the capacities of the soul, and not *just* assertions intended to *sound* persuasive.

Galen eventually did write a discrete commentary on *AWP*: he mentions it in *On My Own Books* (ch. 9.8, Boudon-Millot 2007, 160, line 25), where he refers to *AWP* as *On Places, Airs, Waters*, while suggesting it should instead be called *On Habitations, and Waters and Seasons and Countries*. Galen's Greek commentary is lost, but we have an Arabic translation by Hubayš ibn al-Ḥasan of a Syriac translation by Ḥunayn ibn Isḥāq,[11] which, even in its linguistically mediated form, will be useful as a comparandum for the proto-commentary to the same treatise that we find in *QAM*.[12] As we shall see, Galen's formal commentary on *AWP* suggests a continuity of thought and some retrospective explanation of why he had chosen the particular passages from *AWP* for discussion in *QAM* that he did.

The move in *QAM* from Aristotle on physiognomy to Hippocrates on correlations between environment and character, as we noted, is not particularly smooth, especially since the explanatory pathways of each testimony are different. Physiognomy, on the one hand, takes the appearance of a body as a *sign* of a particular character (with no commentary on *how* that character was produced—which, it is worth remembering, is *supposed* to be Galen's topic). The Hippocratic argument, on the other hand, holds that characters are *formed by* external factors such as climate and geography. At the beginning of chapter 8, Galen quotes the famous passage from *AWP* about the differences between Asians and Europeans:[13]

> ἔπειτα προελθὼν ἐπὶ πλέον περὶ τῶν αὐτῶν ὡδί πως διεξέρχεται· 'τὴν Ἀσίην πλεῖστον διαφέρειν φημὶ τῆς Εὐρώπης ἐς τὰς φύσιας τῶν ξυμπάντων τῶν τε ἐκ

11 Ḥunayn evidently had begun to make an Arabic translation from his Syriac version as well, but left its completion to his pupil Ḥubayš. A manuscript containing the Arabic translation of Galen's commentary on *AWP* was not discovered until 1970; see Sezgin (1970), 37, 124, and Sezgin (2001) (*non vidi*). See Bergsträsser (1925), 35 with more recent detail about the history of the text in Ulmann 1977, Wasserstein (1982), 4–7, Noja (1984), Jouanna (1988), 237–243, and Strohmaier (1993) and (2004), and now Lamoreaux (2016), 104. For the Hebrew translation of the Arabic translation in a fifteenth-century manuscript, see Wasserstein (1982), 93–100.

12 On Galen's commentaries in general, see Manetti and Roselli (1994) and Hanson (1998). I use the term 'commentary' here in the broader sense described by Jouanna (1988, 237), to refer to Galen's substantive exegesis of Hippocratic passages, not just commentary on Hippocratic textual problems.

13 Müller (1891), p. 57, line 21–p. 58, line 8; 4.798–799 K.

〈τῆς〉 γῆς φυομένων καὶ τῶν ἀνθρώπων· πολὺ γὰρ καλλίονα καὶ μείζονα πάντα γίγνεται ἐν τῇ Ἀσίῃ· ἥ τε χώρη τῆς χώρης ἡμερωτέρη καὶ τὰ ἤθεα τῶν ἀνθρώπων ἠπιώ〈τερα καὶ εὐοργητό〉τερα. τὸ δὲ αἴτιον τούτων ἡ κρῆσις τῶν ὡρέων.' τὴν κρᾶσιν εἶναι αἰτίαν φησὶν οὐ μόνον τῶν ἄλλων ὧν διῆλθεν ἀλλὰ καὶ τῶν ἠθῶν.

Then, discoursing further on the same theme, he [Hippocrates] continues: 'I state that the difference between Asia and Europe, in the natures, both of everything that grows out of the earth, and of the people, is a very great one. For all grow much finer and bigger in Asia. For the land is gentler and the characters of the people kinder and better-tempered. And the cause of this is the mixture of the seasons.' He states mixture to be the cause, not just of the other things which he has discussed, but also of the character traits.

Galen picks up on the last sentence of the Hippocratic quotation: 'And the cause of this [the 'kinder and gentler' natures of Asians] is the mixture of the seasons'. Galen knows this calls for comment, and seems to sense the logical problems he is introducing when he explains that Hippocrates' 'view is that different mixtures of the seasons differ from each other in respect of hotness and coldness, dryness and wetness'. Singer (2013, 396, n. 114) notes how Galen tacitly conflates this sense of external, environmental *kráseis* with the more specific, 'theoretically loaded' sense at work in *QAM* (and elsewhere, such as in *Mixtures*). There is, after all, a major conceptual difference between the idea that the mixtures of the *body* causally account for the nature of the soul, and the idea that the mixtures of *environmental phenomena* do.

This conflation underlies the rest of his discussion, which piles on one passage from *AWP* after another. Indeed, it is a relentless barrage of citations, all in the service of essentially the same basic point. It is common enough, of course, for Galen to lay on multiple citations, interspersed with commentary showing how they support his point—*QAM*, in particular, abounds with quotations from Plato and Aristotle as well. But even so, the number of passages Galen cites here from *AWP* (there are 13 in all within these few pages of the one chapter), and their sequential presentation seems more marked than Galen's usual practice. At 4.799.10 K., he alludes to the fact that he had already 'set down together a *large number of quotations*' (παμπόλλας ῥήσεις) in his commentary on the *Nature of Man*, intended to show that the mixtures of environmental elements are the cause of people's character traits.[14] But he still feels the need to

14 *QAM* 11 (Müller 1891, p. 58, lines 8–17; 4.799 K.):

reiterate: 'But in the words following the present quotation, too, *his teaching is the same*'. It is striking that, despite the fact that Galen made his point at the opening of chapter 8 with his initial quotation from *AWP*, he feels the need to keep citing *so many* passages that say the same thing. We may note the cataloging mode with which he introduces each quotation, from 799 K. to the end of 801 K.:

—And so he goes on: bravery ... could never take root in such a nature ....

διὰ τοῦτ᾽οὖν ἐφεξῆς φησι 'τὸ δὲ ἀνδρεῖον ... οὐκ ἂν δύναιτο ἐν τῇ τοιαύτῃ φύσει ἐγγίγνεσθαι.'

MÜLLER 1891, p. 58, lines 19–20; 4.799 K.

—And, conversely, he writes a little further on in the same work: '... the fact that Asiatic men are less warlike than Europeans and gentler in their character traits is caused mainly by the seasons ...'

καὶ μέντοι κατωτέρω πάλιν ἐν ταὐτῷ γράμματι τάδε γράφει· '... ὅτι ἀπολεμώτεροί εἰσι τῶν Εὐρωπαίων οἱ Ἀσιηνοὶ καὶ ἡμερώτεροι τὰ [τε] ἤθεα, αἱ [τε] ὧραι αἴτιαι.'

MÜLLER 1891, p. 59, lines 4–5; 4.799–800 K.

—However, he adds a bit further on: 'You will also find some individual differences between Asiatic people ... and the changes in the seasons are responsible for these to, as I have stated above.'

καὶ μέντοι καὶ μετ᾽ ὀλίγα πάλιν οὕτως εἶπεν· 'εὑρήσεις δὲ καὶ τοὺς Ἀσιηνοὺς διαφέροντας αὐτοὺς ἑωυτῶν ... τούτων δὲ αἱ μεταβολαὶ αἴτιαι τῶν ὡρέων, ὥσπερ μοι εἴρηται ἐν τοῖσι προτέροισι'

MÜLLER 1891, p. 59, lines 9–10; 4.800 K.

I *set down together a very large number of quotations* to this effect in the work in which I display [the fact] that he maintains the same belief regarding the elements in *Nature of Man* and in all his other works. But in the words following the present quotation, too, *his teaching is the same*, as he writes as follows concerning the well-mixed land, which, he states, makes people's character traits well-mixed too ...

παμπόλλας ῥήσεις παρεθέμην ἐν τῇ πραγματείᾳ, καθ᾽ ἣν ἐπιδείκνυμι τὴν αὐτὴν φυλάττοντα δόξαν αὐτὸν περὶ [τε] τῶν στοιχείων ἔν ⟨τε⟩ τῇ περὶ φύσιος ἀνθρώπου βίβλῳ καὶ κατ᾽ ἄλλα πάντα συγγράμματα. ἀλλὰ καὶ κατὰ τὰς ἑπομένας ῥήσεις τῇ προκειμένῃ *ταὐτὸν διδάσκων* ὡδὶ γράφει περὶ τῆς εὐκράτου χώρας, ἣν καὶ τὰ τῶν ἀνθρώπων ἤθη ποιεῖν φησιν εὔκρατα·

— … later on, when the discussion turns to the inhabitants of Europe …

… κατωτέρω τοῦ συγγράμματος, ἡνίκα περὶ τῶν τὴν Εὐρώπην οἰκούντων ὁ λόγος αὐτῷ γίγνεται …
MÜLLER 1891, p. 59, line 14; 4.800 K.

—In another passage, further on, he again writes …

καὶ μετὰ ταῦτα πάλιν ἐν ἑτέρᾳ ῥήσει γράφει ταυτί …
MÜLLER 1891, p. 59, line 17; 4.800 K.

The last passage quoted above (Müller 1891, p. 59, line 17) Galen proceeds to offer an extensive quotation from *AWP* (Jouanna 2003, p. 244, line 11–p. 246, line 4), in which the Hippocratic author notes that *nómos* can also play a role in shaping character traits. This is an important point for Galen, and he quickly explains it as if he is explicating a lemma (here the word *nómos*) in a commentary:[15]

νόμον εἴρηκε [δὲ] δηλονότι τὴν νόμιμον ἐν ἑκάστῃ χώρᾳ τοῦ βίου διαγωγήν, ἣν δὴ καὶ τροφὴν καὶ παιδείαν καὶ συνήθειαν ἐπιχώριον ὀνομάζομεν, οὗ καὶ αὐτοῦ μεμνήσομαι πρὸς τὸν ὀλίγον ὕστερον εἰρησόμενον λόγον. ἐν γὰρ τῷ παρόντι προσθεῖναι ταύτας ἔτι βούλομαι τὰς ῥήσεις αὐτοῦ· 'ὅσοι δὲ ὑψηλὴν οἰκέουσι χώρην καὶ λείην καὶ ἀνεμώδεα καὶ ἔνυδρον, εἶεν ἂν εἴδεα μεγάλοι καὶ ἑωυτοῖσι παραπλήσιοι, καὶ ἀνανδρότεραι καὶ ἡμερώτεραι ⟨τούτων⟩ αἱ γνῶμαι·'

By 'regulation' [*nómos*] here he evidently means the regular upbringing in each country, which we also refer to as nurture, education and local habituation; and to this, indeed, I will return a little further on in the argument. For now, I want to add a few more quotations yet. 'The inhabitants of high, flat, windy, and well-watered land will be tall in stature, and similar to each other, and they will be less brave, and gentler, in their tempers.'

Galen is eager to pursue this topic, but he does not allow himself to get distracted by it just yet. He promises to get back to it soon, he says, but for now, 'I want to add a few more quotations yet … (ἐν γὰρ τῷ παρόντι προσθεῖναι ταύτας ἔτι βούλομαι τὰς ῥήσεις αὐτοῦ·)', which he then proceeds to do.

15 Müller (1891), p. 60, line 14–p. 61, line 3.

At Müller (1891), p. 61, line 10 (4.802 K.), it is as if Galen realizes he is going overboard:

> καὶ [τί γὰρ] ἵνα μὴ πολλῶν αὐτοῦ μνημονεύσω ῥήσεων, ἐφεξῆς ἐρεῖ 'εὑρήσεις γὰρ ἐπὶ τὸ πολὺ τῆς χώρης τῇ φύσει ἀκολουθέοντα καὶ τὰ εἴδεα τῶν ἀνθρώπων καὶ τοὺς τρόπους'.
>
> Well, to avoid having too many quotations from [Hippocrates], consider what he says next: 'You will find, for the most part, that the features of human beings, and their habits, are consequent on the nature of the land.'

With his quotation of *AWP* (from Jouanna 2003, p. 247, lines 1–4), Galen seems on the verge of wrapping up his extended adversion to Hippocrates with a grand summation, but he cannot seem to stop himself. His reiteration that '… of course, [Hippocrates] has often stated in [*AWP*] that the difference between the lands themselves is in terms of the hot, cold, wet and dry …' evokes from him not just one more quotation from *AWP*, but three—substantial passages which serve to restate the claim that Hippocrates also felt that not just character traits, but intellectual faculties as well depend on mixtures (Müller 1891, p. 61, line 16–p. 64, line 2; 4.802–804 K.).

Finally at the beginning of chapter 9, Galen draws his discussion of *AWP* to a close, with a statement which, on the face of it, anyway, does not seem quite accurate:[16]

> Ἱπποκράτης μὲν ⟨οὖν⟩ ἐπιδείξας ἐν ὅλῳ ⟨λόγῳ⟩ τῷ περὶ ὑδάτων καὶ ὡρῶν κράσεως ⟨ἑπομένας⟩ ταῖς τοῦ σώματος κράσεσι τὰς τῆς ψυχῆς δυνάμεις …
>
> Hippocrates, then, displays throughout his entire discussion of the mixture of waters and seasons that the soul's capacities (not only those in the spirited and desiderative parts of it, but also those in the rational) depend on the mixtures of the body …

As we noted earlier, the move from the mixtures of the environment to those of the body is not explicit in the Hippocratic treatise, nor, as Singer (2013, 400, n. 131) also points out, is Galen warranted in ascribing to Hippocrates a tripartite Platonic soul, as he does here. Galen calls Hippocrates in the same sentence

16 Müller (1891), p. 64, line 3–6; 4.804–805 K.

'the witness most worthy of all to be trusted' (ἁπάντων ἀξιοπιστότατός ἐστι μάρτυς, Müller 1891, p. 64, line 8; 4.805 K.), as if slightly uneasy with the claims for him he had just made. He follows this with an even more logically problematic claim, namely that he does not need to fall back on the mere authority of Hippocrates, since one can 'see that his demonstrations are secure …':[17]

> ἐγὼ δ' οὐχ ὡς μάρτυρι πιστεύω τἀνδρὶ τοῖς πολλοῖς ὡσαύτως ἀλλ' ὅτι τὰς ἀποδείξεις αὐτοῦ βεβαίας ὁρῶ, διὰ τοῦτο γοῦν καὶ αὐτὸς ἐπαινῶ τὸν Ἱπποκράτην τίς γὰρ οὐχ ὁρᾷ τὸ σῶμα καὶ τὴν ψυχὴν ἁπάντων τῶν ὑπὸ τοῖς ἄρκτοις ⟨ἀνθρώπων⟩ ἐναντιώτατα διακείμενα τοῖς ἐγγὺς τῆς διακεκαυμένης ζώνης;

> For my part, I do not trust the man as a witness, as most people do; rather, I see that his demonstrations are secure, and for this reason, then, I too praise Hippocrates. For who does not observe that the bodies and the souls of people in the northern regions have a quite opposite disposition to those of people near the fiery zone?

Needless to say, Galen's casual observations about 'ethnic temperaments' prove nothing about a causal relationship between environment, bodily mixtures and behaviour.

Galen's apparent misrepresentation of Hippocratic psychology as Platonic or his apparently tendentious deployment of *AWP* in *QAM* is not, I would suggest, malicious or careless sleight of hand. Rather, Galen seems to adduce his passages from *AWP* because he thinks the Hippocratic passages actually do support his argument with an underlying logic he has just not taken the time to explain in this context. The barrage of Hippocratic passages in quick succession is reminiscent of a commentary, and as such we might expect them to be *interpreted* here in the light of the main thesis of *QAM*. But the immediate goal where they occur within *QAM* is the exegesis of Galen's *own* ideas, not those of Hippocrates; or to put this another way, any exegesis of Hippocrates along the way can only be included in order to add support to Galen's arguments in *QAM*. Presumably there *is* a logic in Galen's mind that satisfactorily connects his idea that the 'capacity of the soul follow the mixture of the body' with Hippocrates' conclusion that '… the features of human beings, and their habits, are consequent (ἀκολουθέοντα) on the nature of the land' (*AWP* 2.90 L., Jouanna 2003, 248, lines 8–10), but further elaboration of this would have to wait until he wrote his actual commentary on *AWP*.

17 Müller (1891), p. 64, lines 11–16; 4.805 K.

Some illumination on this point emerges when we consult the Arabic version of Galen's commentary on *AWP*.[18] Galen here maintains his specific interest in the relationship between *environmental* mixture and human character, but he also alludes several times to *QAM*, despite its own focus on *internal*, bodily mixtures. In these passages of the commentary, the logic can be as frustrating as it was in *QAM*. At one point in the commentary Galen explains a passage from *AWP* (Jouanna 2003, p. 197, lines 3–4)[19] about the balanced mixture of the land, saying simply that the balanced mixture 'of the land' shows that the mixtures of the inhabitants' bodies are also balanced:

قال جالينوس: إنّ هذا ممّا يدلّ على اعتدال بلادهم، فيعتدل لذلك مزاجات أبدانهم. وقد بيّنت ذلك بقول أشرح من هذا في كتابي الذي عنونته بأنّ «قوى النفس تابعة لمزاج البدن».

Galen says: This is something that indicates that their land is balanced, so that the mixtures of their body are balanced. I have explained this more fully than here in my book to which I have given the title *That the Capacities of the Soul Follow the Mixture of the Body*.

Commenting on ch. 16 of *AWP* on the differences between Asians and Europeans, (Jouanna 2003, 244–245), the commentary has:

قال جالينوس: إنّ هذا القول بيّن واضح، وذلك أنّه قال إنّ علّة الغضب وتيهان العقل هو اختلاف الأزمنة. فإذا كان المزاج مستويا، كانت غرائز الناس معتدلة. فمن هٰهنا ينبغي أن نعلم أنّ رأي بقراط هو هذا: أنّ قوى النفس تتبع مزاج البدن.

Galen says: These explanations are transparent and clear. For he says that the cause of anger and confusion of mind is the difference of the seasons.

18 I am deeply grateful to Professor G. Strohmaier for sharing with me his Arabic edition and German translation of Galen's *Commentary on Hippocrates' 'Airs, Waters, Places'*, which he is currently finalising for the *Corpus Medicorum Graecorum*; all quotations adduced here are taken from his edition. For assistance with the Arabic text, I thank Professor Peter E. Pormann, who systematically checked my English translations of Strohmaier's German versions against the Arabic source. I am also indebted to Professor Aileen Das for her helpful comments on an early draft of this chapter.

19 In fact, the lemma does not really translate the Greek of *AWP* 5.4. The Arabic lemma has, 'Hippocrates says: These people do not become quickly angry or excited (قال بقراط: إنّ هؤلاء لا يغضبون سريعا ولا يحتدون)', extrapolated from 'λαμπρόφωνοί τε οἱ ἄνθρωποι ὀργήν τε καὶ σύνεσιν βελτίους εἰσὶ τῶν προσβορείων (The people [here] are clear-voiced and better in temperament and intelligence than those who facing the north …)'.

> When the mixture is well-proportioned, the dispositions of the people are balanced. Therefore, we should know that the opinion of Hippocrates is this, that the powers of the soul follow the mixture of the body.

Galen does not mention *QAM* here, but it is clear from the last clause that he has it in mind. Once again, he equates external environmental mixtures with internal bodily mixtures as if it would be obvious to anyone.

In the other instance where he refers to *QAM* directly, commenting on the famous chapter 24, again on Asians and Europeans, the commentary has:

> وليس أنّ النفس تنقاد وتتبع مزاجات البدن فقط، كما بيّنت ذلك في كتاب على حدته، لكنّها مختلفة أيضا بحال اختلاف الأزمنة. وذلك أنّ البرد الشديد يصيّر الناس أهل شجاعة اضطرارا. وقد ذكر بقراط ذلك حين قال ...

> Not only does the soul tie itself to, and follow, the mixtures of the body, *as I have shown in a separate book*, but it also changes with the seasons. For extreme cold necessarily makes people brave. Hippocrates mentioned this when he said ...

There is a bit of an exegetical loop on this point: *QAM* is invoked here to help explain Hippocrates, whereas within *QAM* itself, as we saw, Hippocrates was invoked to explain Galen's ideas. There is still not much of an actual argument here for a necessary connection between environmental mixtures and those of the body.

A little further in the commentary on this chapter of *AWP* (24.8), however, we do finally see that Galen seems to have thought about this problem, and here he offers an explanation for the explicitly *causative* movement from external to internal mixtures, and then from internal mixtures to character traits. Galen is here commenting on the Hippocratic passage at 24.7: 'And so these [i.e., the seasons] cause the greatest change to human nature.[20] Next comes the land, in which one takes one's nourishment, and then waters (Μέγισται μὲν οὖν εἰσιν αὗται τῆς φύσιος αἱ διαλλαγαί, ἔπειτα δὲ καὶ ἡ χώρη ἐν ᾗ ἄν τις τρέφηται καὶ τὰ ὕδατα)'. Galen explains that the Hippocratic term *phýsis* should be understood as an 'equivalent of the mixtures and also of the forms of the body (*badala mizāǧāti l-abdāni wa-l-ṣuwari ayḍan*)'. And he continues:

---

20 See Jouanna (2003), 248: 'These things cause the greatest changes experienced by human nature (Voilà donc ce qui cause les plus grandes differences que connaisse la nature [humaine]. Viennent ensuite le pays dans lequel on se nourrit, et les eaux.)'.

وأمّا البلاد فلها في الأبدان قوّة ثانية بعد المزاج لأنّ الناس يغتذون بنباتها ثمّ بعدها بالمياه. [...] وهذه الأغذية ممّا يوافق مزاج الأبدان، لأنّه يتولّد منها الكيموسات التي في أبداننا. فمنها ⟨ما⟩ يولّد دما كثيرا ومنها ما يولّد مرّة صفراء ومنها ما يولّد بلغما ومنها ما يولّد مرّة سوداء. والمياه أيضا ممّا يوافق مزاج الأبدان.

> ... The land has an effect on the body that is secondary [in rank/importance] to mixture, because people feed on its plants; after [land comes the effect of] water ... [*a description follows of different plants, fruits and grains that people eat*]. These foods correspond to the mixture of the body, since the humours of our body are generated from them. Some produce a lot of blood, some produce yellow bile, some produce phlegm, and some produce black bile. Water also corresponds to the mixture of the body.

This is the statement, finally, that we wanted to hear in his discussion of *AWP* in *QAM*, something that spelled out Galen's thinking behind his conflation of environmental and bodily mixtures: the argument may not be completely satisfying (e.g., it works well enough for food and water, but less clearly for climate and topography), but we can at least see that the missing step in his proto-commentary in *QAM* is that airs, waters, and places affect bodily mixtures because they *get inside the body* and assimilate themselves materially to those mixtures. The discussion of the passages from *AWP* in *QAM*, then, reads as if it were a kind of rehearsal for the actual commentary he would eventually write. We can see here again, as well, the hermeneutic loop we noted earlier in which Galen adduces passages from *AWP* to corroborate his argument in *QAM*, but in the later *commentary* on *AWP explains* some of *these* passages on the strength of *his* arguments presented in *QAM*.

It is always risky to attempt to get inside the mind of an ancient author, but I close simply by suggesting that, although Galen seems mostly content in *QAM* to line up all the passages from *AWP* in order to bask in the Hippocratic glow of authority, we seem also to catch a glimpse of Galen, while attempting to align Hippocratic views with his own, in the process of discovering deeper implications of *AWP* for his position on the interaction of body and soul, taking mental notes while writing *QAM* of details he would want to flesh out later when he came to write a full and dedicated commentary on that work.

CHAPTER 9

Commenting beyond the Commentary: Galen's Exegetical Strategies in *Difficulties in Breathing*

Daniela Manetti

As Wesley Smith already remarked in his important essay: 'The work on *Abnormal breathing* is pivotal in Galen's literary career and his Hippocratism'.[1] This paper aims at bringing to the fore the intention and the structure of the treatise and its relationship with Galen's running commentaries of Hippocrates.

Galen himself informs us that he wrote *On Abnormal Breathing* or *Difficulties in Breathing* (as I will call it from now on) at the beginning of a long season of Hippocratic exegesis. We can therefore date it to approximate AD 175. I shall not dwell on how other scholars have dated it,[2] but it is undeniably linked to Galen's Hippocratic commentaries, as the following passage from his *My Own Books* makes clear:[3]

> οὔτ' ἄλλο τι τῶν ὑπ' ἐμοῦ δοθέντων φίλοις ἤλπισα πολλοὺς ἕξειν οὔτε τὰ τῶν Ἱπποκρατείων συγγραμμάτων ἐξηγητικά· τὴν ἀρχὴν γὰρ ἐμαυτὸν γυμνάζων ἐγεγράφην εἰς αὐτά ποθ' ὑπομνήματα, καθάπερ ἐποίησα τῆς ἰατρικῆς θεωρίας ἁπάσης καθ' ἕκαστον μέρος ἐμαυτῷ παρασκευάσας οἷς ἅπαντα τὰ κατὰ τὴν ἰατρικὴν τέχνην ὑφ' Ἱπποκράτους εἰρημένα περιέχεται διδασκαλίαν ἔχοντα σαφῆ τε ἅμα καὶ παντοίως ἐξειργασμένην.
>
> I did not expect that many people would come into possession of one or more of the pieces that I had written and given to friends, much less that those texts would include those devoted to exegesis of the works of Hippocrates. At the beginning, I had written some commentaries on this subject as an exercise, just as I did for each area of the medical theory: I provided for myself essays containing all of Hippocrates' doctrines on the art of medicine, presented in instructive manner that would be both clear and comprehensive.

1 Smith (1979), 119.
2 Ilberg (1889); Bardong (1942); Peterson (1977).
3 Galen, *My Own Books* 9; Boudon-Millot (2007), p. 159, lines 10–18.

© DANIELA MANETTI, 2021 | DOI:10.1163/9789004470200_011

As examples of this production he lists immediately afterwards, *Critical Days*, *Crisis*, *Difficulties in Breathing*, and the long treatise in 14 books, *Therapeutic Method*; all these works are apparently presented as the result of his personal study of the Hippocratic doctrine.

Let us consider in slightly greater detail the information that Galen gives here about the destination and circulation of his works. If Galen can be believed, he mostly either writes for a few friends or just to further his own studies.[4] In fact Galen often states that he composed various works for private use, either for himself or to give them to a friend or pupil. The case of private use implies a conception of writing as an 'exercise', an essential part of one's cultural and educational training,[5] whereas the second typology reveals a fairly common characteristic, namely the semiprivate circulation of texts or, in some sense, their circulation through personal channels of communication.[6] For Galen, the difference between private and public works was not so much in the degree to which the text was polished, but rather in the intended readership, be it a single individual or the 'average' reader.[7] Unlike published works, texts composed for friends often lacked both title and authorship information, and could therefore be more easily be appropriated by dishonest persons.

In fact even if Galen wrote *Difficulties in Breathing* for himself, as he says in his later work, it is by no means less elaborated in its composition. Galen outlines very clearly why he decided to pen this work and for whom. First, he seeks to fill a gap in the contemporary scientific literature, as there exists no treatment on the difficulty of breathing, even though many authors wrote extensively on respiration and the pulse in general:[8]

4 He wrote a *sýnopsis* of the Platonic dialogues (of which there remains, in an Arabic translation, that of the *Timaeus*); a *sýnopsis* of the works of Heraclides of Tarentum (*My Own Books* 12.1–2, 3), but also of his own works (*Synopsis on Pulses*). He wrote commentaries on Aristotle as an exercise at the request of friends or for a limited circulation and expert readers (*My Own Books* 14.9).

5 On the composition of works as an 'exercise', see Galen, *My Own Books*. 2.4, 3.7, 14.9; they include the first commentaries on Hippocrates, *Seizures* and *Breathing difficulties* (9.1) and the commentaries on Aristotle (14.14). I discussed these issues Manetti (2015), 1186–1190.

6 Similarly, in *Dispelling Sorrows*, Galen (ch. 21) reports the story of the great fire of AD 192 which ravaged Rome and destroyed all his books. He speculates that if the fire had broken out two months later, all his works would have had two copies, one in Campania, and the other sent to his friends in Pergamon for delivery to the public libraries (διπλᾶ γὰρ ἐγέγραπτο πάντα τὰ πρὸς ἔκδοσιν ἤδη). This shows that Galen relied on personal channels for the circulation of his works.

7 This distinction between published and unpublished writings enabled Galen to identify and justify the 'incomplete' texts of Hippocrates; see Gurd (2011), 171–174.

8 *Difficulties in Breathing* 7.763.18–764.13 K.

> … καί τοι γράψαντος Ἱπποκράτους ἐν τοῖς περὶ τῶν Ἐπιδημιῶν, ὥσπερ τινὰ μύωπα, τὰς διαφορὰς τῶν δυσπνοιῶν, ὑφ' οὗ νυττομένους αὐτοὺς ἐχρῆν ἐξεγερθῆναί ποτε τοῦ βαθέος ὕπνου, καὶ ζητῆσαι, τίς ἐφ' ἑκάστης αὐτῆς ὁ πεπονθὼς τόπος, καὶ τίς ὁ τρόπος τῆς διαθέσεως, καὶ τίς ἡ αἰτία, καὶ εἰ παραλέλειπται ταῦτα τελέως ὑφ' Ἱπποκράτους ἤ τινα μὲν εἴρηται πρὸς αὐτοῦ τινα δ' οὔ; καὶ ποῦ τῶν συγγραμάτων καὶ πῶς; ἆρά γε τελέως καὶ σαφῶς ἢ ἐλλιπῶς τε καὶ οἱονεὶ σπερματικῶς; οὐδὲν γὰρ τούτων ἐζήτησεν οὐδείς, οὔτ' αὐτοῦ τοῦ πράγματος ἀξίως τῶν θ' Ἱπποκρατείους ἑαυτοὺς ὀνομαζόντων, ἐξηγητικά τε γραφόντων ὑπομνήματα τῶν συγγραμμάτων αὐτοῦ, τὸν περὶ τῆς δυσπνοίας οὐδεὶς τελέως ἐπεξῆλθε λόγον.

> … although Hippocrates wrote about the different cases of difficult breathing in the *Epidemics*—in the manner of the horsefly: they [physicians who have neglected to write on the topic of difficult breathing] should have been stung by it and waken up from their deep slumber to investigate the following questions: which is affected part in case of each [breathing difficulty]? what is the nature of the affection? what is its cause? has Hippocrates completely abandoned the topic or does he mention some aspects and says nothing about others? and in which works and how has he treated them in a complete and clear way or in an inadequate and more or less elementary manner? None of these people has inquired into any of this, certainly not in a manner that reflects the importance of the subject. And although they call themselves Hippocratics and write commentaries explaining his [sc. Hippocrates'] works, none of them has provided a complete account about breathing.

Here Galen traces the ideal process of analysing any subject related to Hippocrates: first the medical analysis according to Galenic standards such as the 'affected part (*peponthṑs tópos*)', the 'nature (*trópos*)', and the 'cause (*aitía*)'; secondly whether Hippocrates has omitted it or has given some information, in which work and in what way he tackled it; and lastly the textual explanation: whether Hippocrates' treatment is complete and clear, or is lacunose and scattered casually.

But even the Hippocratic physicians, who habitually wrote commentaries, did not engage in addressing the difficulty of breathing. Thus Galen sets himself the task of collecting everything Hippocrates said in his works on this topic, not only to explain Hippocrates' ideas (*gnṓmē*), but also to give a correct demonstration of the truth. Galen proposes to give a demonstration of the theory of difficult breathing in the first book, and to explain Hippocrates' statements on the subject in the second. The third book is not mentioned here, probably because he wrote it later.[9]

Galen clearly states that he explained the theoretical underpinnings in his works on respiration and pulse, such as *Causes of Breathing* and *Use of Breathing*,[10] and *Function of Pulses* and *Causes of Pulses*. His method is one of 'division (*dihaíresis*)', starting from very general premises and then consequently organizing the subject-matter systematically: given the three components of the process of respiration (breathing in, pause, breathing out), he classifies all the possible variants according to time and space. Only later does he indicate that the differences (*diaphoraí*) which he sets out were already known to Hippocrates, as well as the technical terminology. Already in this part, he thus takes Hippocrates' texts as a model; his definitions of the different kinds of breathing difficulties are all drawn from the *Epidemics*, as we will see later.

Even if he is writing for himself, Galen repeatedly hints at a background of lively discussions with adversaries, usually named 'sophists', with whom he engaged in battles, probably on public occasions.[11] Furthermore, at the beginning of the third book he explicitly aims at two levels of reading public. Galen repeats that in the first book he has offered all that a physician needs to know about difficult breathing, in the second and third book he explains what Hippocrates said in *all* his works:[12]

> ὥστε τοὺς μὲν αὐτῶν τῶν ἔργων τῆς τέχνης μόνον ἐφιεμένους, μηδὲν δ', ὡς αὐτοί φασιν, πολυπραγμονεῖν ἀξιοῦντας ὑπὲρ τῶν τοῖς παλαιοῖς εἰρημένων, ἔχειν ἅπαν ἱκανῶς ὃ σπουδάζουσιν ἐκ τοῦ πρώτου λόγου· τοὺς δὲ καὶ τὴν Ἱπποκράτους γνώμην ἐπιμαθεῖν ὀρεγομένους τε ἅμα καὶ δυναμένους, ἐκ τῶνδε τῶν γραμμάτων ἀναλέγεσθαι.
>
> Therefore those concerned only with the practical applications of the art (*téchnē*), who think it unnecessary to toil, as they say, about what the ancient said, have everything they need for their efforts in the first book. Those, however, who aspire to learn Hippocrates' opinion and are able to do so should gather it from these writings.

He goes on to explain that the desire to know what 'the best (*aristoí*)' said is common to all who love beauty (the *philókaloi*), but he is aware that many

9 7.764.13–765.6 K.

10 See 7.761.3–763.16 K.

11 See 7.759.16–760.2 K.; as usual he polemizes against those who abandon the traditional terms; 7.792.5–7; 798.7–9 K.; cf. also 7.828.15–829.2 K.

12 7.888.8–889.1 K.

people are stressed by multiple commitments and have no time for beauty. It is for them that Galen has composed the first book, separating theory from the Hippocratic texts. But the others, the *philókaloi*, must read the subsequent books in the correct order, because in the second book he has explained Hippocrates' opinion (*gnṓmē*), or choice (*prohaíresis*), that is, Hippocrates' intention in writing, and then he dwelt on all the case histories in *Epidemics* 1 and 3; now, in the third book, he will do the same with *Epidemics* 2 and 6. He will also add, if necessary, quotations from the other genuine works by Hippocrates, such as *Prognostic, Aphorisms, Airs Waters Places,* and *Regimen in Acute Diseases.* Finally, Galen also mentions the possibility of citing works which were attributed to Euryphon, Thessalus or Polybus (7.891.9–10 K.).

In conclusion, Galen uses the same rhetorical tools when writing a text for himself or for publication; the cause of writing and the intended readership are inescapable motives. But I do not think that the picture of the audience is mere forgery: Galen deals with texts he has at hand and wants his readers to be able to check his arguments and comments on Hippocrates in their own text. This is clear from his extreme precision in quoting several Hippocratic passages.[13] Galen gives account of this in chapter 9 (7.869.17–870.5 K.):[14]

> καὶ διὰ τοῦτο μηνύομεν ἡμεῖς ἐν τίνι τε τῶν βιβλίων ὁ ἄρρωστος, ὑπὲρ οὗ ποτ' ἂν ἑκάστοτε διαλεγόμενοι τύχωμεν, γέγραπται καὶ πόστος ἐστὶν, ἢ ἀπὸ τῆς ἀρχῆς ἢ ἀπὸ[15] καταστάσεως ἀριθμοῦντι, πρὸς τὸ μὴ καταμελεῖν[16] διὰ ταῦτά[17] τινα καὶ περὶ τὴν ἀνεύρεσιν ὀκνοῦντα ἢ ἀβασανίστως ἡμῖν πιστεύειν, ὅπερ οὐ βουλόμεθα, ἢ ὑποπτεύειν ὥς τι[18] καὶ[19] παρεγγράφοντας[20] ἡμᾶς, ὃ δὴ πολλοὶ τῶν

13 Cf. 7.841.14 K., in citing the case of the wife of Dealces, after the first sentence he mentions the immediately following passage as ἑξῆς and at 842.6 K. he mentions another, not contiguous, passage saying καὶ μικρὸν ἔτι προελθὼν ὧδέ πως γράφει; 7.865.17: the boy from Meliboea is the last of *Epidemics* 3; 866.2 K.: Anaxion is the eighth patient from the *loimṓdēs katástasis*; 7.866.5 K.: the wife of Dealces is eighth after Anaxion and fifteenth from the *loimṓdēs katástasis*, 7.869.10 K.: Pythion is the third from the *loimṓdēs katástasis*, etc.

14 Kühn's text is corrupt, and there is no modern edition; Minor (1911) edits only two passages. The text presented here is based on my collation of three manuscripts, previously described by Minor (1911, 1–28): Barocc. gr. 220 (13th cent.; B); Vat. Reg. gr. 175 (14th cent; V); and Oxon. Canon. gr. 44 (15th cent.; C); I thank Luigi Orlandi for his help.

15 ἀπὸ] τῆς add. C.

16 καταμελεῖν] BCR : καταμέλλειν Kühn.

17 διὰ ταῦτά] BR Kühn : om. C.

18 ὥς τι] correxi : ὥστε BCR Kühn.

19 καὶ] CR Kühn : om. B.

20 παρεγγράφοντας] C : παραγράφοντας BR Kühn.

ἐξηγησαμένων ἐποίησαν. ἀλλ' ἐκεῖνοι μὲν διὰ τοῦτο σιγῶσι τὰ βιβλία καὶ κατακρύπτουσιν ἑκόντες, ἐξ ὧν ἂν ἑκάστοτε παραγράφωσι τὰς λέξεις, ἡμεῖς δὲ οὐκ αὐτὰ μόνον, ἀλλὰ καὶ τοὺς τόπους αὐτοὺς καὶ τὰ κεφάλαια μηνύομεν, ὑπὲρ τοῦ ῥᾷον εὑρίσκειν τὸ βουλόμενον[21]· ἴσμεν γὰρ ὅτι βεβαιοτέραν πίστιν ὧν λέγομεν ἕξουσιν οἱ πᾶν ἀναγνόντες τοῦ βιβλίου τὸ χωρίον, ἐξ οὗ τὴν ῥῆσιν παραγράφομεν.

For this reason we indicate in which book the patient about whom we happen to speak is described. We also provide the number of the patient, counting either from the beginning [of the book] or from the 'constitution (*katástasis*)'. Therefore, nobody should be negligent and believe us without examination, because he takes a long time to find [the exact reference]. We do not want this. Nor should he be left with a suspicion that we have added material, as many commentators do. The latter do not refer to the books for this very reason and deliberately conceal the passages, on the basis of which they copy the text each time. We mention not only the books, however, but also the actual places and the chapters, so that one can easily find what one wants. In effect we know that those who read the whole context of the book from which we add the passage will have a much more solid trust in what we say.

Galen most definitely wants his readers to have the opportunity to check his own quotations in their copy, so that they do not suspect him of forgery and can grant him 'more solid trust (*bebaiotéra pístis*)'. Even if this is a tool designed for polemics in the argument against his adversaries, I still think that it directly reflects the contemporary reading practice of Hippocrates' texts, when a teacher selects from his own copy passages of the author he is examining, while the students also have the same text in front of them.

Extreme familiarity with Hippocrates' text is always evident and present. Galen is aware that he is producing a kind of exegesis of Hippocrates, a 'new' exegesis, never addressed before, as we have seen. At the beginning of the second book he cites a definition of exegesis as 'the unfolding of an obscure expression (ἀσαφοῦς ἑρμηνείας ἐξάπλωσις)', attributing it to 'one of the ancients' (7.825.3–826.4 K.):

ὅδε μὲν ὁ λόγος ἐξήγησίς ἐστι τῶν ὑφ' Ἱπποκράτους περὶ δυσπνοίας εἰρημένων … ἔστι μὲν οὖν ἡ ἐξήγησις ὥς πού τις τῶν παλαιῶν εἶπεν 'ἀσαφοῦς ἑρμηνείας

21 τὸ βουλόμενον] C : τὸν βουλόμενον B : τὰ βουλόμενα R. Kühn.

> ἐξάπλωσις'· ἡμεῖς δ' οὐ τοῦτο μόνον ἐοίκαμεν δράσειν, ἀλλ' ὅτι καὶ ἀληθῶς ἔχει πάντα τὰ περὶ δυσπνοίας ὑπ' αὐτοῦ γεγραμμένα μαρτυρήσειν, οὐ μὴν ἀποδείξειν οὐδὲν αὐτῶν ἐν τῷδε τῷ γράμματι, ἀλλ' εἰς τὸ προηγούμενον τούτου βιβλίον ἀναπέμψειν, ἐν ᾧ χωρὶς ἀποδείξεως οὐδὲν εἴρηται.
>
> This book is an explanation of what Hippocrates said about the difficulty of breathing … Explaining is, as an ancient author said, the 'unfolding of an obscure text'. We will probably not only do this, but also testify that everything written by him on difficult breathing (*dýspnoia*) is true. We shall not, however, demonstrate this in the present book, but rather refer back to the previous book, in which nothing was said without demonstration.

Such a definition, based on the metaphor of 'unfolding', provides a good illustration of how Galen rewrites and adjusts Hippocrates to his opinion and to that of his contemporaries by adapting and integrating Hippocrates' language and doctrines. This constitutes the type of exegesis commonly applied in the literary and philosophical tradition, both in continuous commentaries and in treatises.[22]

But in the case of *Difficulties in Breathing* other factors combine to orient Galen's composition. First of all there is the desire to pay homage to the ancient medical tradition. A very revealing passage follows the definition of exegesis (7.826.7–14 K.):

> ἐπεὶ δ' ἐκεῖνος (ὁ πρῶτος λόγος) ἐτελειώθη μετὰ τῶν προσηκόντων συλλογισμῶν, ἐν τῷδε τῷ γράμματι τὸν εὑρετήν τε καὶ οἷον πατέρα τῶν δογμάτων τιμήσομεν, αὕτη καὶ δικαία τέ ἐστιν ἅμα καὶ πρέπουσα τοῖς ὁτιοῦν ἀγαθὸν ἐξευροῦσι τιμή, μήτε κατακεκρύφθαι τὰ εὑρήματα αὐτῶν μήτ' ἀγνοεῖσθαι τοῖς ἀνθρώποις, ἀλλ' αὐτά τε φαίνεσθαι τήν θ' εὑροῦσαν αὐτὰ μέθοδον γίγνωσκεσθαι. Οὕτως γὰρ αὐτοῖς καὶ τὸ θαυμάζεσθαι κατὰ τὴν ἀξίαν ὑπάρξει.
>
> Since this [first book] was completed with adequate arguments, we shall honour the inventor and the father, as it were, of these doctrines in the present book. This is a well deserved and appropriate honour for those who have discovered good things. Their discoveries should neither be concealed nor disregarded by men, but rather they should be clearly vis-

22 See Manetti (2015), 1188–1190.

> ible and the method by which they were found should be known. In this manner, they will also be appropriately admired.

Galen reflects a cultural background that is very similar to the observations put forward by Vitruvius in the preface to the seventh book of his work *On Architecture* (pr. 1 and 3 tr. Morgan 1914, 3–4):

> 1: Maiores cum sapienter tum etiam utiliter instituerunt per commentariorum relationes cogitata tradere posteris, ut ea non interirent, sed singulis aetatis crescentia voluminibus edita gradatim pervenirent vetustatibus ad summam doctrinarum subtilitatem. Itaque non mediocres sed infinitae sunt his agendae gratiae quod non invidiose silentes praetermiserunt, sed omnium generum sensus conscriptionibus memoriae tradendos curaverunt.
>
> 3: Itaque quemadmodum his gratiae sunt agendae, sic contra qui eorum scripta furantes pro suis praedicant sunt vituperandi, quique non propriis cogitationibus scriptorum nituntur, sed invidis moribus aliena violantes gloriantur, non modo sunt reprehendendi, sed etiam, quia impio more vixerunt, poena condemnandi.

> 1: It was a wise and useful provision of the ancients to transmit their thoughts to posterity by recording them in treatises, so that they should not be lost, but being developed in succeeding generations through publication in books, should gradually attain in later times to the highest refinement of learning. And so the ancients deserve no ordinary, but unending thanks, because they did not pass on in envious silence, but took care that their ideas of every kind should be transmitted to the future in their writings
>
> 3: So, while they deserve our thanks, those, on the contrary, deserve our reproaches, who steal the writings of such men and publish them as their own; and those also, who depend in their writings, not on their own ideas, but who enviously do wrong to the works of others and boast of it, deserve not merely to be blamed, but to be sentenced to actual punishment for their wicked course of life

Both in Vitruvius and in Galen, the necessity of paying homage to the ancient tradition is likewise due to the presence of those who ignore it or appropriate ancient texts without saying so, or falsify the ancients' texts in many ways. So Galen's aim is essentially to defend Hippocrates against omission or misunderstanding of his doctrine. This differs little from the motive that induced Galen, shortly afterwards, to write running commentaries on Hippocrates' works.

What distinguishes the work discussed here from the running commentaries is the *explicit* systematic bias: in addressing the subject 'difficulty of breathing' Galen has inserted it into a diaeretic systematic framework, which he is inclined to present as already Hippocratic. This becomes clear when in the third book he compares the two parallel passages of *Epidemics* 2.3.7 and *Epidemics* 6.2.3 (texts as cited by Galen):

> *Epidemics* 2.3.7 (5.108.17 L.; 7.891.13–15 K.):
> πνεῦμα σμικρὸν πυκνόν· μέγα ἀραιόν· σμικρὸν ἀραιόν· ἔξω μέγα, εἴσω σμικρόν· τὸ μὲν ἐκτεῖνον, τὸ δὲ κατεπεῖγον· διπλῆ εἴσω ἐπανάκλησις, οἷον ἐπεισπνέουσιν· θερμὸν ψυχρόν.
>
> Breathing: frequent, small, large, infrequent. Large exhalation, small inhalation; one stretched out, the other hurried. Double inspiration like people breathing in successively; hot, cold.
>
> SMITH 1994 modified
>
> *Epidemics* 6.2.3 (5.278.6 L.; 7.895.18–896.3 K.)
> πνεύματα μικρὰ πυκνά, μεγάλα ἀραιά· μικρὰ ἀραιά, μεγάλα πυκνά· ἔξω μέγα, εἴσω μικρόν· εἴσω μέγα, ἔξω μικρόν· τὸ μὲν ἐκτεῖνον, τὸ δὲ κατεπεῖγον· διπλῆ εἴσω ἐπανάκλησις, οἷον ἐπεισπνέουσιν· θερμὸν ψυχρόν.
>
> Breathing: shallow and rapid; deep and intermittent; shallow and intermittent; rapid and deep. Out large, in small; in large, out small. One prolonged, another hurried. Double inspiration like people breathing in successively; hot, cold.
>
> SMITH 1994

The more complete version of *Epidemics* 6 is the right one, according to Galen, and it is evident to all the interpreters that Hippocrates used the logical method of *dihaíresis* (7.894.18–895.3 K.):

> ὅτι μὲν γὰρ ἐκ διαιρέσεως λογικῆς εὑρίσκειν ἐπιχειρεῖ (*sc*. Ἱπποκράτης) τὰς διαφορὰς ἁπάσας τῶν δυσπνοιῶν, τοῦτο μὲν καὶ τοῖς ἐξηγησαμένοις αὐτοῦ τὰ βιβλία δοκεῖ, καὶ πάντῃ ῥᾴδιον εἶναι νομίζω συμβαλεῖν.
>
> That Hippocrates is aiming to find all the different types of difficult breathing (*dýspnoia*) on the basis of a logical division is the opinion of the commentators of his books and it is, in my view, remarkably easy to understand.

Here in *Difficulties in Breathing*, as in works like *Anatomy of Hippocrates*, *Critical Days* and so on, the intention is to find confirmation of Hippocrates' doctrine, filtered by Galen's reorganization, in all the texts attributed to Hippocrates.[23]

On the other hand, Galen has knowledge of a Hippocratic tradition that had long been structured as a corpus, that is to say, as a set of works with different degrees of authenticity. It was something very concrete and had a sort of unity. Although originally the object of a longstanding critical debate, by the time of Galen, it had attained a relative stability: there was a recognized canon and a selection of Hippocratic texts (the most genuine works: *tà gnēsiótata*) had become a key reference matter in the medical curriculum.

Galen's concept of the Hippocratic Corpus in *Difficulties in Breathing*, even if limited to its subject matter, appears to be very similar to the first part of the works actually used by Erotian (first century AD) in writing his *Glossary* of the Hippocratic words.[24] The reading order of the Hippocratic books in Erotian's glossary is *Prognostic*, *Prorrhetic* 1, *Use of Liquids*, perhaps *Regimen* (but this is doubtful), *Epidemics*, *Aphorisms*, followed by *Airs, Waters, Places* and *Regimen in Acute Diseases*, just to quote some works also present in *Difficulties in Breathing*. The core of the Hippocratic Corpus in *Difficulties in Breathing* is similarly constituted, comprising *Prognostic*, *Prorrhetic* 1, and *Epidemics*. Galen draws useful parallels to other 'genuine' works as well, such as *Aphorisms, Air Waters Places*, *Regimen in Acute Diseases*, and *Joints*.

It is remarkable that *Prorrhetic* 1 is quoted in *Difficulties in Breathing* as Hippocratic without a shadow of doubt: this was the current opinion and only later did Galen try to correct this situation, arguing against the Hippocratic authorship, when he wrote the commentary on the treatise.[25] In any case Galen's personal position concerning the authenticity of individual works did not influence his treatment in any way: although convinced that *Epidemics* 4 was definitely spurious, against the current opinion which attributed it to Hippocrates' son Thessalus, Galen nevertheless quotes and comments on some passages of *Epidemics* 4 in detail in the third book.[26]

---

23 On *Anatomy of Hippocrates*, see Garofalo (1994), 1797.

24 Roselli (2000), 182.

25 Roselli (2015). Galen seems to consider *Prorrhetic* 1 genuine also because he says at the end of the work (7.959.16 K.) 'We have analysed, however, almost all the genuine works in this book (καίτοι σχεδὸν ἡμεῖς πάντα διήλθομεν ἐν τῷδε τῷ λόγῳ τὰ γνήσια).' In any case, he only quotes two passages from the *Prorrhetic*: 1.16 at 7.791.12 K., and 1.44 twice, at 7.800.15–16 and 7.863.8–10 K.; it therefore played only a marginal role.

26 7.949.5–13, 951.13–955.11 K.

At the ends of the second and third books, Galen hints at the possibility of continuing his analysis of difficult breathing and commenting on the works attributed to Euriphon, Thessalus and Polybus. They probably constituted the second category of 'Hippocratic' texts, which Galen examined after 'the most genuinely Hippocratic texts', to use Rebecca Fleming's definition.[27] These were written by close associates, certainly Thessalus and Polybus; it is quite likely that Euryphon is present here also because the biographic tradition had connected him to Hippocrates.[28]

The specific topic of the treatise, namely difficult breathing, means that the *Epidemics* occupy a privileged place in it, as they contain many relevant case histories. Already at the beginning of the second book (chapter 3), does Galen establish a connection between *Prognostic* and the patients of *Epidemics* 1. He quotes and explains the case of Philiscus, the first patient, of Silenus and of the wife of Dromeades;[29] in all these cases, Hippocrates mentioned the symptom of 'deep and intermittent breathing (*pneûma méga araión*)'. Galen quotes *Prognostic* 5: 'deep and intermittent breathing indicates delirium (μέγα δὲ ἀναπνεόμενον καὶ διὰ πολλοῦ χρόνου παραφροσύνην σημαίνει, cf. 2.122.12–13 L.)'; he thus confirms that this kind of breathing is a sign for delirium.[30] Galen notices the difference in language that is connected with the general tone of the *Prognostic*—Hippocrates explains things in general terms (καθ' ὅλου) here—, whilst he deals with specifics (κατὰ μέρος) in the *Epidemics*, cf. 7.840.5–12 K.

Galen's arguments often target individuals. First, some sophists say that they have never seen a patient with 'deep and intermittent breathing (*pneûma méga araión*)', to which Galen objects that they are not real physicians, because they only 'sit around inside (ἔνδον καθέζονται)' rather than go out and treat patients. Such breathing, Galen points out, reveals delirium as also confirmed by *Prognostic*; moreover, Hippocrates never mentions deep and intermittent breathing without referring to delirium.

From chapter 4 onwards, Galen directs his arguments against those who deny the relationship between deep and intermittent breathing and delirium. First, they claim that Hippocrates is inconsistent just because he diagnoses delirium in some patient who do not suffer from deep and intermittent breath-

27 Flemming (2008), 341–342.

28 Soranus, *Life of Hippocrates* 5 (Ilberg 1927, p. 176, lines 6–7). As far as we know, only *Regimen* was attributed possibly to Euryphon together with Phaon, Philistion or Ariston; see Galen, *Commentary on Hippocrates' 'Regimen in Acute Diseases'* 1.17 (ed. Helmreich 1914, p. 135, line 3).

29 2.682.5–684.9; 684.11–688.8; 708.7–710.11 L.

30 7.831.6–12 K.

ing. Then they object that some patients affected by delirium do not breath in this way. Galen refutes these objections first with a general methodological argument: deep and intermittent breathing is only 'particular (ἴδιον)', but not 'inseparable (ἀχώριστον)' from delirium. In other words, the link between such breathing and the delirium is not reciprocal. Galen then repeats that Hippocrates only claimed that such breathing is an instrument for recognising delirium, as Galen himself as a respectful interpreter of the Hippocratic text had stated (834.6–11 K.):

> ὁ μὲν γὰρ τὸ μέγα καὶ ἀραιὸν πνεῦμα παραφροσύνης εἶναί φησι γνώρισμα, τά τε πρὸς ἡμῶν λεγόμενα ταὐτὸ τοῦτ' ἐπαγγέλλεται, μηδὲν παραχαραττόντων ἡμῶν μηδὲ μεταποιούντων ὧν ἐκεῖνος ἔγραψεν, ἀλλὰ τὰς ἐξηγήσεις καὶ τὰς ἀποδείξεις μόνας προστιθέντων.
>
> He says that deep and infrequent breathing is a sign of delirium. Our arguments confirm this opinion, as we neither corrupt nor change anything he wrote, but only add explanations and demonstrations.

The good interpreter, then, does not change anything of the Hippocratic text but only adds exegesis and demonstration.

Moreover, Galen endeavours to defend Hippocrates against the accusation of inconsistency; he explains that in many cases the patient suffered two different pathological situations (*diathéseis*). Galen then begins to quote several passages from the *Epidemics*, starting with Pythion of Thasus in *Epidemics* 3 (the second Pythion, 3.112.14–116.13 L.) and continuing with the wife of Dealces (3.142.6–146.6 L.), in order to show that these patients suffered from more than a single pathological situtation (*diáthesis*), that of delirium.

Galen alternates verbatim quotations with paraphrase and exegesis of individual sentences, occasionally explaining the meaning of an individual word or expression. Throughout this section he freely selects the passages, commenting only on the parts that are relevant for his argument. This enables him to return later to the same passages, thereby extending his commentary to include what he had omitted. An interesting case in point is that of the expression 'as though recollecting (ὥσπερ ἀνακαλουμένῳ)' that occurs in the case of Philiscus: Galen merely quotes it at 7.827.12 K., but then explains it at 7.844.16 K., commenting on the wife of Dealces. Another example is the expression 'with long intervals (διὰ χρόνου)' attested in the same case history (the wife of Dealces). Galen says (7.844.16–17 K.): 'It would also be right to explain what the expression "*dià chrónou*" means (τί ποτ' οὖν ἐστι τὸ "διὰ χρόνου" καὶ δὴ τοῦτ' ἐξηγήσασθαι δίκαιον)' and engages in a comparative analysis of the expressions διὰ χρόνου and διὰ τέλεος ('throughout'), the latter present here (3.142.8; 2.146.5 L.) and also in the case history of Philiscus (2.684.9 L.). He invokes the Hippocratic usage, with numerous quotations, to conclude that the two expressions do not have the same meaning (ch. 6; 7.844.16-848-13 K.).

Galen has moved progressively from the theorical discussion about Hippocrates' doctrine towards the analysis of the diction of the Hippocratic text and now (ch. 7) to address the complete analysis of the histories in *Epidemics* 1 and 3, he feels obliged to state a general premise on the subject of Hippocrates' writing intention. It is the famous parallel between Hippocrates' and Thucydides' manner of describing phenomena, drawing on a lost work by Galen, *The Plague of Thucydides*.[31]

> δοκοῦσι γὰρ οἱ παλαιοὶ πάντα τὰ τοῖς νοσοῦσι συμβαίνοντα γράφειν αὐτὸν ὥσπερ καὶ τὸν Θουκυδίδην. ἔχει δ' οὐχ οὕτως, ἀλλ' αὐτὸ δὴ τοῦτο τὸ ἐναντιώτατον ὑπάρχει τοῖς Ἱπποκράτους γράμμασι πρὸς τὰ τοῦ Θουκυδίδου. ὁ μὲν γὰρ πάντα γράφει τὰ καὶ τοῖς ἰδιώταις γνώριμα, μηδὲν ὅλως αὐτῶν παραλιπών, ὁ Θουκιδίδης, ὁ δ' Ἱπποκράτης ὀλίγα μὲν τούτων ὅσα πρὸς τὴν ὅλην διάθεσιν, καθ' ἣν ἐκινδύνευσεν ὁ κάμνων διαφέρει, πάμπολλα δ' ἄλλα τοῖς ἰδιώταις παρεωραμένα, τεχνικὴν δὲ πάνυ καὶ ἀκριβῆ τὴν διάγνωσιν παρεχόμενα καὶ δυνάμενα πολλάκις καὶ αὐτοὺς τοὺς ἀρίστους ἰατροὺς λαθεῖν.
>
> The ancients thought that he [sc. Hippocrates] wrote down everything that happened to the patients in the same way as Thucydides. But this is not the case; rather Hippocrates' writings are diametrically opposed to those of Thucydides. The latter, that is, Thucydides, noted all the things that are known to laypeople and did not omit anything. Hippocrates, however, only noted a few of these, namely those relevant to general condition in which the patient happened to be, but also very many things that are overlooked by laypeople, but provide [indications] for a professional and exact diagnosis; these things can sometimes even escape the notice of the very best physicians.

As a practitioner of the art of medicine, Hippocrates did not describe all the symptoms in the individual patients: rather, he focused on what was not obvious, was rare, and had a technical meaning and was often unknown even to the most advanced physician. This premise would permit Galen to focus his commentary on what Hippocrates omitted, but Galen needed to make an explicit

31 The quotation is at 7.850.11–851.3 K.; see also Biagini (2007) on this work.

mention of another premise, namely the current opinion of his time concerning the authenticity of the *Epidemics* (chapter 8; 7.854.8–855.14 K.).

The statement serves to justify the sequence of Galen's discourse, which starts with the genuine *Epidemics* 1 and 3, and continues with those attributed to Thessalus (books 2, 4, 6) and, finally, with the later *Epidemics* 5 and 7, and the other Hippocratic works. In chapters 8–9, Galen sets out his manner of justifying what Hippocrates has omitted, using the cases of Anaxion of Abdera (3.124.2–4 L.) in *Epidemics* 3, and then the boy of Meliboea and the already mentioned wife of Dealces and Pythion.

He comments on these selected passages using the same tools as the running commentaries: he poses a problem (*zḗtēma*) and solves it; he paraphrases the text so as to rewrite it in more Galenic language; he identifies particular syntactic constructions (for instance a construction *apò koinoû*) or semantic features and so on. His duty as an interpreter, he says, is to add what is lacking in the text through his commentary. But he provides very precise references to the Hippocratic text on which he is commenting, as noted earlier.

From chapter 10 to 13, Galen reads through and explains the case histories of *Epidemics* 1 and 3, following strictly the order of the text; in his comments he always justifies that Hippocrates omitted to note certain types of difficult breathing. He even suggests that in the strange case of Crito in *Epidemics* 1 (2.704.7 L.), who died unexpectedly the second day, perhaps Hippocrates did not observe the difficulty in breathing, because physicians usually do not come close to mad people (7.877.13–15 K.).

When comparing these ad-hoc comments with the later lemmatic commentaries on *Epidemics* 1 and 3, one discerns some differences, although Galen adhered to the same exegetic method. For *Epidemics* 1, the running commentary often refers to *Difficulties in Breathing* and sometimes summaries its content. Galen quotes and comments on more text in *Difficulties in Breathing* than in the commentary, which has very short lemmas. For *Epidemics* 3, Galen pursues different aims in his running commentary from those in *Difficulties in Breathing*, because he inveighs against the bad commentators (Sabinus in particular) there.[32]

In the third book, Galen analyses difficult breathing as described in the other books of *Epidemics* and other genuine works by Hippocrates. As we have seen already, he compares the two parallel passages of *Epidemics* 2.3.7 and 6.2.3.

32 On Galen's approach to the *Epidemics* in the commentaries on *Epidemics* 1 and 2, see van der Eijk (2012). The situation seems different from that of the surgical texts, treated in *Therapeutic Method* and in the commentaries, insofar as Witt's (2012) reconstruction is plausible. See also Jouanna in this volume.

He finds the model description of *dýspnoia* in *Epidemics* 6, which fits very well in his systematic bias. But he cannot consider that the shorter version of *Epidemics* 2 results from an omission by Hippocrates himself; it would be an unacceptable logical inconsistency. Rather, Galen thinks that it was probably the fault of the first copyists who made a mistake. Galen believes that one should explain omissions in a Hippocratic text in terms of textual transmission by using the tools of philology. In the case of *Epidemics* 2, the ancient mistake was perpetuated up to his own time for two reasons: partly because of a general indifference to ancient texts, but also because it was the practice among ancient editors not to modify a text that was attested in the same version in all the ancient manuscripts. Instead, they usually considered it sufficient to put a sign to show that something was missing at that point. Galen was probably alluding here to the Alexandrian editorial practice of using diacritical signs with different meanings when editing the text (7.819.16–832.16 K.).

Galen was in general conservative and, even although he considered *Epidemics* 2 to have been corrupted by bad omissions, he did not feel that it was correct to add missing elements to the text of *Epidemics* 2. He was aware that some copies did contain the addition of some of the omitted words, but he respected the ancient tradition when it was fundamentally univocal on some point, as the following passage illustrates (7.896.14–17 K.):

> πολλαχόθι μὲν οὖν εὑρίσκειν ἔστι καὶ προσγεγραμμένον τοῦτο τὸ λεῖπον ἀλλ' ἐν τοῖς πλείστοις καὶ ἀξιοπιστοτάτοις τῶν ἀντιγράφων παραλέλειπται, καὶ οὐδὲν τοῦτό γε πρὸς τὸ παρὸν διαφέρει.
>
> In many copies you may find that something which was missing has actually been added, but in the most trustworthy exemplars it is omitted, and certainly for the present context this makes no difference at all.

However, Galen did allow minor corrections of the text which change only a few letters, but essentially he felt that the process of correcting the text is only the final step of an intelligent interpretation which, following the Alexandrian tradition, has no need to alter the copy of the author on which he comments. This was Galen's firm belief and it explains why he would later express such admiration for the famous correction of Heraclides of Tarentum, who corrected 'ΟΥΡΑΙ (tails)' into 'ΘΥΡΑΙ (doors)'.[33]

33 *Epidemics* 2.2.20; Vagelpohl (2016), p. 343, lines 6–10.

Galen then returns to *Prognostic* 5, which he had used at the beginning to confirm Hippocrates' statements in the stories of *Epidemics* 1 and 3. But, as he has just established that the passage of *Epidemics* 6 is the complete logical description of *dýspnoia*, he feels obliged to explain why the general treatment in *Prognostic* 5 is not as complete as *Epidemics* 6. He devotes considerable effort to this (chapters 4–9) and, to solve the apparent problem, he resumes the argument of Hippocrates' habit, already addressed in the second book, namely Hippocrates' writing intention or *prohaíresis*. He talks again about Hippocrates' tendency to be brief while saying great things, expressing differently the same ideas that he had already mentioned when he compared Hippocrates to Thucydides, namely that Hippocrates omits the obvious and chooses to mention what is rare and relevant for the medical art.

Even though Galen often repeats the same motives, I do not agree completely with Smith's opinion (1979: 121) that 'Galen's argument is impromptu and poorly structured: he is clearly working out its shape as he goes along'. In a work written for oneself, the argument is by nature weakly structured in some points, but the general plan of *Difficulties in Breathing* is very clear. Galen aims to reconstruct Hippocrates' system of the difficulties in breathing by quoting many different passages not only from *Epidemics*, but also from *Prognostic*, *Regimen in Acute Diseases* and *Joints*. This is Galen's declared goal from the start. But in doing so he also reconstructs Hippocrates' authorial identity on the basis of the works which were then considered the 'most genuine works by Hippocrates' or members of his circle. Actually Galen provides Hippocrates with a clear plan in composing a 'corpus' of works with an internal logical sequence, as is clear from the passages at 7.924.5–17, 927.1–4, and 938.14–17 K.:

> καὶ δὴ ὥσπερ ἐξεπίτηδες διατέμνων αὐτὰ τὸ μὲν ἕτερον ἐν Προγνωστικῷ γράφει ταῖς ὀλεθρίαις συνάγχαις προσεῖναι λέγων, τὸ δὲ δεύτερον ἐν τῷ Περὶ ἄρθρων, ἐν μὲν τῷ Προγνωστικῷ τὴν ὀρθόπνοιαν, ἐν δὲ τῷ Περὶ ἄρθρων τὸ κερχνῶδες· ἄμφω δὲ ἐν τῷ Περὶ διαίτης ὀξέων ἐς ταὐτὸν ἤγαγεν, οὕτως γράψας ὁ Ἱπποκράτης 'οἱ δ' ὑπὸ τῆς ὀρθοπνοίας καὶ τοῦ ῥέγχους ἀποπνιγέντες'. ὃ γὰρ ἐν τῷ Περὶ ἄρθρων κέρχνον, τοῦτ' ἐνταῦθα ῥέγχος ὠνόμασε. χρῆται δὲ καὶ ἀλλαχόθι τῶν συγγραμμάτων ἀμφοτέροις τοῖς ὀνόμασιν, ὡς ταὐτὸν δυναμένοις δηλοῦν. ἐπειδὴ οὖν οὕτως ἐπιμελῶς αὐτὸς ἐν τῷ Περὶ διαίτης περὶ πάσης γενέσεως πυκνοῦ πνεύματος διεξῆλθε, θαυμαστὸν οὐδὲν εἰ μόνον τὸ κεφάλαιον αὐτὸ τοῦ παντὸς λόγου γέγραφεν ἐν τῷ Προγνωστικῷ.
>
> He certainly divided them (the types of *dýspnoia*) deliberately: he describes the first [type] in the *Prognostic* and says that it is connected to fatal angina, and the second in *Joints*; in the *Prognostic* 'upright breathing

> (*orthóphoia*)' [when one can only breath whilst standing up], and in *Joints* 'hoarse breathing (*kerchnôdes*)'. Hippocrates unifies the two in *Regimen in Acute Diseases* by using the expression 'those who suffocate owing to "upright breathing (*orthópnoia*)" and "cavernous breathing (*rénchos*)"'. He used the term 'hoarseness (*kérchnos*)' in *Joints*, which is the same as the term 'cavernous breathing (*rénchos*)' used here. Elsewhere in his writings he employs both terms as well, because they can mean the same thing. Since he examined in such a meticulous manner the whole genesis of frequent breathing, it is hardly surprising that he only summarises the whole account in the *Prognostic*.

> καὶ ὅτι τελέως αὐτὴν [*sc.* τὴν τοῦ πυκνοῦ πνεύματος εἰς τὰς ἐν αὐτῷ διαφορὰς τομὴν] ἔφθασεν ἐν τούτῳ τῷ βιβλίῳ (*sc.* τῷ Περὶ διαίτης ὀξέων) γεγραφέναι, διὰ τοῦτο ἐν τῷ Προγνωστικῷ ταχέως περιέδραμε, ὡς πρὸς εἰδότας ἤδη τὸ σύμπαν οἷον ἐπιτομήν τινα τοῦ λόγου ποιησάμενος.

> Since he had previously given a full written account of [how to divide thick breath into its various different types] in this book (that is, *Regimen in Acute Diseases*), he offered only a very brief overview in the *Prognostic*; for he addressed himself to those already knowing everything, thus writing something like a short summary.

> ἐν μὲν τοῖς τῶν Ἐπιδημιῶν τὴν εἰς ἁπάσας τὰς κατὰ μέρος δυσπνοίας διαίρεσιν τιθέμενος, ἐν δὲ τῷ Προγνωστικῷ καὶ τοῖς Ἀφορισμοῖς τὸ πρὸς τὴν χρείαν ἐπεῖγον.

> … setting out in the *Epidemics* the entire division of the particular types of difficult breathing, but in the *Prognostic* and the *Aphorisms* that which is more oriented towards the useful.

The systematic bias plays a preeminent role in *Difficulties in Breathing* up to the end[34] but it is accompanied by such a lively sense of Hippocrates' diction—and more generally of the 'literary' aspects of Hippocrates as an author—that it marks the beginning of Galen's exegetical work on Hippocrates which will redefine and correct the status of many works in the Hippocratic Corpus.

---

34 In chapters 11–13, after solving the interpretation of *Prognostic* 5, Galen adds a lexical appendix to the subject of difficult breathing, dwelling on the use of *pneûma* and related adjectives *pneumatías*, *pneumatṓdēs*, used very frequently in *Epidemics*, with the meaning of 'difficult breathing' and 'having difficulties of breathing'.

The form of *Difficulties in Breathing* is generally classified as a 'systematic treatise' on a certain subject (*sýngramma*) and not a commentary (*hypómnēma*), but the exegetical methods and the cultural premises shared by Galen are very close to those of his later commentaries. I would adopt the definition now suggested by Elizabeth Craik in her paper in this volume and claim that *Difficulties in Breathing* can be defined as a 'quasi-commentary'.

CHAPTER 10

Types of Cranial Injuries in the Hippocratic *Wounds in the Head* in Light of the Ancient Commentary Tradition

Mathias Witt

The present paper focusses on fairly specific problems of text and content in an outline of skull injuries from the Hippocratic treatise *Wounds in the Head*, the oldest classification of skull injuries known in medical history. As will be shown, some of the textual problems of this description can be understood better by examining the ancient commentary tradition on the passages in question, even though only a few bits and pieces of this tradition have come down to us. Before discussing the Hippocratic types of skull injuries and the way Galen and others interpreted them, a succinct overview needs to be given on what treatises of Galen's include surgical commentary. As I observed elsewhere,[1] Galen is providing commentary on the Hippocratic surgical writings in books 3–6 of his main therapeutic work, the *Method of Healing*.

Along with giving a more or less systematic overview on how to treat lesions of different tissue types, books 3–6 of the *Method of Healing* were meant to be a 'synthetic' basic commentary on Hippocratic surgical works: books 3 and 4 provide a commentary for the Hippocratic *Ulcers* and book 6 (second part) gives a commentary on the Hippocratic *Fractures* and *Wounds in the Head*. Books 5 and 6 (first part) are likely to have been intended (at least partly) as commentary or supplements to the lost Hippocratic treatise *Deadly Wounds*.[2] Immediately after completing the first half of the *Method of Healing* (books 1–6) in around 175 A.D., Galen started to write a series of lemmatic commentaries on Hippocratic writings, the first of which were his four commentaries on Hippocrates' *Fractures*, *Joints*, *Ulcers* and *Wounds in the Head*.

Galen's plan to write lemmatic commentaries on Hippocratric treatises is already announced in the first section of the *Method of Healing*.[3] According to

1 Witt (2012).
2 See Witt (2012), 88–103.
3 See Witt (2012), 106–107.

© MATHIAS WITT, 2021 | DOI:10.1163/9789004470200_012

him, the 'synthetic' commentary given in this work was intended for beginners, to teach the principles of therapy, whereas the lemmatic commentaries were aimed at providing in-depth-commentary for advanced learners when reading the Hippocratic surgical treatises.

With respect to tissue lesions, the Byzantine compilers clearly preferred the *Method of Healing* to Galen's lemmatic surgical commentaries. This is most probably due to the fact that, in the respective sections of the *Method of Healing*, the instruction is given more systematically and succintly; this is a a preferable format for making excerpts. Only for more specific information (e.g., special types of injury, like the type of lesions of the head) the compilers had to excerpt Galen's lemmatic commentaries. This predominance of the *Method of Healing* may also be a reason why eventually Galen's commentaries on the Hippocratic *Ulcers* and *Wounds in the Head* got lost.

Some fragments of them are however preserved in Oribasius' *Medical Collections*: six fragments from the commentary on *Ulcers* and fifteen fragments from the commentary on *Wounds in the Head*.[4] The most important passage of the latter commentary focusses on the Hippocratic classification of head wounds. This fragment of Galen's commentary will be analysed in the present paper, since it contibutes to understanding and interpreting the respective Hippocratic paragraphs which seem to have been problematic to a certain extent already for ancient readers. Except for this fragment of Galen, no other ancient lemmatic commentary on this passage is preserved. Passages in Heliodorus (in Oribasius), Soranus and Paul of Aegina, however, seem to reflect hellenistic Hippocratic exegesis as well, and thus equally provide a kind of "synthetic" commentary on this passage from *Wounds in the Head*.

1 Hippocratic Types of Cranial Injuries

As the context clearly indicates, the cranial injuries described in the Hippocratic *Wounds in the Head* are injuries sustained in war and combat, caused by arrowheads and by various kinds of blunt or sharp missiles. To this date, little scholarship has been devoted to Hippocratic types on skull injuries.[5] The

4 For a collection of fragments see Witt (2014).
5 For a comparison of some of these types with corresponding ancient Egyptian lore see Keyser (2013), 44–46.

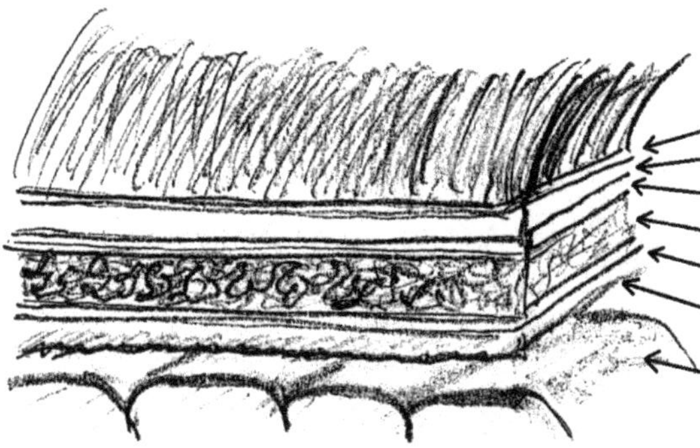

FIGURE 10.1 Anatomy of the Skullbone

fairly broad description and classifiction of the types of injury extends over six chapters (3–8), which is almost a third of the treatise. A proper understanding of these types is thus essential for understanding the treatise as a whole. Along with a description of them, a numbering is included which is clearly not an interpolation of late antique or medieval times. It was known to Galen (see below), but is certainly of a much older date, probably going back to the author of the Hippocratic treatise. In its transmitted form, the numbering is, however, problematic due to some confusion at its end. Furthermore, one of the types of injury (φλάσις) is problematic from a medical point of view and the others (especially the ἕδρα) are not easy to understand, either. Already in ancient times the readers of this text seem to have been faced with these problems as will be illustrated in the following argument, by an examination of the reception of the problematic passages of the treatise in the works of Galen, Heliodorus, Soranus and Paul of Aegina. This reception has not previously been fully taken into account by editiors of this text or by historians of medicine. In order to understand the classification properly, a somewhat lengthy discussion of the text, along with illustrations of the modes of injury, is unavoidable.

In the Hippocratic text, the main forms of cranial injury are addressed in chapter 3. The clasification proper, however, starts only from chapter 4 onwards. The author states that there are types (τρόποι) and subtypes (ἰδέαι) of injuries. The given numbering clearly applies only to the τρόποι (cf. the wording: εἷς οὗτος τρόπος, etc.). These forms of injury are the following, in the order in which they are presented:

(1) ῥωγμή (chapter 4). This is a simple fracture of the skull. It is noteworthy that the Hippocratic author does not use the common word for bone fracture here, κάτηγμα, as one might expect. This shift of terminology is due to the fact that κάτηγμα is used in a much broader sense in this treatise, in the sense of

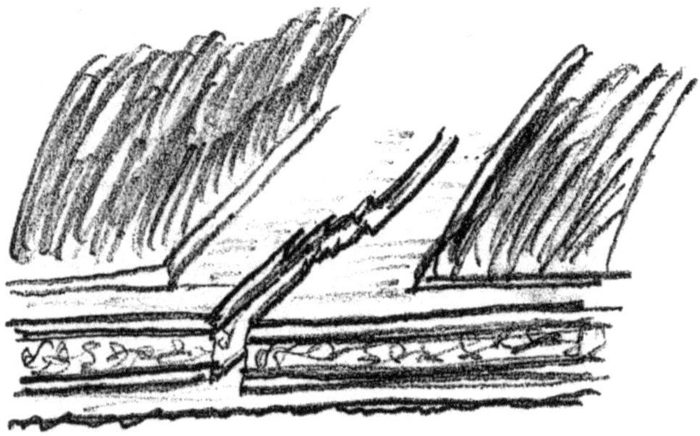

FIGURE 10.2A Linear Fracture: Pure ῥωγμή
Note: In this caption and the following ones, the skin and hair covering the bone lesion is removed, so that the latter one can be fully shown.

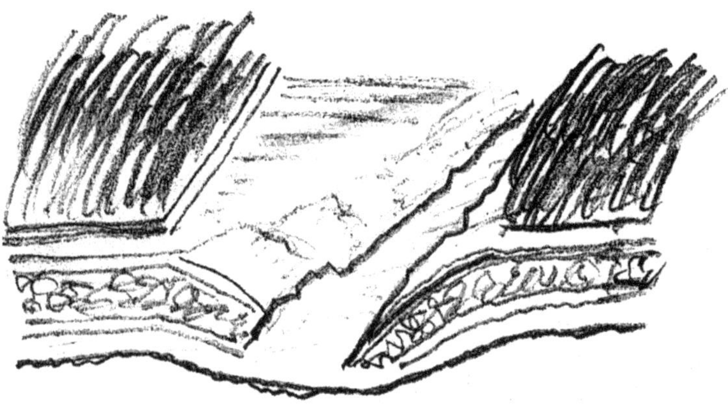

FIGURE 10.2B Linear Fracture with Depressed Margins: ῥωγμή + φλάσις

'injury', so that a fracture proper needed to be referred to with another word.[6] That a ῥωγμή designates any linear complete dissolution of continuity of the skullbone, regardless what the shape or geometry of a ῥωγμή might be, can be concluded from the third form of injury (see below).

The author seems to suggest that a pure ῥωγμή (Fig. 10.2a) does not exist. He stresses that it is in actual fact always asociated with a φλάσις, a depression of bone on the margins of the fracture zone (Fig. 10.2b). From a modern (med-

6 Hanson (1999), 100, previously observed by Withington (1928, p. 19, n. 2) with respect to κάτηξις.

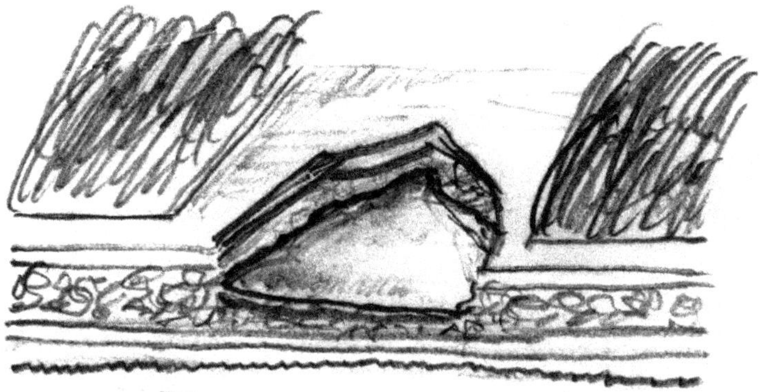

FIGURE 10.3A Depressed Fracture (Infraction of External Layer) [Theoretical Form]

ical) viewpoint this is true only for fractures that occur directly within the zone of impact, a zone, that, moreover, needs to be rather small (e.g. when caused by weapons or smaller objects). If, in contrast, the zone of impact is broad, no depression occurs, nor does it in contrecoup fractures (see below).

(2) A pure φλάσις is the second type of injury discussed (chapter 5). It is explicitly described as a depression of bone that occurs 'without fracture' (this remark is most problematic). It is said to vary in depth and either go 'through the whole bone' or just a part of it. These variations are called ἰδέαι by the author.

Concerning a pure φλάσις, several ways of explaining this type of injury may be considered. The bone of the skullcap consists of three layers (see fig. 10.1): an outer and an inner layer (table) of compact bone as well a layer of spongy bone between the two tables (the so-called 'diploe'). There are impression fractures of the outer layer into the diploe with the inner layer remaining intact (fig. 10.3a). These impression fractures can indeed vary in depth and are less dangerous since the continuity of the bone remains intact and the meninges and the brain are not exposed. It is possible that by φλάσις such a lesion was meant: this indeed constitutes a dent without a fracture proper (linear fracture), since the inner layer remains intact and only the upper two layers of bone are focally depressed. If we follow this explanation we must suppose that the Hippocratic author regarded an infraction and superficial depression of bone as something other than a fracture proper (ῥωγμή); this supposition seems rather doubtful. A second problem is that, usually, the inner layer gets crushed as well in such injuries (fig. 10.3b), since it is much more fragile than the outer layer. Only a few cases without a fracture of the inner layer are reported.[7] Such hidden infractions of the inner layer

7 Ganz (2018), 30.

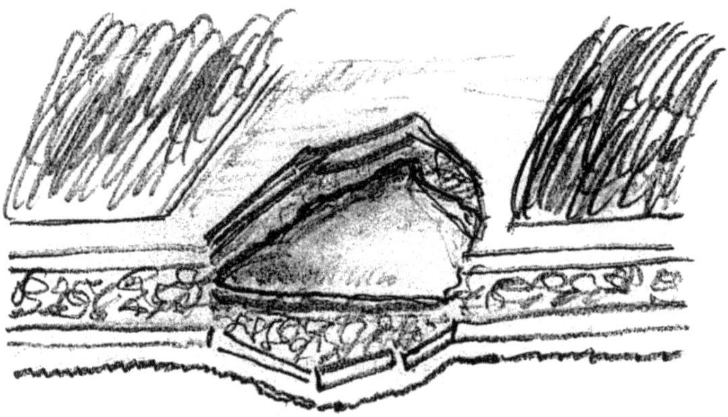

FIGURE 10.3B Depressed Fracture (Infraction of Both Internal and External Layers) [Usual Form]

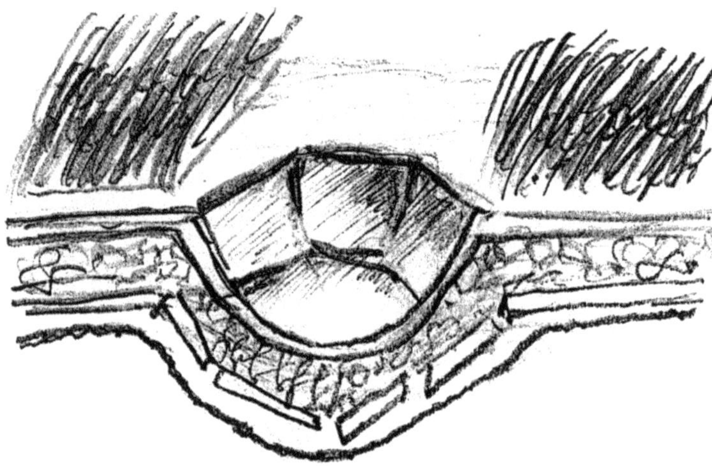

FIGURE 10.3C Depressed Fracture (All Layers)

were not known to physicians until modern radiography and high resolution CT imaging became available. This second observation should not, therefore, present an obstacle to interpreting the Hippocratic mode of injury in this way.

If we follow this interpretation, a φλάσις going 'through the whole bone' would be a depressed fracture of all layers of bone (fig. 10.3c). One can hardly speak of an injury 'without fracture' in this case, since this mode of injury entails fissures on the surface of the bone as well as in its depth. The fact that in the first mode of injury, a linear fracture with depressed margins (ῥωγμή + φλάσις), the depressed margins are necesssarily not perfectly smooth, but would also have more or less extended infractions of their surface, could be a hint

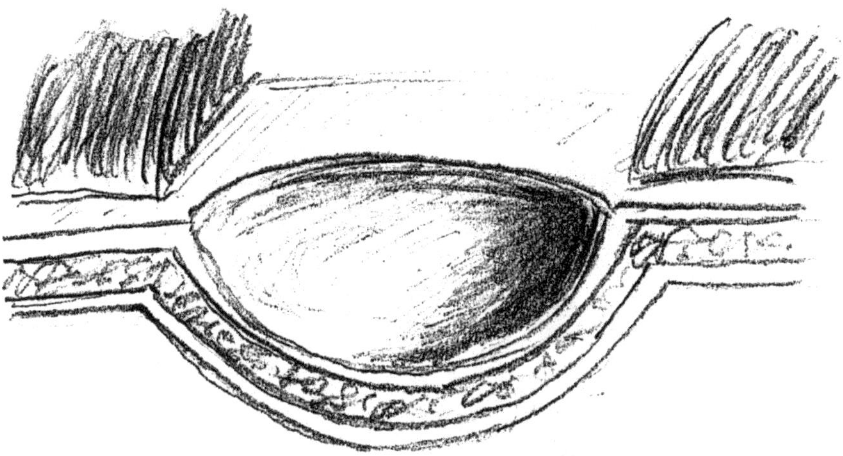

FIGURE 10.4 Ping Pong Fracture

that 'without fracture' is not to be understood in a strict sense. It could rather mean 'without full-thickness fissures of the bone'.

However, a second approach of explanation for a pure φλάσις might be considered: in children of early age, where the skullcap is not yet ossified, an injury usually leads to a dent of the skull without a fracture proper. There is no fissure whatsoever involved so that this form would perfecly fit the Hippocratic remark that it is an injury 'without fracture'. This mode of skull deformation is, in today's terminology, called 'pond fracture' or 'ping-pong fracture' (fig. 10.4). The visual analogy of a locally deformed ping-pong ball led to this name, as did the tendency of these fractures to remodel spontaneously.

It seems that antique authors understood the Hippocratic φλάσις this way. This is suggested by the fact that in later times a ping-pong fracture was indeed usually referred to, with an almost identical term, as θλάσμα (see below). At first it might seem rather odd that this form of injury had been addressed by the Hippocratic author, since he does not mention in chapter 5 that this form of injury can occur only in children. However, in chapter 18, he addresses war wounds in infants. It should be differentiated, he states, whether in infants a ῥωγμή and φλάσις, a pure φλάσις or a ἕδρα (associated with φλάσις, ῥωγμή or both) has occurred. Hence it becomes clear that by φλάσις a pond fracture could well have been meant. However, the author's remark (ch. 5) that this form of injury either extends 'through the whole bone' or only parts of it would be odd. For in any case of 'ping-pong fracture', the whole bone is deformed so that such a remark would be pointless.

As a third possibility of interpreting this type of lesion, one could assume it to be a collective diagnosis that comprises both slighter forms of depressed

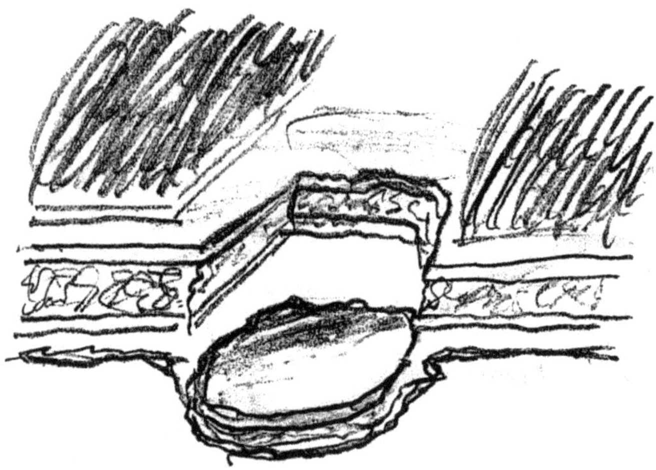

FIGURE 10.5
ἔσφλασις

fracture and a ping-pong fracture proper. Hence the ambiguity could be explained that on the one hand a 'pure' φλάσις without fracture is said to exist and, on the other hand, compound forms are described (e.g. ῥωγμή + φλάσις) in which the φλάσις is necessarily caused by an inward crushing of bone and thus entails several tiny fractures in this crushed area.

Finally, (fourth possibility) one could assume that a φλάσις has no equivalent in modern medicine, as Hanson (1999, 102) did who regarded it as a 'catch-all diagnosis for patients who did poorly in the absence of demonstrable skull damage'. Thus it would be a rough equivalent to the modern concept of brain commotion or an intracerebral bleeding. This thesis seems highly questionable. Elsewhere the Hippocratic author carefully examines the bone after the injury by using rasps and observing how it absorbes black ink, in order to trace fractures and distinguish them from physiological structures like cranial sutures. The remark that a φλάσις can either go 'through the whole bone' or only parts of it, presupposes a posttraumatic examination and would be pure fantasy in case of a φλάσις being merely a hypothetical type of injury, as postulated by Hanson.

The next, third, Hippocratic type of skull injury does not provide any problems for interpretation. An ἔσφλασις (chapter 6) is, according to the author, a depressed fracture with a fragment of bone that has been separated from the surrounding skull as a result of fractures (ῥωγμῇσιν) and displaced inwards (fig. 10.5). It is thus a compound injury consisting of a circumscribed fracture and an inward depression of the broken-off fragment.

By this remark it becomes clear that ῥωγμή refers not only to single linear fractures, but also to any geometries of fractures, round, oval and square.

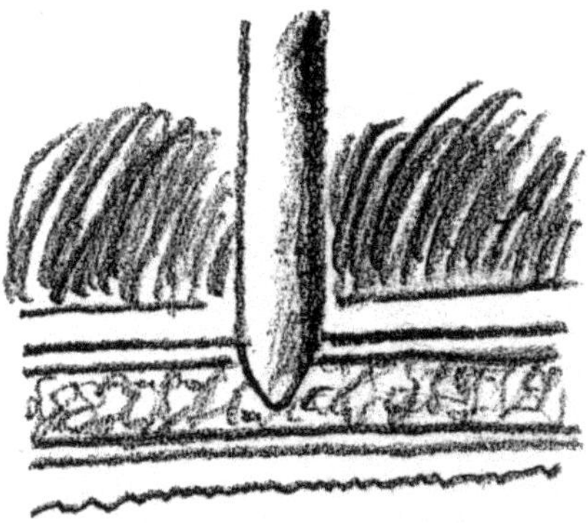

FIGURE 10.6A
Incomplete Buttonhole Fracture: Superficial ἕδρα

Again there are several ἰδέαι of this type of fracture, depending on the size of the fragment and the depth of depression. Considering the previous statement of the author, that a ῥωγμή is invariably connected with a φλάσις, one might doubt whether ῥωγμή (+ φλάσις) can be clearly differentiated from an ἔσφλασις. An ἔσφλασις, however, presupposes a broken-off fragment of bone (ἀπορρηγνύμενον). In a ῥωγμή (+ φλάσις) only the borders of the fracture zone are depressed.

In chapter 7, the next type of skull injury, (4) ἕδρα, is outlined. This chapter presents several textual difficulties. According to the definition given, a ἕδρα constitutes a (complete or incomplete) buttonhole fracture in which the weapon may or may not remain stuck within the bone.[8] A characteristic of the ἕδρα is that the surrounding bone remains in its natural position. There are both superficial and deep forms of a ἕδρα. The depth is just a parameter in the sense of an ἰδέα: In superficial forms that may range from scratches to craters (fig. 10.6a), only the superficial bone layers are perforated. In deep forms, however, (fig. 10.6b, buttonhole fracture proper) the whole bone is. In *Wounds in the Head*, chapter 9, the author states that perforation (διακοπή) and ἕδρα are the same. It is doubtful whether διακοπή is a synonym for ἕδρα in general. It certainly only refers to the deep forms in which the bone is completely perforated. Thus, this remark is to be understood in the sense that every διακοπή is a ἕδρα, but not every ἕδρα a διακοπή (superficial ones are not).

In the transmitted text, a plain ἕδρα is only defined after compound forms (ἕδρα + ῥωγμή + φλάσις [Fig. 10.6c] and ἕδρα + φλάσις [Fig. 10.6d]) have been introduced. In these compound forms, the φλάσις involved is certainly not a φλάσις in which the bone remains intact. Rather, due to the impact, inevitably

8 Withington (1928, 4) remarks that a ἕδρα results 'from a prick to a gash' and thinks that this terminological vagueness was the reason that this term was not used by later authors any more;

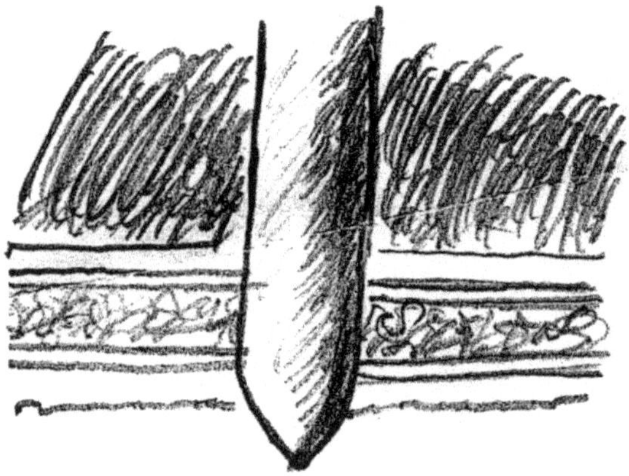

FIGURE 10.6B
Buttonhole Fracture: Complete
ἕδρα, διακοπή

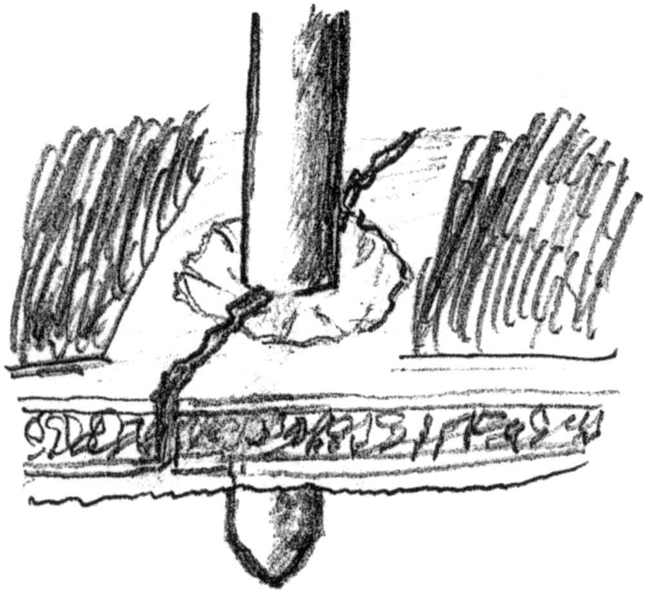

FIGURE 10.6C
ἕδρα + ῥωγμή + φλάσις

more or less superficial fissures are affiliated with it. Again the reader is faced with the paradox (as before in fractures) that this φλάσις is different from the pure φλάσις, described to be a form of injury without fracture.

The first textual problem in this paragraph concerns the sequence in which the forms of injury are introduced as well as their numbering: (a) ἕδρα + ῥωγμή

see also Hanson (1999), 100. Golder (2001, 157) erroneously interprets a ἕδρα as a compound injury of a fracture and a contusion. Ganz (2018, 30) equally erroneously interprets a ἕδρα as a focally depressed fracture.

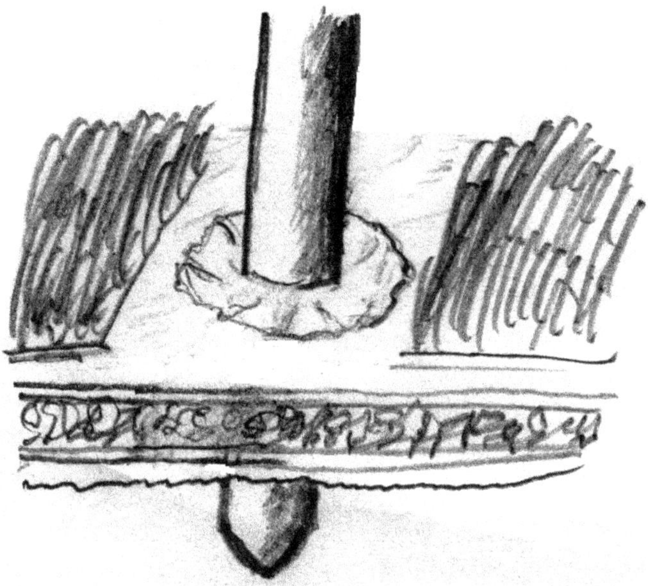

FIGURE 10.6D
ἕδρα + φλάσις

+ φλάσις ('fourth type'), (b) ἕδρα + φλάσις ('fifth type'), (c) plain ἕδρα (without number). Unlike this chapter, all the other follow the sequence: definition of a form of injury, pathogenesis, subtypes (ἰδέαι). Most editors, however, leave the seemingly confused arrangement of chapter 7 as transmitted. Only Reinhold and Kühlewein rearrange the text and place the definition of ἕδρα at its beginning. Withington (1928, p. 17, n. 2) also regards the definition of a plain ἕδρα as 'obviously out of place', but leaves the Greek text as found in the manuscripts. Even with this rearrangement, the order remains confused and somehow unpleasing, in that it starts with the plain form, follows with the most complicated and finally reaches that second to the most complicated. In this case, one furthermore had to assume that the numbering of the last two forms of injury as forth and fifth type was posterior to the postulated textual corruption so that one would have to delete these numbers as well. This would end up in a series of textual manipulations that can hardly be justified. Hanson (1999, 104) argues for the arrangement as it is transmitted in the manuscripts: it would then be an anticlimax from the most complicated to the simple form (a view previously advocated by Rutgers [1849, 54] and Ermerins [1859–1864, vol. 1, p. 376]). Of course, if we assume this, we lack an explanation why the author deviates from the structure of all other chapters, starting with a definition of the respective type of injury. Considering chapter 3 which immediately refers to a ἕδρα and its complication by a ῥωγμή and φλάσις, we might assume that the term ἕδρα was so well known that it was not really in need of an explanation. If the author starts with a simple ἕδρα in chapter 3 and ends with a simple ἕδρα in chapter seven, this could be a deliberate rhetorical device, a ring-composition to mark the beginning and the end of the section in which the forms of injury are defined. If there was no need of defining a ἕδρα, one could even asume that the definition of the simple ἕδρα was an interpolated gloss. This could explain why a number is lacking. However, with this hypothesis, chapter 7 would be incomplete and only addressing compound injuries with the ἕδρα, whereas it was explicitly stated in chapter 3 that a plain ἕδρα without ῥωγμή or φλάσις does exist.

The second major textual problem concerns the numbering of the 'subtypes' of the ἕδρα. That both compound forms (type four and five just mentioned) were indeed regarded as forms in their own right, not only as a subspecies of the ἕδρα, is clearly confirmed by the following sentence of chapter 7 (3.208.4–7 L.):

> Ἐν δὲ τῷ τρόπῳ ἑκάστῳ πλέονες ἰδέαι γίγνονται· καὶ περὶ μὲν φλάσιός τε καὶ ῥωγμῆς, ἢν ἄμφω ταῦτα προσγένηται τῇ ἕδρῃ, καὶ ἢν φλάσις μούνη γένηται, ἤδη πέφρασται, ὅτι πολλαὶ ἰδέαι γίνονται καὶ τῆς φλάσιος καὶ τῆς ῥωγμῆς.
>
> In every single type [τρόπος] several forms occur, both concerning the φλάσις and the ῥωγμή, if both of them accompany the ἕδρα, and if only a φλάσις accompanies it, it has already been stated that many forms of both the φλάσις and the ῥωγμή occur.

'In every single type' clearly points back to the fourth and fifth types described, not to the first and second, the pure ῥωγμή and φλάσις. This remark seems to have been overlooked by those who question the numbering of the ἕδρα 'subtypes' (Littré, Withington, Hanson); it clearly underlines that the compound forms are types (τρόποι) in their own right, as was already correctly remarked by Rutgers (1849, 54) and Ermerins (1859–1864, vol. 1, p. 376).

The last form of cranial injury (5) is presented in chapter 8. According to the description, this is a fracture that comes about at another place of the skull than the one where the primary impact occurred (fig. 10.7). This injury is not provided with a name of its own. In today's medical terminology it is called contrecoup fracture.[9] Strangely, it is called the 'seventh' type in the manuscript tradition with type 6 missing in the transmitted text. One could ask whether

9 For a succinct overview on the ancient history of the contrecoup fracture, see Witt (2015) and (2014), p. 67, n. 47.

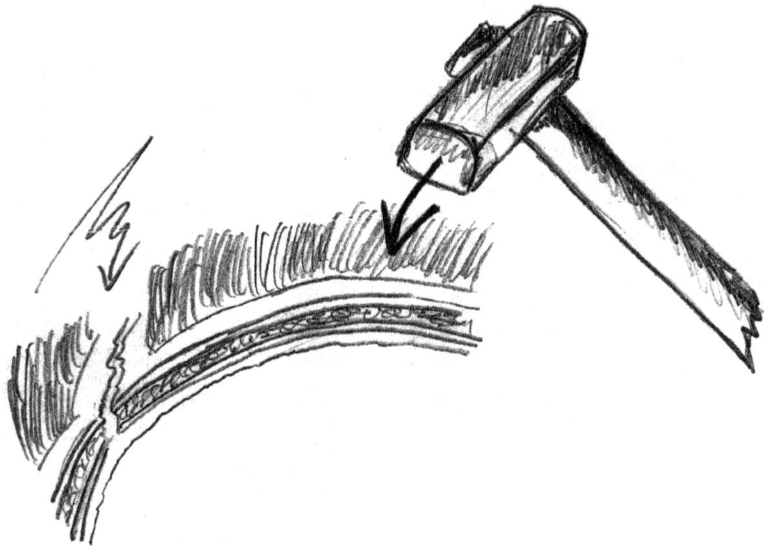

FIGURE 10.7 Contrecoup Fracture (Hellenistic Term: ἀπήχημα—'Echo Fracture')

the author of the text regarded the contrecoup fracture as a τρόπος at all. If not, the numbering as seventh τρόπος would be a later interpolation. Given that a contrecoup fracture is nothing else than a fissure, only occurring in another place, one could rather regard it as an ἰδέα of a fissure. The author does not, however, speak of a fissure here, but more generally of an 'injury'. Thus this paragraph could be meant as a sort of general postscript to the types of injuries mentioned before, without aiming at establishing a new type of injury, even if, from a medical viewpoint, it must be a fissure. Since the next paragraph starts with 'τοῦτον τρόπον τῆς κατήξιος (this mode of injury)', one is inclined, however, to regard the countercoup fracture as a τρόπος as well.

2 Problems of the Hippocratic Modes of Injury

The editors of the treatise *Wounds in the Head* follow different approaches of dealing with the discrepancies of numbering. Kühlewein is most purist of all and refuses to change the text of the manuscript tradition. He leaves 'type number 5' with the first ἕδρα subtype, number 7 with the contrecoup fracture and thus accepts that there is no 'type number 6' in the text. Likewise, Hanson leaves number 7 with the contrecoup fracture, but then follows an addition by Ermerins (1859–1864, vol. 1, p. 376) and Rutgers (1849, 54), who add number 6 (ἕκτος οὗτος τρόπος) to the second subtype of the ἕδρα. This, however, contradicts Hanson's (1999, 102) remark at another place where he speaks of 'five types of skull injury listed in De capitis vulneribus'. Older editors (Cornarius, Littré, Pétrequin und Withington), undertook more substantial alterations of the text in order to restore the logic of numbering: in the contrecoup fracture they changed the transmitted number 7 to 5 and deleted number 5, transmitted with the first variant of the ἕδρα.

Littré (3.207.3 L.) and Withington (1928, 5) hold the view that the numbering of subtypes of the ἕδρα goes back to a glossator or later scribe, respectively. This assumption, however, clearly contradicts the passage quoted above, in which the ἕδρα subtypes are expressly addressed as τρόποι in their own right, unless one assumed that the word τρόποι was added here by the later scribe as well: Ἐν δὲ τῷ τρόπῳ ἑκάστῳ πλέονες ἰδέαι γίγνονται· καὶ περὶ μὲν φλάσιός τε καὶ ῥωγμῆς, ἢν ἄμφω ταῦτα προσγένηται τῇ ἕδρῃ, ... Littré argues with the context that the author of *Wounds in the Head* intended to number only major types and not subtypes. Withington, in contrast, briefly refers to Galen who is explicitly talking of five forms of skull fractures in his commentaries: in a fragment of his lost commentary on *Wounds in the Head*, transmitted in Oribasius, and in another passage in his commentary on *In the Surgery*. Apart from Withington's short remark, Galen's commentary on the Hippocratic forms of skull injury has not been taken into account so far. A further analysis of these passages is, however, interesting since they are witnesses of the manuscript tradition of *Wounds in the Head* that Galen used and that evidently predates the one of the manuscripts available today.

3 Commentary by Galen and Others

Excerpts of Galen's lost commentary on the Hippocratic *Wounds in the Head* are preserved in chapter 46.21 of Oribasius' *Medical Collections*. This chapter is headed 'From the writings by Galen on Fractures in the Head (Ἐκ τῶν Γαληνοῦ περὶ τῶν ἐν κεφαλῇ καταγμάτων)'. It is composed of excerpts from Galen's *Therapeutic Method* 6.6, his lost commentary on *Wounds in the Head* and a few other excerpts (e. g. Galen's *Simple Drugs*), as the scholia indicate.[10] Oribasius' chapter starts with an excerpt from Galen's lost commentary on *Wounds in the Head*. According to the scholia, this excerpt belongs to a commentary on the first sentence of chapter 3 of *Wounds in the Head*, that is, the opening sentence on the treatise's section of injuries of the head: 'From the (treatise) *On Wounds*

10 On the scholia to Oribasius see Witt (2014), 39–44.

in the Head, from the lemma: 'the ἕδραι […] of the sharp' (ἀπὸ τοῦ Περὶ τῶν ἐν τῇ κεφαλῇ τρωμάτων, ῥητοῦ· αἱ δ' ἕδραι […] τῶν ὀξέων).'[11] Thus, Galen is giving a sort of 'overview commentary' on chapters 3–8 of *Wounds in the Head*. According to him, there are indeed not seven, but five Hippocratic types of skull injury: 'The affections of the head bones which are provoked by an external blow are five in total: ἕδρα, φλάσις, ῥωγμή, ὦσις, ἔσφλασις· ….' In this sentence, the order of the modes of injuries is not the one given in chapters 4–8 where they are numbered as first, second etc. τρόπος (1. ῥωγμή, 2. φλάσις, 3. ἔσφλασις, 4. ἕδρα + …). Rather Galen follows the order given in the first sentence of chapter 3 where all major types of skull injury are outlined, starting with ἕδρα and ending with ἔσφλασις: 'The ἕδραι of the sharp and light weapons occur in the bone in their own right, without a ῥωγμή, φλάσις or ἔσφλασις which is directed inwards … (Αἱ δὲ ἕδραι τῶν βελέων τῶν ὀξέων καὶ κουφοτέρων, αὐταὶ ἐπὶ σφῶν αὐτέων γινόμεναι ἐν τῷ ὀστέῳ, ἄνευ ῥωγμῆς τε καὶ φλάσιος, ἢ ἔσω ἐσφλάσιος …)'. Surprisingly, Galen's commentary also has a form named ὦσις, which is never mentioned in the Hippocratic treatise as it has come down to us. A comparison of the words 'ἢ ἔσω ἐσφλάσιος' in the quotation just given and 'ὦσις, ἔσφλασις' in the fragment of Galen's commentary suggests textual corruption. Galen could have read ἢ ὤσεως ἢ ἐσφλάσιος here, with ἢ ὤσεως being an explanation for the preceding φλάσιος, perhaps originally a gloss, that was incorporated into the main text later. Later copyists could have read Η ΩΣΕΩΣ as Η ΩΣ ΕΩΣ which later could have become Η ΕΣΩ, as we have it today.

A careful comparison between the Hippocratic *Wounds in the Head* and Oribasius suggests the need for another emendation, this time of Galen (in Oribasius). It would be odd that Galen, starting with ἕδρα and otherwise keeping the exact sequence of the forms of injuries as given in the first sentence of *Wounds in the Head*, chapter 3, had just inverted ῥωγμή and φλάσις. Thus in the sequence ἕδρα, φλάσις, ῥωγμή, ὦσις, ἔσφλασις in Oribasius, φλάσις and ῥωγμή should be inverted.

But let us return to ὦσις. Since in the Hippocratic text no ὦσις can be found, we need to raise the question what Galen meant by ὦσις. According to the definition of ὦσις given a little later by Galen, in the fragment of his lost commentary, by this term he designates a ping-pong fracture in children:[12]

> ἐὰν δὲ βαρὺ μὲν ᾖ τὸ πλῆττον, ὀξύτητα δ' ἔχον οὐδεμίαν, ἤτοι γ' ὦσις γίνεται μόνη τοῦ πληγέντος ἢ καὶ ῥωγμὴ σὺν αὐτῇ, ὦσις μὲν ἐπὶ τῶν μαλακῶν ὀστῶν,

11 The brackets are added here to mark the omission in the Hippocratic quotation within the scholion (an omission not indicated by the scholiast).

12 Oribasius, *Medical Collections*, 46.21.2 (ed. Raeder 1931, p. 227, line 35–p. 228, line 2).

> ὁποῖα τὰ τῶν παίδων ἐστί, ῥωγμὴ δ' ἐπὶ τῶν σκληρῶν τε καὶ ξηρῶν, ἐπὶ δὲ τῶν μέσων τὴν φύσιν ἀμφότερα.
>
> If the hitting object is heavy, but devoid of sharpness, then either an ὦσις of the bone that was hit alone occurs, or it is accompanied by a fracture. An ὦσις occurs in soft bones like those of children, a fracture in hard and dry ones; in bones whose quality is in between, both forms of injury occur.

It is equally unclear in what way an ὦσις is meant to differ from a φλάσις. There is no explicit definition of a φλάσις in Galen. Whether Galen deliberately left it out in his commentary or whether this omission results from a condensation of the excerpted text by Oribasius cannot be determined. A little earlier Galen merely states that a φλάσις is due to the heaviness of the weapon. In this context he describes the effect made by the heavy weapon by the verb ὠθεῖν:[13]

> ἡ μὲν γὰρ φλάσις[14] γίνεται διὰ τὸ βάρος τῶν πληττόντων, ἡ δὲ διαίρεσις διὰ τὴν ὀξύτητα· συνελθόντων δ' ἐς ταὐτὸν ἀμφοτέρων τῶν αἰτίων, ἔσφλασις γίνεται, τῆς μὲν ὀξύτητος τοῦ πλήττοντος διαιρούσης τὸ ὀστοῦν, τοῦ βάρους δ' ὠθοῦντος εἴσω τὸ διῃρημένον.
>
> The φλάσις comes about because of the heaviness of the hitting objects, the division because of the sharpness. If both qualities occur together in the same object, an ἔσφλασις results with the sharpness of the hitting object splitting the bone and its heaviness pushing the divided parts inwards.

Might one therefore conclude that ὦσις and φλάσις are the same? But why did Galen mention them as different τρόποι then? Just in order to follow the (probably corrupt) text of *Wounds in the Head*, chapter 3?

Paul of Aegina understood ὦσις and φλάσις as synonyms. His chapter 6.90 is entitled 'On Fractures in the Head (Περὶ τῶν ἐν τῇ κεφαλῇ καταγμάτων)'. It consists of excerpts from Heliodorus' χειρουργούμενα (in Oribasius' *Medical Collections* 46.12–15), Soranus' *Signs of Fractures*, and at least one unknown source. At the beginning the types of cranial injuries are listed (Hellenistic, not Hippo-

13 Oribasius, *Medical Collections*, 46.21.2 (ed. Raeder 1931, p. 227, lines 31–35).

14 In Oribasius' *Medical Collections* and Paul of Aegina's *Medical Handbook*, Hippocratic Attic rather than Ionic terms appear (e.g., θλάσις, ἔσθλασις, instead of φλάσις, ἔσφλασις). Since in his commentaries on Hippocratic writings Galen uses Hippocratic terms in their Ionic forms (Witt [2014], p. 65 with n. 39), the Ionic forms in Oribasius' passage quoted above were restored to reflect Galen's putative original wording.

cratic forms). In this context Paul states that a φλάσις only occurs in infants (ἐπὶ δὲ τῶν νηπίων καὶ θλάσις[15]). In a later passage, which is an excerpt from an unknown source, φλάσις is explained by the synonym ὦσις. For Paul (or rather the source he excerpted), φλάσις and ὦσις are synonyms, the former more technical than the latter:[16]

> ἡ δὲ θλάσις οὐκ ἔστι διαίρεσις τοῦ ὀστέου, καὶ ταύτῃ ἄν τις εὐλόγως οὐδὲ κάταγμα φαίη τὴν τοιαύτην διάθεσιν, ἀλλ᾽ ἔστιν ὦσις καὶ οἷον κάμψις ἐπὶ τὰ ἔνδον τοῦ κρανίου κοιλαινομένου χωρὶς τοῦ λυθῆναι τὴν συνέχειαν, καθάπερ ἐπὶ τῶν χαλκῶν τε καὶ ὠμοβυρσίνων ἀγγείων ἔξωθεν πληττομένων γίνεται.
>
> The θλάσις is not a division of the bone, and for this reason one might reasonably not even call this form of injury a fracture. But it is an ὦσις and a sort of bending inwards. Hereby the skullbone is scooped out without a dissolution of its continuity as it happens in vessels of bronze and raw leather that are hit from outside.

Did Paul (or rather his source) have the same text of *Wounds in the Head* with the gloss ἢ ὤσεως as Galen apparently did? The remark εὐλόγως οὐδὲ κάταγμα φαίη seems to echo the Hippocratic author's statement that a φλάσις comes about without a fracture. Interestingly, also Soranus (*Signs of Fractures* 9) uses the analogy of leather or lead vessels (δερμάτινοι ἢ μολύβινοι λήκυθοι) to illustrate how a ping-pong fracture comes about. However, Soranus uses the word θλάσμα (not θλάσις), which was the standard term for a ping-pong fracture in Hellenistic times.[17] Paul employs the more old-fashioned word θλάσις here, perhaps because he is excerpting a Hippocratic who was reluctant to use modern terminology and rather adhered to the more traditional Hippocratic terms.[18] Or this excerpt could come from a commentary on the Hippocratic *Wounds in the Head*—perhaps even from a section of Galen's lost commentary dealing with φλάσις—that was not excerpted by Oribasius. For it is a characterisic of Galen to use consistently the rather old-fashioned and out-of-date Hippocratic

15 See the previous note.

16 Paul of Aegina, *Medical Handbook*, 6.90.2 (ed. Heiberg 1924, p. 137, lines 1–5).

17 Cf. 7.38.12–16, 19.432.16–19 K.; and the chapter Περὶ θλάσματος from Heliodorus' χειρουργούμενα in Oribasius' *Medical Collections* 46.17.1.

18 For the nosological concept of sympathy, the Hippocratic physician Sabinus (quoted by Galen 17a.519.12 K.) uses, for example, the traditional Hippocratic term κοινωνία, apparently in order to avoid the more common, but stoically connotated word συμπάθεια. In a similar vein, in his *Method of Healing* (e.g. 10.257 K.) Galen prefers the Hippocratic πεπαλαιομένος and κακοήθης to χρονικός, a term coined by the Methodist school of medicine; see Witt (2014), p. 49, n. 18.

terminology when commenting on Hippocrates. This can also be observed in the fragments of his lost commentary on *Wounds in the Head*. For example, he uses the term εἴσθλασις in it. As technical term for a type of cranial injury this word only occurs in the Hippocratic *Wounds in the Head* and in the fragments of Galen's lost commentary on *Wounds in the Head*. Elsewhere in medical litterature the common term for this type of injury is ἐμπίεσμα.[19]

Turning back to the θλάσις, Paul continues to distinguish between two different forms of θλάσις, one that goes through the whole bone (εἰσὶ δὲ τῆς θλάσεως δύο διαφοραί· ἢ γὰρ δι' ὅλου τοῦ πάχους ἑαυτοῦ θλᾶται τὸ ὀστέον) and another one that does not (ἢ οὐ δι' ὅλου). This is clearly an echo of the Hippocratic *Wounds in the Head* where the same distinction was made, speaking of the ἰδέαι of a θλάσις (καὶ διὰ παντὸς τοῦ ὀστέου, καὶ ἧσσον ἐς βαθὺ, καὶ οὐ διὰ παντὸς τοῦ ὀστέου). This could be a further indication that Paul excerpted this passage from a commentary on the Hippocratic *Wounds in the Head*. The two different forms that are mentioned in Paul are, however, a somewhat strange interpretation of the Hippocratic text. The first seems to be a deformation of the whole skullbone in the sense of a ping-pong fracture since it was stated before that it only occurs in infants and moreover the analogy with bronze and leather vessels was established as well. The second variant, in contrast, is a completely different type of injury that is not at all ping-pong fracture, but a superficial lesion of the skull, going down just to the diploe: ἢ οὐ δι' ὅλου, ἀλλὰ κατὰ τὴν ἐκτὸς μένον πυκνὴν ἐπιφάνειαν ἄχρι τῆς διπλόης. This is the form that seems to be the one that the Hippocratic author had in mind when speaking of θλάσις, as I tried to demonstrate above (see fig. 10.3a). Of course, this form is not limited to children, but can occur in anybody. So the previous remark that a θλάσις occurs 'in children (ἐπὶ δὲ τῶν νηπίων)' does not make any sense with reference to the second variant. Apparently two different attempts of the exegetical tradition of explaining the Hippocratic θλάσις merged here in a somewhat awkward and contradictory way and thus misguidedly became two ἰδέαι of a θλάσις. According to some people, Paul continues, the contrecoup fracture was considered as a mode of cranial injury:[20]

> τινὲς δὲ ταύταις ταῖς διαφοραῖς καὶ τὸ ἀπήχημα προστεθήκασιν, ὅπερ ἐστὶ κατ' αὐτοὺς ῥῆξις κρανίου κατὰ τὰ ἀντικείμενα τῶν πεπληγμένων γινομένη μερῶν.

---

19 This term is transmitted in Soranus, *Signs of Fractures* 6; Heliodorus (quoted by Oribibasius, *Medical Collections* 46.14); and Paul of Aegina 6.90. Only the Herophilean Demetrius used ἐμπίεσμα in the sense of θλάσμα (= contrecoup fracture), according to Soranus, *Signs of Fractures* 9; see also Michler (1968), 55.

20 Paul of Aegina, *Medical Handbook*, 6.90.2 (ed. Heiberg 1924, p. 137, lines 10–12).

> To these different forms (of injury) some people also added the echo fracture which is—according to them—a breaking of the skullbone which occurs in the parts opposite to those which were hit.

That only some considered it as a separate form might be a hint that in ancient editions there was no number given in *Wounds in the Head* chapter 8 where this type of fracture is described. Had there been a consistent numbering, there would not have been any problem with this mode.

Galen's second mention of the different modes can be found in his commentary on *In the Surgery* (18b.672.9–673.1 K.). Since a critical edition of this treatise does not yet exist, the text is given according to Anastassiou and Irmer (1997–2012, vol. 2.1, p. 453) who have collated the extant manuscripts. The Greek text is transmitted in just two manuscripts, Parisinus gr. 1849 (14th. cent.) and the Marcianus gr. Z 279 (= 705) (15th cent.) There is also an Arabic version (Scor. arab. 845, 12th cent.) that was edited by Lyons (1963). This version is, however, incomplete. It only starts at 18b.738.4 K. and therefore cannot be used for establishing the present text.

> κἀν τῷ Περὶ τῶν ἐν τῇ κεφαλῇ τραυμάτων αὐτὸς διῆλθε τοὺς τρόπους, καθ' οὓς αἱ πληγαὶ γίγνονται, κατὰ τήνδε τὴν ῥῆσιν· 'τιτρώσκεται δὲ ὀστέον τὸ ἐν τῇ κεφαλῇ κατὰ τοσούσδε τρόπους' (3.194.11 L.). καὶ ἐφεξῆς πάλιν· 'τῶν δὲ τρόπων ἑκάστου πλείονες ἰδέαι γίγνονται τοῦ κατάγματος ἐν τῇ θλάσει' (3.194.12–196.1 L.). καὶ μετὰ ταῦτα πάλιν· 'θλασθείη ⟨δ'⟩ ἂν ὀστέον μένον ἐν τῇ αὐτοῦ φύσει, καὶ ῥωγμὴ τῇ θλάσει οὐκ ἂν προσγένοιτο ἐν τῷ ὀστέῳ οὐδεμία. δεύτερος οὗτος τρόπος' (3.200.8–10 L.)· εἶτ' ἐφεξῆς ἄλλον εἰπὼν ἐπιφέρει· 'οὗτος τρίτος' (3.204.4 L.)· καὶ πάλιν ἐφεξῆς· 'πέμπτος οὗτος τρόπος' (3.208.1 L.)· ἀπορώτατος οὗτος φαίνεται.

> In *Wounds in the Head* he also discussed the modes in which the blows come about, saying: 'The skulbone is injured in the following number of modes.' After this, he said: 'And for each mode several subtypes of injury occur in the θλάσις.' Later he said: 'The bone may be indented and stay in its natural position; and no fracture may accompany the θλάσις in the bone. This is the second mode'. After that he talks about another mode and adds 'this is the third mode' and after that, he said 'this is the fifth mode'. This mode seems to be the most difficult to understand.

We learn from this passage that Galen knew a numbering amounting to five τρόποι. Interestingly, number 4 is missing in his outline—Kühn adds 'τέταρτος οὗτος τρόπος' which does not appear in the manuscripts. Whether Galen did not have number 4 in his text or whether he just did not regard it necessary to mention number 4 remains unclear. In the manuscripts that have come down to us we have indeed a version in which, due to a textual loss (*saut du même au même*), mode 5 is missing. But we lack manuscript evidence for a missing mode 4. From the present passage we only know that Galen knew ῥωγμή and φλάσις as modes 1 and 2. About the other modes we are less explicitly informed. That he regarded ἕδρα and ἔσφλάσις als separate modes can be inferred from the abovementioned fragment of his commentary on *Wounds in the Head*.

The concluding remark ἀπορώτατος οὗτος φαίνεται can be found in both manuscripts of Galen's commentary. It may either go back to Galen himself who would thus be confessing to be unable to make sense of mode 5. Or it could be a marginal gloss of a scribe that slipped into the main text. In the transmitted text of *Wounds in the Head*, number 4 is the compound injury ἕδρα + ῥωγμή + φλάσις and number 5 ἕδρα + φλάσις, as shown above. If Galen indeed only had mode 5 in his text with number 4 missing, it seems fairly understandable that he considered this compound mode as ἀπορώτατος.

It remains however unclear why, in his commentary on chapter 3, Galen lists ὦσις as another mode of injury. For there is no passage in the Hippocratic text that could be regarded as a matching description for this mode of injury. Galen must have identified it as a textual corruption. Or did he not want to mention this corruption out of reverence for the transmitted text in order to conceal the shortcomings of the text and possibly the inconsistencies of the Hippocratic author?

The question whether Galen had a numbering in chapter 8 (contrecoup fracture) might be answered by going a little further in the fragment of Galen's commentary on *Wounds in the Head*. According to his general aim in writing commentaries, firstly, to supplement the connective explanations 'left out by Hippocrates' in his bachylogic style and, secondly, to supplement the newer tradition,[21] the second part of commentary is devoted to the more recent terminology for additional forms of cranial injuries that had been described since the Hippocratic *Wounds in the Head*.

The first post-Hippocratic form outlined ist the ἀποσκεπαρνισμός (see fig. 10.8), a loss of substance caused by the tangential cut of a sharp weapon with the rest of the bone remaining in its place. Therefore it is likened to the ἕδρα by Galen since a loss of substance only occurs in the zone of injury, whereas the surrounding bone remains intact and stays in its place.

21 See Witt (2012), 116–118.

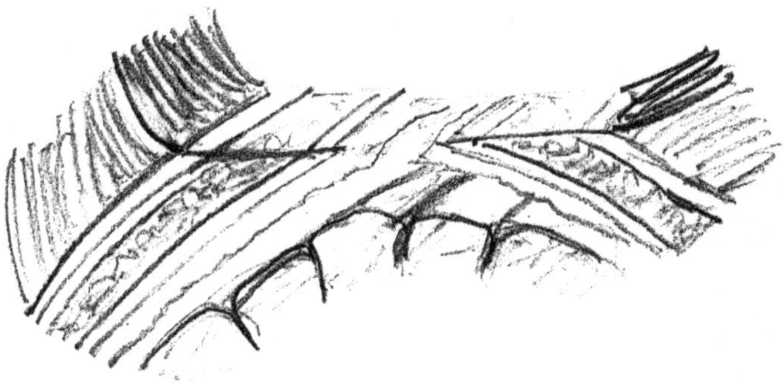

FIGURE 10.8
ἀποσκεπαρνισμός

FIGURE 10.9
ἐγγείσωμα

Two further forms of injury presented by Galen are compound forms, as he says (σύνθετον … τὸ πάθος), consisting in a ῥωγμή plus a φλάσις. In the first of these compound forms, a fractured piece of bone 'dives' under the opposite margin of bone as one tectonic plate under an adjacent one. Since this form resembles a cornice it was called by the 'younger surgeons (ὑπὸ τῶν νεωτέρων χειρουργῶν)' a 'cornice fracture (ἐγγείσωμα)' (fig. 10.9).

If by means of shear forces a vault-like elevation of fragments resulted, this type of injury was named vault fracture or καμάρωσις (fig. 10.10).

Finally, Galen adds a mode of injury that is called 'echo fracture (ἀπήχημα)'. An echo fracture is one in which the fracture does not occur at the zone of impact, but at another place, according to Galen's definition: 'The remaining mode of injury that is called echo fracture by them is a fracture which does not come about in the part that was hit, but in another one. (λοιπὸν δὲ τὸ κληθὲν ὑπ' αὐτῶν ἀπήχημα ῥωγμή τίς ἐστιν, οὐ κατὰ τὸ πληγὲν μέρος, ἀλλ' ἐν ἑτέρῳ γινομένη)'. Of course, this is the same as the contrecoup fracture, outlined in chapter 8 of

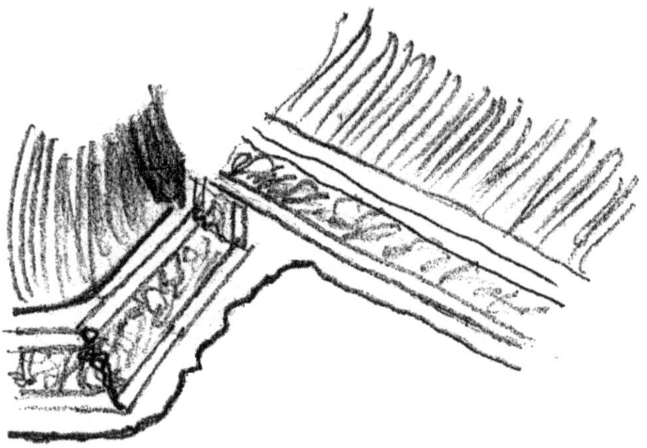

FIGURE 10.10
καμάρωσις

Wounds in the Head (fig. 10.7), just with an Alexandrian name attached to it. It is unclear why Galen lists this form at the end of a section of his commentary beginning with 'τῶν δ' ἄλλων παθῶν τῆς κεφαλῆς ... (Of the other affections of the skull ...)', just as if it had not been mentioned in the Hippocratic treatise. Did he do so because this form of injury had no numbering in his edition? Or was perhaps the passage as a whole missing? Or did he just do so because there was no authentic Hippocratic name for it? Similarly Paul of Aegina remarks that 'some people' added the echo fracture to the modes of cranial injuries (τινὲς δὲ ταύταις ταῖς διαφοραῖς καὶ τὸ ἀπήχημα προστεθήκασιν). This also suggests that the contrecoup fracture was not universally regarded as a Hippocratic mode of cranial injury in its own right.

4 Conclusions

As a result of this short overview of ancient commentary on *Wounds in the Head* the following may be concluded. The numbering of the cranial injuries is original, as is the numbering of subtypes of ἕδρα, since these compound forms are adressed as τρόποι in the running text as well. Galen had a text with five τρόποι. His last one (number 5) was probably the second subtype of the ἕδρα. In Galen's edition the chapter with the ἕδρα (chapter 7) may have had textual losses or a more confused arrangement than today. The chapter with the contrecoup fracture was probably not numbered as a separate τρόπος in ancient editions; maybe this whole chapter is even a later interpolation.

In chapter 3 Galen may have had a text reading 'ἢ ὤσεως ἢ ἐσφλάσιος' rather than 'ἢ ἔσω ἐσφλάσιος', as we read it today. Probably ἢ ὤσεως is a gloss that slipped into the text. This gloss hints at certain difficulties in understanding the φλάσις type of injury, which is confirmed by the exegetical tradition. Instead of pointing at the textual corruption, Galen explains ὦσις as if it was a separate type of injury, probably to conceal the shortcomings of the Hippocratic text.

How should future editors of this treatise proceed? It seems justified to leave the unusual order of chapter 7 as transmitted (from the most complicated to the simplest form of ἕδρα). It remains, however, within the purview of the editor to decide whether to delete the numbering of the contrecoup fracture as number 7. This would result in a numbering Galen and his contemporaries are supposed to have had, ending with the second subtype of ἕδρα. Alternatively the editor could add mode 6 with the simple ἕδρα (as Ermerins did) and leave mode 7 with the contrecoup fracture. This would create a logical text structure which may however be anachronistic since we do not know by whom and at what point of time number 7 was introduced. The ancient commentary tradition suggests that this last numbering does not go back to the Hippocratic author.

CHAPTER 11

Galen's Surgical Commentaries on Hippocràtes

Amneris Roselli

Galen wrote about the anatomy of bones in the treatise *Bones for Beginners* (which belongs to the so-called 'minor anatomical works'); he also discussed bones in his short work *Movement of Muscles* and in the two major anatomical and physiological treatises, *Anatomical Procedures* and *Usefulness of the Parts*. As far as we know, he never wrote a work on bone injuries; he touched on this subject only in a few pages of the sixth book of his therapeutic treatise *Method of Healing*, where he dealt with both fractures of the limbs (chapter 5; 10.424–444 K.) and lesions of the skull (chapter 6; 10.444–455 K.), but not with dislocations.[1] Therefore, the two commentaries on Hippocrates' *Fractures* and *Joints* (18b.318–628 and 18a.300–767 K. respectively) together with the commentary on *Surgery* appear to be the only extensive and comprehensive documents of Galen's doctrine in the field of orthopaedics and bone surgery.[2]

To help us better understand how Galen evaluated the Hippocratic surgical treatises, I shall begin quoting a statement Galen made in *Method of Healing* 6.5 about the content and style of *Fractures*. Having appreciated the accuracy of Hippocrates in distinguishing different kinds of fractures such as '*stalk-like* (*kaulēdón*)', 'splinterlike (*schidakēdón*)', 'radishlike (*rhaphanēdón*)', 'comminuted (*alphitēdón*)',[3] Galen continues commenting on Hippocrates' treat-

1 In books 4–6 of *Method of Healing* Galen deals with the pathologies caused by 'dissolution of continuity' (ἑνώσεως / συνεχείας λύσις). See Manetti-Roselli (1996); and Witt (2012), 73–126. At the end of chapter 5 (10.443.17–444.1 K.), he anticipates a work or a presentation on the treatment of dislocations: 'But I shall say more about instruments in relation to the treatment of dislocations. Similarly, more will also be said about the variety of bandages in those considerations (ἀλλὰ περὶ μὲν ὀργάνων ἐπὶ πλέον ἐροῦμεν ἐν ταῖς τῶν ἐξαρθρημάτων ἰάσεσιν· ὡσαύτως δὲ καὶ περὶ τῆς ἐπιδέσμων ποικιλίας ἐν ἐκείνοις λελέξεται)'. The presentation of this topic is found neither in *Method of Healing* nor elsewhere. Galen could have hinted at the *Cheirourgoúmena* that should have accompanied *Method of Healing* and that he never wrote, as Witt (2012), 120–123 believes, but could also have referred to a commentary on *Joints*. In *Method of Healing* 6, chapter 6, Galen also refers to a future commentary on *Wounds in the Head* (10.444.12–16 K.).

2 For an overview concerning form and content of the two *Commentaries On Fractures* and *On Joints*, see Manetti-Roselli (1994), 1531–1535.

3 10.424.1–14 K. In fact, this specific terminology was unknown to Hippocrates and was introduced by later physicians.

© AMNERIS ROSELLI, 2021 | DOI:10.1163/9789004470200_013

ment of damaged bones and how it relates to contemporaneous bone surgery:[4]

> If the discourse about all the affections [of the body] had been fulfilled (*exeírgasto*) by him in the same way [sc. as clearly and completely as in *Fractures*], the book (*pragmateía*) I just now set forth [*Method of Healing*] would have been brief. But, since he set out the kind of path it is necessary to take for most things, but left the individual matters unfulfilled (*anexérgasta*), it is necessary for me to take some time over those. It is certainly not right to pass over them. But I shall make mention of them under the chief points (*dià kephalaíōn*) of those matters stated completely (*teléōs*) by Hippocrates and add a demonstration for some matters which were stated by him without proof. Further I shall define those matters stated without definition, bring order to those not ordered, and explain more clearly those things that were written not so clearly by him. But if I were to transcribe his statements on each subject, my book (*lógos*) would take the length of an exegetical treatise.[5] And someone will, perhaps, accuse me of prolixity (*makrología*), and reasonably so—one of those who has already reproached me unreasonably (*alógōs*) for this in the case of the third and fourth books [of the *Method of Healing*]. For in those it was necessary for me to quote (*paratheménōi*) many statements of Hippocrates from his book *On Wounds* to show all other doctors what sort of thing it is to write cures of wounds according to method.[6] But in the case of *Fractures*, who is so stupid that he does not praise the teaching as clear (*saphês*) and, at the same time, describing everything in an utterly fulfilling way (*teleṓtata exeirgasménē*)? If, however, one or two were to say that that work is not remarkable, for such people particularly what was said by the Poet (*sc.* Homer) is apposite—'permit those one or two to perish'.

In short, Galen does not need to write extensively about the treatment of fractures, quoting Hippocrates, as he usually does in *Method of Healing*, commenting, adding demonstrations and distinctions, clarifying obscurities, and

4 *Method of Healing* 10.425.1–426.7 K.; translation with modifications by Johnston, Horsley (2011), vol. 2, pp. 183–185.

5 Here my translation differs substantially from the ones of Johnston, Horsley (Loeb 2011) and Witt (2012), 104.

6 In books 2 and 3 of *Method of Healing* Galen quoted extensively the Hippocratic treatise *Wounds* and for these reason he was blamed by some of his readers (10.425.12–426.1 K.).

reordering the Hippocratic text,[7] because every reader of *Method of Healing* can deal on his own with *Fractures*. He is so confident in his exegetical strategy that he boldly takes the risk of losing a couple of readers.

1 Works on Bone Surgery before Galen

The medical literature concerning bone injuries and their treatment was not scarce at all in the Hellenistic period, as proved by the great number of fragments of the Hellenistic surgeons—many of which are quoted by Galen, and by Celsus in the surgical books 7 and 8 of *de medicina*.[8] Galen had touched on all other areas of medical practice and was definitely interested in the theoretical and practical issues related to bone surgery. So why did he not write a separate and substantial work on this topic? The possible answer lies, I think, in the authoritativeness of the Hippocratic treatises *Fractures* and *Joints*—along with *Surgery*, especially for what concerns the doctrine of the bandage, and *Wounds in the Head*. Despite the progress made at the time—especially in the field of medical instruments and reduction tools—the Hippocratic teaching about treatment of bones remained essentially valid. For this reasons, Galen probably thought that the most direct way to know what matters in orthopaedics was still to read the Hippocratic treatises. So, as a faithful follower, he wrote his surgical commentaries with the aim of making the Hippocratic treatises even easier to access and reassessing them in a more systematic way, as requested by the readers of systematic works of his time.[9]

2 Commentaries on *Fractures* and *Joints*

2.1 *Form*

Reading the two commentaries on *Fractures* and *Joints* feels like reading a monograph on bone surgery formally organized under headings taken from

7 All the listed operations are adequate for the exegesis of any text, but 'to reorder the text' fits especially to *Fractures* and *Joints*. The exegetic activities listed in *Method of Healing* provide the guidelines on how to approach the surgical commentaries: mention briefly the topics which Hippocrates covered exhaustively; add demonstrations of the things stated but not proven; define things that lacked a definition; order topics in disorder; and write more clearly those things that were written not so clearly.

8 Michler (1968).

9 On the relation between the author's text and the comment, see Shuttleworth Kraus (2002) and von Staden (2002).

Hippocrates (the lemmas); this sensation is strongly reinforced when we restore the text of the manuscripts *Laur.* 75.7 (L) and *Par. gr.* 1849 (P).[10] Whereas in Kühn's edition the two commentaries *On Fractures* and *On Joints* provide the entire Hippocratic text in the lemmas (in some cases, lemmas happen to be longer than the comment on them), the manuscripts show that those long lemmas are not original, but have been added in the printed editions.[11] Galen's own lemmas are very brief and focus on the crucial points in the Hippocratic text; Galen took them as a starting point to address specific issues and used them as headings separating different thematic issues. Each lemma introduces one of the three major themes of the commentary, namely: anatomy of the injured part of the body (forearm and shoulder; foot; leg and thighbone); simple and compound fractures; and methods of treatment (bandaging, immobilising the limbs, alternative treatments for each kind of injury, especially in *Joints*, postoperative therapy). In other words, Galen usually selected *important* lemmas, not difficult ones as Witt (2012, 111) suggests. I am aware that I am giving an excessively concise synopsis of the topics of the surgical commentaries; they actually clarify some obscurities of the text, especially the lexicon, and some expressions typical of these treatises, such as the notion of *dikaíē phýsis*. Galen, however, very frequently states that Hippocrates' text is clear and accessible (as he does also in *Method of Healing* 6.5), and therefore not in need of exegesis; this allows him to skip large sections of the text.

2.2 *Content*

One of the usual tasks of the commentator of a medical text is to give information about the causes (the *dià tí*) of pathologies that have not been made explicit by the author. In our case, however, this task has been largely fulfilled by Hippocrates himself. In the commentaries on *Fractures* and *Joints* Galen remarks repeatedly that '*he himself* (Hippocrates) stated the cause (αὐτὸς εἶπεν τὴν αἰτίαν)',[12] implying that the Hippocratic text is self-explanatory and not in need of further explanation. Other similar expressions add to this image of Hippocrates' comprehensiveness and clarity, such as '*he himself* showed

10 According to von Staden (2002), 118 and 129, Galen thought of his commentary on the *Aphorisms* as 'more than just a sequence of lemmas and comments': it has been 'shaped by something resembling a plot'; and it 'should be read as a single whole' alongside other systematic treatises. I think this may well be the case here, too.

11 Kudlien (1960); Brockmann (2006).

12 See *Commentary On Hippocrates' Fractures* 18b.373.6 and 492.13 K.; and *Commentary On Hippocrates' Joints* 18a.390.13, 409.11, and 700.4 K.

you in all that follows (*αὐτὸς* ἐνεδείξατό σοι διὰ τῶν ἐφεξῆς ἁπάντων)' (18b.340.1 K.); 'this, too, *he himself* taught (καὶ τοῦτ' *αὐτὸς* ἐδίδαξεν)' (18b.383.14 K.); '*he himself* taught the kind of diet that is strick (ἐδίδαξεν *αὐτὸς* ⟨τό τε⟩ τῆς ἀκριβοῦς διαίτης εἶδος)' (18b.406.8 K.); and 'and by means of his own words, *he himself* clearly explained to those paying attention how to use these [instruments] (καὶ τίνα δὲ τρόπον αὐτοῖς προσήκει χρῆσθαι σαφῶς *αὐτὸς* ἐδήλωσε διὰ τῆς ἰδίας λέξεως τοῖς προσέχουσι τὸν νοῦν αὐτῷ)' (18b.479.8–10 K.). Sometimes Galen invites the reader to refer back from the commentary to the Hippocratic text: 'so let us hear the words through which *Hippocrates himself* explains the cause of this (*αὐτὸς* οὖν *ὁ Ἱπποκράτης* ἥντινα λέγει τούτου τὴν αἰτίαν εἶναι διὰ τῆς λέξεως ἀκούσωμεν)' (18b.412.10–12 K.). Despite these repeated stances, Galen was well aware of the fact that Hippocrates did not explain many important things, and as a commentator, he set himself the task of filling these gaps.

When choosing on what themes to focus his exegesis, Galen regularly privileges the criterion of utility (*tò chrḗsimon*) over the need to explain difficult words or variant readings, on which he only touches lightly, see for instance *On Fractures* 338.11–17 K.:

> μένοντος δὲ τοῦ διδασκομένου πράγματος, ὅπως ἄν τις ἀκούῃ, τὸ ζητεῖν ἐπὶ πλέον ὑπὲρ τῶν τοιούτων περιττόν. *ἄχρηστά* τε γὰρ ἅμα καὶ ἀδύνατα[13] τοὐπίπαν ἐστὶν εὑρίσκεσθαι τὰ κατὰ τὰς ἀμφιβόλους λέξεις εἰρημένα, διὸ καὶ παρατρέχειν αὐτὰ χρὴ τὸν τοῦ χρόνου φειδόμενον ὡς ἐχρῆν εἰς τὰ χρήσιμα μᾶλλον ἀναλίσκειν αὐτόν.
>
> However one understands [the meaning of the verb '*aporégei*'], what he teaches remains the same. It is therefore superfluous to investigate these things further. Things that are expressed through ambiguous phrases are both *without benefit* and impossible to find. Therefore, if you want to save time, you have to pass over these things, as one should rather spend time on useful things.

Galen reassesses here the 'conventional' exegetical praxis used for other types of texts, which goes back to the Alexandrian exegesis of Homer and proposes a different track. In the commentary on *Fractures*, and even more so in that on *Joints*, we find some explanations of Hippocratic words, and some discussions of variant readings. Nonetheless, Galen does not seem to be committed to

13 ἀδύνατα scripsi : δυνατά P edd.

providing such philological niceties and the overall part of this kind of exegesis compared to the whole commentaries remains small: the surgical commentaries aim at practical utility, as can be seen from the following quotation:[14]

> Εἴτ' αἰγὸς δέρμα προσαγορεύεται κυρίως ἰξάλη εἴτε κατ' ἄλλου τινὸς ὑποφέρεσθαι δύναται τοὔνομα περιττὸν ἐν τῇδε τῇ διδασκαλίᾳ ζητεῖν. οὐ γὰρ ἐξήγησις λέξεων, ἀλλὰ θεραπεία πρόσκειται παθῶν, εἰς ἣν ἀρκεῖ γιγνώσκειν ὅτι μανὸν οὐ πυκνὸν ὑποτετάσθαι χρὴ δέρμα.
>
> It is superfluous to investigate in this exposition whether the term *ixálē* specifically denotes 'goat leather', or can refer to something else. The task at hand is *not to explain words, but to treat injuries*. For this it suffices to know that the leather you have to put under the limb should be soft rather than hard.

In other words, Galen is here concerned with the modalities how best to treat the patient.

2.3 *Addressee*

Who is the presumed reader of the two commentaries on *Fractures* and *Joints*? Galen addresses the reader as someone who would perform surgery. For instance, in the commentary on *Fractures*, he addresses someone who is about to learn through repeated exercise and through the appropriate questions to the patient how to find the right amount of pressure in a bandage:[15]

> προσέχων γὰρ τὸν νοῦν ἀκριβῶς τῷ ποσῷ τῆς τάσεως ἣν ἐποιήσω περιβάλλων τὸν ἐπίδεσμον εἶτ' ἐρωτήσας τὸν ἐπιδούμενον, ὁποίας αἰσθάνεται τῆς περιβολῆς τῶν ὀθονίων, ἐκ δευτέρου περιβάλλων εἴσει πότερον[16] ἐκλῦσαι δεῖ τὴν τάσιν ἢ ἐπαυξῆσαι· … καὶ μέντοι καὶ πρὶν ἐπ' αὐτοῦ τοῦ τὸ κάταγμα σχόντος ἄρχεσθαι τῆς ἐπιδέσεως, ἔνεστί σοι προγυμνάσασθαι, παιδάριον ὑγιὲς ἐπιδέσαντι πολλάκις ἅμα[17] τῷ πυνθάνεσθαι τὰς ἀρτίως εἰρημένας πεύσεις. ἑτοιμότερος γὰρ οὕτως ἔσῃ πρὸς τὰς ἐν τοῖς κατάγμασι ἐπιδέσεις.
>
> You have to pay careful attention to the amount of tension you applied when dressing the bandage. Ask the patient how it feels when the linen

14 *Commentary On Hippocrates' Fractures* 18b.572.8–12 K.
15 Ibid. 18b.372.2–13 K.
16 πότερον scripsi : ἴσως προτέρῳ K.
17 ἅμα scripsi : ἀλλὰ K.

bandages are put on. When you put on the second layer, you will know whether to loosen or to increase the pressure. […] Before you start bandaging a patient with a fracture, you can practise applying the bandage by putting it repeatedly on a healthy slave and asking him the questions which I have just mentioned. In this way you will be more prepared to apply bandages in the case of fractures.

There is no clear distinction between explanations for a reading and a listening public; within the same commentary both approaches coexist. Galen has mainly physicians in mind who know anatomy and have gained experience through practice; however, he admits that some of his readers or listeners have never seen a skeleton (neither of a human nor of a monkey) for themselves, and have no experience of anatomy, as the following passage on the anatomy of jawbones shows:[18]

Εἴρηταί μοι καὶ πρόσθεν … ὡς[19] εἴ τις οὐ νοεῖ σαφῶς τὰ οὕτως ὑφ᾽ Ἱπποκράτους λεγόμενα, δείκνυσθαι δεῖ τούτῳ πρὸς[20] τοῦ διδάσκοντος ὀστᾶ μάλιστα μὲν ἀνθρώπων, εἰ δὲ μή, πιθήκων. ἄμεινον δὲ μὴ νῦν, ὁπότ᾽ ἀναγιγνώσκει τὰ βιβλία, ταύτην δεῖξιν[21] γίγνεσθαι τῶν ὀστῶν, ἀλλ᾽ ἔμπροσθεν ἐπὶ σχολῆς[22] γεγονέναι. λέλεκται δὲ καὶ ὡς ὑφ᾽ ἡμῶν γέγραπται βιβλίον *Τοῖς εἰσαγομένοις περὶ ὀστῶν*, ⟨ὅτι τε⟩[23] τῷ μέλλοντι συνιέναι τί[24] ἐν τούτοις τοῖς γράμμασιν ὁ Ἱπποκράτης λέγει, προγεγυμνάσθαι βέλτιόν ἐστιν ἐν ἐκείνῳ. καὶ τοίνυν ⟨ὡς⟩[25] ἔμπροσθεν ἔγραψα καὶ νῦν ποιήσω μέσην τινὰ τοῖς θ᾽ ἑωρακόσι καὶ μὴ ἑωρακόσι διδασκαλίαν [ποιησάμενος].[26] οὕτως γὰρ οἵ θ᾽ ἑωρακότες οὐκ ἀνιάσονται τῷ μήκει τῶν λόγων οἵ τ᾽ οὐδ᾽ ὅλως ἑωρακότες οἷον ὑπογραφήν τινα ἕξουσι τῆς ἀκριβοῦς μαθήσεως, ἣν οὐχ οἷόν τε χωρὶς τῆς ἐπὶ τῶν ὀστῶν αὐτοψίας γενέσθαι.

I said earlier […], that if someone does not clearly understand the words of Hippocrates, the teacher should show him the bones—preferably of a human, otherwise, of a monkey. It would be better for this display of the bones not to occur at the moment when one reads the book, but it

18 *Commentary On Hippocrates' Joints*, 18a.425.3–14 K.
19 ὡς P : καὶ K.
20 δείκνυσθαι δεῖ τούτῳ πρὸς P : δείκνυσι καὶ τοῦτο πρὸ K.
21 δεῖξιν scripsi : ἕξιν K.
22 σχολῆς P : χολῆς K.
23 ὅτι τε K : om. P.
24 τί P : δῆλον τί K.
25 ὡς addidi.
26 διδασκαλίαν] K : διδασκαλίας ποιησάμενος P.

> should have taken place beforehand without any time pressure. I have also said that I wrote a book, *Bones for Beginners*, and that it would be better for those who want to understand what Hippocrates says in these [surgical] treatises to learn it as a preliminary training. As I have done in [previous] writings, I shall now provide an intermediate level of teaching (*didaskalía*) for both those who have previously seen [bones themselves] and those who have not. In this way, those who have seen [bones] will not be annoyed by the length of the text, and those who have not seen everything may have some sort of first glance (*hypographḗ*) of the in-depth teaching which cannot take place without seeing the bones for oneself.

Similarly, discussing the anatomy of the vertebrae, Galen says:[27]

> εἴρηται δὲ ἀκριβῶς ἡμῖν ἅπασα τῶν σφονδύλων ἡ σύνθεσις ἐν τῇ περὶ τῶν ὀστῶν εἰσαγωγῇ, καθ' ἣν ἠξίωσα ἀπογυμνάσασθαι τὸν ἀκολουθήσοντα[28] τοῖσδε τοῖς ὑπομνήμασι, τεθεαμένος ἀκριβῶς ἕκαστον τῶν ὀστῶν ὁποῖόν ἐστιν, ἐπ' αὐτῶν μὲν μάλιστα τῶν ἀνθρώπων σκελετῶν, εἰ μὴ πάντως τῶν πιθηκείων.
>
> I have accurately discussed the entire arrangement of the vertebrae in my introduction about bones [i.e., *On the Bones for Beginners*]. If someone wants to follow the thread of this commentary, then he should peruse this introduction by way of preparation. He should also have observed the form of each bone of a human skeleton—or, failing that, of monkeys.

When discussing the shape of the so-called 'Hippocratic bench', Galen insists again on the need to see for oneself:[29]

> ἐφεξῆς οὖν αὐτῷ γράφοντι τὴν κατασκευὴν τοῦ ὀργάνου προσέχετε τὸν νοῦν ἐφαρμόζοντες ἃ λέγει τοῖς τεθεαμένοις, ἐφ' ὃ τεθέασθε βάθρον. μόνη γὰρ δεῖξις σαφηνίζει τὰ τοιαῦτα, καθάπερ εἴρηται καὶ πρόσθεν. ἐπὶ μὲν οὖν τῶν ἀναγιγνωσκόντων παρ' ἐμοὶ τὸ βιβλίον ἑτοίμως ποιοῦμαι παρακειμένου τοῦ ὀργάνου, πολλάκις μὲν αὐτοῦ τοῦ μεγάλου, πολλάκις δὲ καὶ τῶν μιμημάτων αὐτοῦ τινος ἃ διὰ ταύτην μόνην τὴν χρείαν κατασκευάζομεν, ἵνα ἔχωμεν δεικνύναι τοῖς ἀναγιγνώσκουσιν. οὐ γὰρ δὴ δι' αὐτῶν ἐστιν ἐμβαλεῖν ἄρθρον, ἀλλὰ νῦν γε τοῦτο

27 *Commentary On Hippocrates' Joints*, 18a.493.5–11 K.

28 ἀκολουθήσοντα scripsi, cf. lat. percepturus est : ἀκολουθήσαντα P edd.

29 Ibid. 18a.747.14–748.9 K.

μὲν ἀδύνατόν ἐστι πρᾶξαι, τὸ δ' ἐξηγήσασθαί τι τῶν κατὰ τὴν λέξιν ἀσαφῶν δυνατόν, ὅπερ ἔν τε τοῖς ἔμπροσθεν ἐποίησα, καὶ νῦν ἐν τοῖς ἐφεξῆς πράξω.

Next, he [sc. Hippocrates] describes the construction of the instrument [sc. the bench]. Pay attention to his words, and link what he says to what you have seen, namely in the bench that you have already seen. Only the actual display (*deîxis*) makes such things clear, as I said earlier. For those who read the book [sc. *Joints*] with me I can easily do this, because I keep the instrument at hand, either the full-size bench, or a model specifically made for the purpose, so that I can show [it] to those who read [this passage with me]. A joint could obviously not be reduced by means of these models, for this is impossible; it is, however, possible to explain some obscurely worded point, as I did before [sc. in this commentary] and am continuing to do in what follows.

3 The Commentary on the First Lemma of *Fractures*

The commentary on *Fractures* is preceded by a long preface (18b.318–322 K.) in which Galen defines the aim of explaining medical texts and his audience.[30] Yet, throughout his commentary, he does not always adhere to the principles which he himself laid down in the preface.[31] Let us therefore examine in this paragraph the commentary on the first lemma with the aim of verifying concretely the essential lines of Galen's exegesis in the case of the surgical treatises. The lemma itself runs as follows:[32]

Ἐχρῆν τὸν ἰητρὸν τῶν ἐκπτωσίων τε καὶ καταγμάτων ὡς ἰθυτάτας τὰς κατατάσιας ποιέεσθαι.

In dislocations and fractures, the practitioner should make extensions in as straight a line as possible.

The commentary to this lemma occupies thirteen pages in Kühn's edition (18b.322–335 K.) and reveals essential aspects of Galen's exegesis. Galen first deals with some preliminary issues, such as how to handle the Ionic dialect and what terminology is in use for bone and articular lesions (*ágma*, *kátagma*;

30 Manetti, Roselli (1996).

31 Von Staden (2002), 135–136.

32 *Fract.* 1, 3.412.2–3 L.; Kühlewein (1902), vol. 2, p. 46, lines 2–3; tr. Withington (1928), 95.

exárthrēsis, exárthrēma); he also tackles the related problem of the title and the original form of the book: was it one work later divided into two parts (*Fractures* and *Joints*) because of its length, or maybe two separate books from the very beginning? Then Galen turns to the question of authorship: did Hippocrates write *Fractures* and *Joints* or rather Hippocrates' grandfather? Finally, he reflects on the fact that the author discussed fractures and dislocations together. These are all topics that belong in a preface or proem.[33] At this point (18b.325.15 K.) Galen transcribes again the second part of the lemma ('make extensions in as straight a line as possible (ὡς ἰθυτάτας τὰς κατατάσιας ποιεῖσθαι)') and then asks two exegetical and pertinent questions about the issue of 'extension (κατάτασις)': 1) why (*dià tí*) do we have to extend the damaged limb at all? and 2) why must the extension be made in a straight line?

The first question is clearly fundamental, although Hippocrates never broached it; in *Fractures* 1 he rather deals with the position of the extension, 'as straight as possible (ὡς ἰθυτάτας)', and criticises other physicians for erroneously choosing bizarre positions. Hippocrates' failure to discuss this first fundamental question leads Galen to embark on a short digression about Hippocrates' eagerness to say the most important things first and arguing that for this reason every reader must be free to read the Hippocratic text in a different and more suitable order. After this digression Galen returns to the first question of 'why (*dià tí*) it is necessary to extend the damaged limb before setting it in place' and contrasts his own priorities with those of Hippocrates:[34]

> αὐτὸς μὲν γὰρ ὕστερον ἀπορεῖ διὰ τί[35] χρὴ κατατείνειν πρότερον, εἴτε διαπλάττειν μέλλοις τὸ κατεαγὸς ὀστοῦν εἴτ' ἐμβάλλειν τὸ ἐξηρθρηκός. ἐμοὶ δὲ νῦν φαίνεται καιρὸς αὐτῷ σαφηνείας ἔχοντι σκοπὸν τῆς ἐξηγήσεως, …
>
> Hippocrates wonders only later why you have to extend first, whether you are about to reshape a fractured bone or to reduce a dislocated joint. Now seems to me to be the right time to explain this, as I endeavour to be clear.

Galen then refers his readers to his treatise *Movements of Muscles* and summarises some main points in order to explain why extension is necessary: muscles naturally contract if they are severed; in dislocations, when one of the two bones is displaced from its position next to the other, the muscles originating

33 Later Neo-Platonic commentaries will deal with them systematically. Also Ihm (2002), 103 observed that the commentary to the first lemma is a new proem.

34 Galen, *Commentary On Hippocrates' Fractures*, 18b.327.11–15 K.

35 τί P : τίνα K.

at either end of the bone contract. The same also happens with fractures: if the two segments of the fractured bone overlap, the muscles contract, so that they need to be extended first; only then can one reposition the fractured bone avoiding the risk that the two parts come into contact with each other in an incorrect way. Galen ends by summarising his conclusion succinctly (18b.332.1–3 K.): 'It has been demonstrated that the treatment of dislocations and fractures must begin with the extension (ὅτι μὲν οὖν ἀπὸ κατατάσεως ἄρχεσθαι προσήκει τὴν θεραπείαν τῶν ἐξαρθρημάτων τε καὶ καταγμάτων ἐπιδέδεικται).'

Galen then turns to the second question posed by the Hippocratic lemma: why must the extension be made in a straight line? Once again Galen widens his enquiry: the 'straight' position is not only required in extensions, as Hippocrates says here, but in all the four operations in the field of bone surgery: *katátasis* (stretching), *diáplasis* (setting), *epídesis* (bandaging), *apóthesis* (immobilising). The terminology is only partly Hippocratic: among the names of the four operations (*enérgeiai*) neither *diáplasis* nor *apóthesis* are attested in the Hippocratic Corpus; Galen thus silently updates terminology according to contemporaneous technical vocabulary. Moreover, nowhere in the Hippocratic surgical treatises do we find these four operations listed together; Galen adduces them here to give a complete account. He does not, however, dwell on the fact that he is adding something missing in the text and only says that these operations follow one another stressing the fact that a change in the limb's position can affect the final result. Then he concludes (18b.322.15–17 K.): 'It has therefore been demonstrated that there must be one single common position for the four operations (ὅτι μὲν οὖν ἓν εἶναι δεῖ σχῆμα κοινὸν τῶν εἰρημένων τεττάρων ἐνεργειῶν ἐπιδέδεικται)'.

Finally, tackling the question of why the correct position is 'as straight as possible', Galen begins explaining what the straight position entails: the muscles are more relaxed in this position and the patient feels less pain. If, however, the muscle is twisted, the tension is greater, so that the patient feels more pain and may also suffer from spasms. Galen correctly claims that Hippocrates himself adhered to this idea; and this is confirmed by experience (*peîra*): 'experience also shows that this is the least painful position (καὶ μὲν δὴ καὶ ἡ πεῖρα δείκνυσιν ἀνωδυνώτατον εἶναι τοῦτο τὸ σχῆμα)'.[36] Galen thus relies on the two main recognized sources of authority: Hippocrates' account (*historía*) and experience (*peîra*). Later in the commentary he will also argue on the basis of anatomy:[37]

36 Ibid. 18b.334.15–16 K.; see also 18b.467.2 K.

37 Ibid. 18b.368.17–369.2 K.

ὅτι μὲν οὖν ὀδυνῶδές ἐστιν ἡ πεῖρά σε διδάξει. τὴν δ' αἰτίαν τῆς ὀδύνης ἡ φύσις τῶν κινούντων μυῶν τὴν κατ' ἀγκῶνα διάρθρωσιν ἐπιδείξεται.

Experience will teach you that [this position] is painful; the nature of the muscles which move the joint in the elbow will show you the cause for the pain.

and on the basis of logical-deductive reasoning:[38]

ἀλλὰ νῦν γε πρόσεχέ μοι τὸν νοῦν· ὅπως ἂν [ἢ] ὁ λογισμὸς[39] εὑρίσκῃ τὸ προσῆκον, οὐ περιμενεῖς[40] μακρὰν πεῖραν.

Now pay attention to my words: if reason finds what is required, you will not need to wait for a long experience.

In conclusion, the commentary on this first lemma sets out in a systematic way the fundamentals of bone injuries; in doing so, Galen tends to minimize the differences between his exposition and that of Hippocrates: modestly, he 'claims' to anticipate something that will be discussed later by Hippocrates himself; he simply presents in a systematic way what disparate remarks found in *Fractures*. But in fact, he also reminds his audience of the anatomy of bones and muscles and invites them to pay attention to pain as a criterion for evaluating whether an intervention is correctly carried out or not.

4 A Platonic Echo

For a better understanding of Galen's approach to the Hippocratic text, I shall conclude by discussing a passage of the commentary on the lemma 'I am forced to write more on this topic (Ἀναγκάζομαι δὲ πλείω γράφειν περὶ αὐτέου)'.[41] It still belongs to early part of the commentary where Galen explores more general points. Here, Galen exploits the opportunity to recall the didactic principle of freeing the mind of students from errors and prejudices before teaching them new things. Galen states:[42]

38 Ibid. 18b.543.5–7 K.

39 [ἢ] ὁ λογισμὸς scripsi : ἢ ὁ λογικὸς P, ἢν ὁ λογικὸς K.

40 περιμενεῖς scripsi : περιμένει P edd.

41 *Fracture* 1, 3.414.3–4 L., Kühlewein (1902), vol. 2, p. 46, lines 12–13.

42 *Commentary On Hippocrates' 'Fractures'*, 18b.340.1–19 K.

> ἐπεὶ τοίνυν ἐγινώσκετο μὲν ὀρθῶς τοῖς κατ' αὐτὸν ἰατροῖς ὡς χρὴ τὸν ἰατρὸν κατάτασιν ἡγεῖσθαι τῆς συμπάσης θεραπείας τῶν ἐξαρθρωμάτων τε καὶ καταγμάτων, ἠγνοεῖτο δὲ τὸ κατὰ φύσιν σχῆμα, διὰ τοῦτο περὶ πρώτου τοῦδε τὸν λόγον ἐποιήσατο, καὶ πολύ γε μᾶλλον ἔτι διότι τὰ χείριστα τῶν σχημάτων ἔνιοι τῶν ἰατρῶν αἱρούμενοι [ἐρχόμενοι][43] πρὸ τοῦ βελτίστου μοχθηροῖς λόγοις ἑαυτούς τε καὶ τοὺς ἄλλους ἔπειθον. εἰ μὲν ἁπλῶς ἠγνόουν, διδασκαλίας ἂν αὐτοῖς ἀληθοῦς ἔδει· ἐπεὶ δ' οὐ μόνον ἠγνόουν, ἀλλὰ καὶ προσειλήφεσαν οἴησιν γνώσεως, *ἀναγκαῖον ἐγένετο τῷ Ἱπποκράτει πρότερον ἐκκόψαντι τήνδε καὶ καθαρὰν ἐργασαμένῳ τὴν ψυχήν*, οὕτως ἀληθῶς εἰς αὐτὴν ἐντιθέναι τὴν τῶν ἀληθῶν ἐπιστήμην.
>
> Since the physicians of his time recognised correctly that extension belongs to any treatment of dislocations and fractures, but did not know the natural position, he first discussed this matter. An even more important reason for this was the fact that some physicians chose the worst positions instead of the best, persuading themselves and others with flawed reasoning. If they simply lacked knowledge [of this matter], it would have been enough to teach them [the right position]. But since they not only lacked knowledge, but also believed to have knowledge, Hippocrates had *to remove this false opinion first by wiping their souls*, and then put true knowledge of the correct facts into it.

As we have already seen, Galen justified the untidy arrangement of the argument in *Fractures* in psychological terms: Hippocrates had an urge to say the most important things first. Yet he also recalls the pedagogical principle of first expunging false opinions from students' minds and then teach them true knowledge. This principle goes back to Plato's *Phaedrus* 67b: 'it is not licit that a pure thing is touched by something impure (καθαρὸς μὴ καθαρῷ ἐφάψασθαι μὴ οὐχὶ θεμιτόν)' and to another unidentified Platonic quotation: 'you will hurt the impure souls the more you teach them good doctrines (τὰς μὴ καθαρὰς τῶν ψυχῶν ὁκόσα ἂν διδάξῃ χρηστὰ δόγματα μᾶλλον βλάψεις)'. This second quote from Plato can be compared with the Hippocratic *Aphorism* 2.10 'The more you feed the impure bodies, the more you will hurt them (τὰ μὴ καθαρὰ σώματα ὁκόσῳ ἂν θρέψῃ μᾶλλον βλάψεις)'. This pedagogical topos had a long afterlife in the late-antique medical and philosophical introductory literature; and the Hippocratic aphorism became extremely popular in the Neoplatonic medical schools of late-antique Alexandria.[44]

43 P, secl. edd.

44 Examples include the anonymous Alexandrian text *On Medicine*, published by Dietz

The oldest evidence for the link between the *Aphorism* 2.10 and Plato in terms of pedagogy is found in Galen. At the end of the first book of *Simple Drugs*, he outlines the plan of the work and insists on the need to clear before the minds of errors and prejudices (in fact, he devotes two entire books to this task). Only afterwards does he turn to outlining his own theory of simple drugs. To justify his approach, he invokes the authority of both Hippocrates and Plato:[45]

> The first book ends here. In the second, I shall take the example of olive oil and rose oil to show also there that many physicians employ erroneous methods in their practice, deceiving themselves and many others through false reasoning. Once I have done this, I shall move on to the third book of this work and endeavour to explain the rational investigations used to provide a complete description of simple drugs. Then in book four I shall define the powers of all the simple drugs. I would have started with this, had it not been for the fact that nearly all the books of modern physicians are replete with faulty reasoning. These faulty arguments need to be expunged and removed from the learners' soul first (ἐκκαθᾶραί τε καὶ ἀποσκευάσασθαι χρὴ πρῶτον ἐκ τῆς τοῦ μανθάνοντος ψυχῆς), so that they do not impede correct ones. For as Hippocrates said, and as Plato confirmed: not only do you damage impure bodies the more you feed them, but also impure souls; if you offer them nourishing discourses, you not only bring no benefit whatsoever to them, but you also harm them significantly (ὡς γὰρ Ἱπποκράτης φησίν, οὕτω καὶ Πλάτων ἔλεγεν· οὐ μόνον τὰ μὴ καθαρὰ σώματα, ὁπόσῳ ἂν θρέψῃς μᾶλλον βλάψεις, ἀλλὰ καὶ ταῖς ἀκαθάρτοις ψυχαῖς, εἰ τροφίμους προσφέρεις λόγους, οὐ μόνον οὐδὲν ὠφελήσῃς ἂν ἀλλὰ καὶ βλάψεις οὐ σμικρά). Therefore, because many of my friends wanted me to criticise the faulty arguments of modern physicians not just during the social gatherings which we organised and at which we spent time together, but also through this work, I had to spend more time on the

(1834), Usener (1859), Flashar (1962), Roselli (1998) and Kapetanaki, Sharples (2006); the commentaries on the *Aphorisms* by Theophilus and Damascius (Dietz 1834, vol. 2, p. 245, lines 16–19); Palladius' *Commentary on Galen's 'Sects'* (Baffioni 1958, p. 72, line 1); Olympiodorus' *Introduction* (Busse 1902, p. 10, lines 5–8: μὴ καθαρὸν γὰρ καθαροῦ ἐφάπτεσθαι μὴ οὐχὶ θεμιτόν ἐστιν, ὡς ὁ θεῖος Πλάτων φασί, καὶ Ἱπποκράτης τὰ μὴ καθαρὰ τῶν σωμάτων ὁκόσῳ ἂν θρέψῃς μᾶλλον βλάψεις); *Commentary on Plato's 'Alcibiades'* (Westerink 1956, p. 137, lines 6–8 and p. 226, lines 7–9) and *Commentary on Plato's 'Gorgias'* (Westerink 1970, p. 40, lines 23–24); *Explanations on Galen's 'Method of Healing'* (Lorusso 2010, p. 117 lines 1–30); see Anastassiou-Irmer (2012), 75–77.

45 Galen, *Simple Drugs*, 11.456.11–458.6 K.

> first two books, so that by the third the audience would be pure in their soul and able to follow the correct arguments. Let me explain the theoretical principles of the subject before us with which one needs to be familiar, and then list all the powers of each drug. I shall do this in eleven books, each of the same size as this very first one. Since this [first book] has acquired the right size, I shall end it with these words.

When commenting on *Fractures*, Galen did not mention the Hippocratic aphorism nor did he mention Plato, but the allusion to them is absolutely clear. Both in the commentary and in the treatise on *Simple Drugs*, Galen assumed the same pedagogical attitude that he attributed to Hippocrates himself.

5 After Galen

Thanks to Galen's commentaries, *Fractures* and *Joints* became core texts in the medical curriculum on bone surgery.[46] Although unsystematic and at times odd, they remained a source of valid insights into how to practice surgery in the Imperial Age and beyond.

46 See Anastassiou, Irmer (1997–2012), vol. 2.2, pp. 162–166 (Testimonies on *Joints*) and pp. 239–246 (Testimonies on *Fractures*).

CHAPTER 12

Galen and Pseudo-Galen in Conversation: *Epidemics* 2.3.2 and *Aphorisms* 4.5

Véronique Boudon-Millot

As a preliminary caveat, I want to emphasise that I do not intend to comment on the content of the two Hippocratic texts under scrutiny here (*Epidemics* 2.3.2 and *Aphorisms* 4.5), nor to interpret them or to establish their text. Rather, my aim is to study the way in which these two passages were copied and interpreted not only by Galen in his commentaries on the *Epidemics* and the *Aphorisms*, but also in the treatise *Theriac to Piso*. In this latter treatise, the author uses a different text for these two passages than that given in Galen's commentaries, and suggests a completely different interpretation. Therefore, if Galen really is the author, this creates a small mystery that obviously needs to be addressed.

The author of *Theriac to Piso* (14.210–294 K.; Boudon-Millot 2016) mentions the name of Hippocrates five times and includes three verbatim quotations of the Hippocratic text:

- chapter 1.9 (14.213 K.; Boudon-Millot 2016, p. 4, line 21) quoting μηδὲν εἰκῇ ποιεῖν (Hippocrates, *Epidemics* 6.2.12.1; 5.284.1 L.; Smith 1994, p. 230, line 7; Manetti, Roselli 1982, p. 36, line 8);
- chapter 4.13–14 (14.228 K.; Boudon-Millot 2016, p. 17, line 20–p. 18, line 8) quoting Hippocrates, *Epidemics* 2.3.2 (5.104.6–12 L.; Smith 1994, 50; Anastassiou, Irmer 1997–2012, vol. 2.2, p. 165);
- chapter 17.4 (14.285 K.; Boudon-Millot 2016, p. 85, line 17–p. 86, line 2) quotation of Hippocrates, *Aphorisms* 4.5 (4.502 L., also quoted by Galen, *On the Sects for Beginners* 8 [Helmreich 1893, p. 20, lines 8–9; 1.89.17 K.]).

The author of *Theriac to Piso* moreover refers to Hippocrates in two other instances without an explicit citation:

- chapter 11.8 (14.252 K.; Boudon-Millot 2016, p. 53, line 14): reference to *Epidemics* 6.2.4 (Smith 1994, 72) in the context of Hippocrates' advice to provoke an outburst of anger in weak patients, in order to cure their lethargy by the vigour of the anger;
- chapter 16.12 (14.281 K.; Boudon-Millot 2016, p. 82, line 1): the author of *Theriac to Piso* confuses the famous 'plague' of Athens described by Thucydides, which originated in Ethiopia (the Abyssinia of the Arabs) and lasted from 430 to 429, with another plague that came from the North and prob-

© VÉRONIQUE BOUDON-MILLOT, 2021 | DOI:10.1163/9789004470200_014

ably happened during the years 419–16. This latter plague is mentioned in the *Embassy* (9.418.4–5 L.) as 'a plague proceeding through the countries of the Barbarians, which lie beyond Illyria and Paeonia (ὁκότε λοιμοῦ ῥέοντος διὰ τῆς βαρβάρου, ᾗ ὑπέρκειται Ἰλλυριῶν καὶ Παιόνων)'.

Yet, when the author cites Hippocrates explicitly, as he does in the two passages in *Epidemics* 2.3.2 and *Aphorisms* 4.5, he does not give the same version of the Hippocratic text as that in Galen's commentaries. In a case like this, one can always argue that the variations, if they do not result from the textual tradition (which is always a possibility), can be explained by the fact that Galen did not always use the same copy of Hippocrates throughout his career.[1] Nevertheless, in this case we are actually dealing with two different authors. As a matter of fact, *Theriac to Piso*, as I have already tried to demonstrate elsewhere, is the work of an *archiatrós* who lived a short while after Galen, and whose work was integrated into the Galenic corpus at a very early stage, probably at the turn of the third to fourth century AD.[2] Our purpose therefore is to use *Theriac to Piso* to recover a different interpretation of the Hippocratic text than that provided by Galen in his commentaries and to resuscitate a reading of the Hippocratic text not attested elsewhere based on the author of *Theriac to Piso* (whom I shall from now on refer to as Pseudo-Galen).

1 *Epidemics* 2.3.2

We will first look at a difficult and controversial passage from *Epidemics* 2.3.2. This passage has been transmitted through a direct and indirect manuscript tradition that presents multiple important differences. The abundant material available to edit and interpret this passage seems not to have been addressed before. It includes:

---

1 In his edition of *On the Nature of Man*, J. Jouanna (2002) discusses certain differences between the lemmas in Galen's commentary and passages he quotes elsewhere in *Elements According to Hippocrates* and *Doctrines of Hippocrates and Plato*. These differences can be explained as resulting from a reconstruction of the lemmas under the influence of the Hippocratic tradition. Jouanna remarks (p. 107, n. 3) that in certain cases 'it is possible that throughout his career Galen did not always use the same copy of *On the Nature of Man*'. Similarly, P. de Lacy (1996, 206) writes that '[i]t is quite possible that the text of *De natura hominis* used by Galen for *In Hippocratis De natura hominis comm.* was different from the text he used for *De elementis*'.

2 For arguments in favour of a apocryphal character of *Theriac for Piso*, see Boudon-Millot (2021), and my edition of the treatise (Boudon-Millot 2016). See also the arguments given by Leigh (2016), although they are not always coherent.

- The Hippocratic text edited by Littré and Smith (= Hipp).[3]
- Galen's *Commentary on Hippocrates' 'Epidemics' 2*, which has only been preserved in Arabic, first translated into German by Pfaff (Wenkebach, Pfaff 1934, p. 265, lines 10–22) and more recently edited and translated into English by Vagelpohl (2016, p. 457, lines 8–16) (= Gal^{ar}).
- The *Commentary on the Epidemics 2* falsely attributed to Galen (= PsGal^{com}), compiled in Latin by Rasarius from authentic passages and other ancient sources. It was edited for the first time in Latin in Venice for the Juntine press in 1586. John Sozomen of Cyprus, the librarian of Venice, reconstructed it in 1617 in Greek, and René Chartier (1679, vol. 9) and Kühn (17a.401.3–10 K.) reproduced this Greek version in their complete works of Galen. Littré, who considered it to be authentic, then quoted it in his critical apparatus under the abbreviation 'Gal'.[4]
- to these, we should add the passage in *Theriac to Piso* as it is transmitted through numerous Greek manuscripts and also preserved in an Arabic translation (= Ar); the Arabic translation, however, only provides loose paraphrase of the text and is therefore of no use here.

This leaves us with three main witnesses: the passage in the direct tradition; the passage of Galen in the commentary preserved in Arabic; and the quotation of the passage in *Theriac to Piso*. An analysis of these witnesses allows us to clarify the persisting editorial problems, even if we cannot solve them, as well as to revive, so to speak, the ghost of a new interpreter of Hippocrates, who has hitherto remained concealed: the anonymous author of *Theriac to Piso*. Let us begin by quoting these three main witnesses. The passage in the Hippocratic *Epidemics* 2.3.2 runs as follows, and I have put in bold the problematic words and expressions that I am going to discuss below:[5]

> Φαρμάκων δὲ τρόπους ἴσμεν, ἐξ ὧν γίνεται ὁκοῖα **ἄσσα** (ἅσσα Smith)· οὐ γὰρ πάντες ὁμοίως, ἀλλ' ἄλλοι ἄλλως **εὖ κεῖνται** (κέονται Smith)· καὶ ἄλλα ὅσα (ἄλλοθι Smith) πρωϊαίτερον ἢ ὀψιαίτερον **ληφθέντα**· καὶ οἱ διαχειρισμοί, οἷον ἢ ξηρᾶναι, ἢ κόψαι, ἢ ἑψῆσαι· καὶ **τὰ τοιαῦτα ἐῶ** τὰ πλεῖστα, καὶ **ὁκόσα** ἑκάστῳ, καὶ ἐφ' οἷσι νουσήμασι, καὶ ὁπότε τοῦ νουσήματος, ἡλικίην, εἴδεα, δίαιταν, ὁκοίῃ ὥρῃ ἔτεος, καὶ ἥτις καὶ ὁκοίως ἀγομένη, καὶ τὰ τοιαῦτα.

3 See the forthcoming edition by R. Alessi in the Collection des Universités de France, whom I thank for generously sharing the critical apparatus of the Hippocratic lemma under discussion.

4 On this false commentary, see Wenkebach in Wenkebach and Pfaff (1934), p. xxiii, n. 1 and Fortuna (2012), 308.

5 5.104.6–12 L.; Smith (1994), 50; Anastassiou, Irmer (1997–2012), vol. 2.2, p. 165.

Smith and Littré both provide a translation of this passage:

> We know the characteristics of drugs, from what ones come what kinds of things. For they are not all equally good, but different characteristics are good in different circumstances. In different places medical drugs are gathered earlier or later; also the preparations differ, such as drying, cruschin, boiling, and so on (I pass over most things); and how much for each person and in what diseases and when in the disease, in relation to age, appearance, regimen, what kind of season, what season and how it is developing, and the like.

> (Des médicaments évacuants). Nous connaissons la nature variée des médicaments évacuants, par laquelle ils produisent tels et tels effets; car tous ne conviennent pas semblablement, et les uns conviennent dans un cas, les autres dans un autre. Il y a encore les différences qui résultent de l'administration anticipée ou tardive; il y a les manipulations telles que dessécher, piler, cuire. J'omets beaucoup d'autres remarques du même genre: ainsi quelle dose pour chacun, dans quelle maladie, à quelle époque de la maladie, l'âge, l'habitude du corps, le régime, la saison de l'année, quel en est le caractère, quelle elle est, comment elle marche, et autres choses semblables.

Galen provides the following version of the lemma in his commentary:[6]

> قال أبقراط: وضروب الأدوية التي منها تكون قد نعلم أنها هذه: كيف هي **وما هي** فإنها ليست كلها متشابهة لكن تركيب بعضها على خلاف تركيب البعض. فإنّ هذا أيضا قد يكون منه اختلاف، ومن أن يتقدم في تناولها أو يتأخر، وفي صنعتها أيضا مثل أن تجفف أو أن تطبخ أو أن تدق وما أشبه ذلك. **وأدع ذكر ما هو أكثر من ذلك** وكم لكلّ واحد وفي أيّ الأمراض ومتى من المرض وبحسب السنّ والسحنة والتدبير والوقت من السنة أيّ وقت هو وكيف يجري أمره وما أشبه ذلك.

> Hippocrates said: **And** we know what these kinds of drugs consist of, how and **what they are**. They are not all similar but some have a different composition than others. They also differ in the following, for example

6 Galen, *Commentary on the Epidemics* 2.2.12.1; Vagelpohl (2016, p. lines 456, 7–12 [text] and p. 457, lines 8–16 [translation]).

> whether they are taken earlier or later, and also in their preparation, for example whether they are dried, boiled or crushed and so forth—**I shall not mention more of this**—, how much for each one, for which diseases, when during the disease, relative to age, appearance, regimen, what the season is, how it is progressing and the like.

The author of *Theriac to Piso* gives this version of the Hippocratic text, for which I also quote my previous French translation and a new English one:[7]

> **Οὕτω** φαρμάκων **δὲ** τρόπους ἴσμεν ἐξ ὧν γεγένηται ὁκοῖα **ἄττα**. οὐ γὰρ πάντες ὁμοίως, ἀλλ' ἄλλοι ἄλλως **σύγκειται**, καὶ ἄλλα ὅσα πρωϊαίτερον ἢ ὀψιαίτερον **ληφθέντα**, καὶ οἱ διαχειρισμοί, οἷον ξηρᾶναι, ἢ κόψαι, ἢ ἑψῆσαι, καὶ τὰ τοιαῦτα. **ἐῶ τὰ πλεῖστα [μειώσῃ πλείω]**. καὶ **ὁκοῖα** ἑκάστῳ, καὶ ἐφ' οἷσι νοσήμασι, καὶ ἐφ' ᾧ τε τοῦ νοσήματος, ἡλικία, ἰδέα, καὶ δίαιτα, ὁκοῖα ἡ ὥρη ἔτεος, ὁκοίως ἄγομεν, καὶ τὰ τοιαῦτα.

> **Ainsi**, à propos des modes d'action des médicaments, **nous savons** d'où vient qu'ils (*sc.* les médicaments) soient tels ou tels, car ils (*sc.* leurs modes d'action) ne sont pas tous semblables, mais **se présentent** les uns d'une façon et les autres d'une autre: car il en est **que l'on récolte** de façon plutôt prématurée ou plutôt tardive; et aussi pour les opérations telles que dessécher, piler ou cuire, et les autres choses de la sorte. **J'omets la plupart**; et quels médicaments pour chacun, et pour quelles maladies et pour quel moment de la maladie, âge, constitution et régime, quelle est la saison de l'année, comment nous la passons, et les autres choses de la sorte.

> **Thus**, about the kinds of effect of drugs **we know** how they [sc. the drugs] come to be like this, because they [sc. the kinds of their effects] are not all alike, but the effects of drugs **appear** to be different from one another. For some of them **are harvested** rather early or rather late; and also for manipulations, such as drying, crushing, boiling, and other similar things. **I omit most**; and what drugs for each, and for what diseases, and for what moment in the [course of the] disease, the age, constitution or regimen, what season in the year, how we spend it, and other such things.

7 Pseudo-Galen, *Theriac to Piso* 14.14 (14.228–229 K.; Boudon-Millot 2016, p. 17, line 20–p. 18, line 8).

Finally, we also have the evidence of the Arabic translation of *Theriac to Piso*, edited by Richter Bernburg (1969, 27–28 [text], 66–67 [translation]), which, however, deviates from the Greek at times:

قد **ينبغي أن نتعرف** الوجوه التي تتصرف عليها الأدوية، وذلك أنه ليس كل دواء نافعا لكل إنسان بل لكل إنسان دواء من الأدوية المؤلفة فينبغي أن ننظر في الدواء الذي **يسقاه** المريض إلا بعد صنعته[8] بزمان، ومنها ما يجوز أن **يسقاه** وهو قريب العهد، ومنها ما لا ينبغي أن يسقاه الشاب، ومنها ما لا يسقى في زمان الصيف. فعلى هذه الطريق ينبغي أن يكون فحصنا عن الأدوية قبل استعمالنا إياها.

> We **must know** the different ways in which drugs behave. For not every drug is useful for every person, but each person has a [specific] compound drug. Therefore we must look at the drug which **is administered** to the patient only some time after its production. Other drugs **can be administered** near in time [of production]. Others should not be administered to young people. Others yet should not be administered during the summer. In this way we should examine drugs before using them.

The context of this quotation is chapter 4 of *Theriac to Piso*, where the author lists truly astonishing properties of certain simple medicines (καὶ θαῦμα τοῖς ὁρῶσι τὸ τοιοῦτον εἶναι δοκεῖ), which can be both dangerous and useful at the same time. According to the author, their efficiency depends on:

- which parts are used (seeds or leaves), for example in the case of aloe vera, the leaves cause intestinal problems, whereas the seeds may cause constipation.
- the method of cooking and whether one uses the gravy or the meat, as in the case of old roosters and sea snails: their gravy causes intestinal problems, but their meat causes constipation.
- the method of administering (external, or internal via the mouth); for instance, aloe and copper filings dry the skin when applied externally, but have a purgative effect when ingested.
- the method of preparation, as in the case of milk: in the form of whey, it relaxes the stomach, but in the form of cheese, it constipates.
- to whom it is administered or who ingests it, as in the case of hemlock or hellebore: certain animals (such as starlings and quail) can eat it, but it kill humans.

8 صنعته] coni. Pormann: ضيعته Richter-Bernburg.

– the parts of the body (lung, bladder, liver, kidney etc.) on which certain plants have a specific useful or harmful action; for example, agrimony is very useful for the liver, and myrobalan for the spleen, whereas sea slug cause ulcers in the lungs, and Spanish flies in the bladder.

The author of *Theriac to Piso*, moreover, boasts to have thoroughly reviewed other medicines appropriate for other parts of the body 'so as to use them appropriately in each condition (οἰκεῖα φάρμακα, ἅπερ ἡμεῖς, ὡς ἔφην, ἀκριβῶς ἐξετάζοντες οὕτως ἑκάστῳ τῶν παθῶν τὴν κατάλληλον προσφορὰν ποιούμεθα).'

The context of the passage is therefore clearly one of simple drugs, and of substances capable of curing certain parts of the body and certain symptoms. In these matters, as in all others, Pseudo-Galen claims to have the eminent Hippocrates as his master (διδασκάλῳ καὶ τούτων, ὥσπερ καὶ τῶν ἄλλων ἀπάντων, Ἱπποκράτει τῷ ἀρίστῳ χρώμενοι), who developed 'the art of medicines as thoroughly as possible as one can see from his numerous writings and particularly in what he says in book 2 of the *Epidemics* (ὅτι γὰρ ἀκριβεστάτην τὴν περὶ τῶν φαρμάκων τέχνην πεποίηται καὶ ἐξ ἄλλων πλείστων ὑπ' αὐτοῦ λεγομένων ἔστιν ἰδεῖν, μάλιστα δὲ ἐξ ὧν φησιν ἐν τῷ δευτέρῳ τῶν ἐπιδημιῶν).' Yet, in my edition of the passage,[9] the Hippocratic quotation presents various problems and has been interpreted in different ways.

Galen gives us the same information in his commentary on the *Epidemics* 2.3.2, where he identifies a number of textual problems and lists the various ways in which the different commentators tried to solve them. The first is the question of what is the beginning of the Hippocratic lemma and, consequently, what is the beginning of its citation in *Theriac to Piso*? In his commentary, which has only been preserved in Arabic (Gal^{ar}), Galen notes (Vagelpohl 2016, p. 456, line 13) that some used to write *qad naʿlamu annahā*, (ἴσμεν, 'we know'), but that others wrote *li-naʿlama annaha*, which Vagelpohl (2016, p. 457, line 17), translates as 'so that we know'. I think, however, that we have to take the verb as a jussive (*li-naʿlam*) and understand it to mean 'let us know that'. These Hippocratic words introduce (simple) information in the first case, and in the latter, a kind of advice. Yet, it seems to me that this variant reading in the Arabic renders the Greek words οὕτω ἴσμεν 'thus we know'. It turns out that the author of *Theriac to Piso* has preserved exactly such a reading. He begins his quotation with the adverb οὕτω, which, according to Pseudo-Galen, does not serve to introduce Hippocrates' words,[10] but constitutes the first word of the lemma.

9 Boudon-Millot (2016), p. 17, line 20–p. 18, line 8; see especially the critical apparatus.

10 Contrary to what the punctuation of the old manuscript *Laurentianus Plut* 74, 5 (12th century) seems to indicate, in which the period is placed after οὕτω: μάλιστα δὲ ἐξ ὧν φησιν ἐν τῷ δευτέρῳ τῶν ἐπιδημιῶν οὕτω. φαρμάκων δὲ κτλ.

Thus, we find the first difference between the two authors in the fact that Galen chooses to begin the lemma in his commentary with φαρμάκων, while Pseudo-Galen begins his citation with οὕτω.

Moreover, in the same commentary, Galen explains that some scholars link the Hippocratic lemma to the preceding sentence by adding 'and (δὲ or τε)' and thus read φαρμάκων τε (as one finds it in the Hippocratic manuscripts) or φαρμάκων δὲ (as in the case of the author of *Theriac to Piso*), while others disagree with such a connection and consider the lemma to be completely independent from what precedes it.[11] In writing φαρμάκων δὲ, the author of *Theriac to Piso* has chosen the first option, that of coordination. He thus follows Galen, who begins the lemma with the Arabic '*wa-* (and)', although it is impossible to know whether Galen read φαρμάκων τε (as in the tradition going back directly to Hippocrates) or φαρμάκων δὲ (as the author of *Theriac to Piso*). In this case, Galen and the author of *Theriac to Piso* partly adopt the same solution.

The second problem is how to translate τρόπους: as 'species' or 'genus' as opposed to 'way' of 'mode'.[12] In the Arabic version of his commentary, Galen gives τρόπους a meaning close to γένη (genus or kind)[13] and understood this term to refer to 'the kinds (τρόποι) of medicine of which we know their components', when talking about compound drugs. For Galen, the Hippocratic phrase refers to a particular category of compound drugs, namely purgatives. This interpretation has been adopted by Littré in the title which he adds before this paragraph, namely '*Des médicaments évacuants* (On purgatives)'.

The author of *Theriac to Piso*, however, understands τρόπους to refer in this context to 'the effects of drugs.' He avoids the term later on by using the word 'natures (φύσεις)' instead. As he explains immediately afterwards, by using these words Hippocrates wants us to know 'the nature' of drugs (παραινῶν καὶ τὰς φύσεις τῶν φαρμάκων εἰδέναι). This quotation is found in the middle of a chapter of *Theriac to Piso* devoted to, as we have seen, the particular effect of individual substances and thus relates to the nature of simple drugs only; this is the second difference between Pseudo-Galen and Galen.

We find another difference in the fact that in his commentary Galen divides the rest of the lemma using three interrogative pronouns after ἴσμεν: 'what they consist of, how they are, and what they are,'[14] corresponding to the Greek ἐξ

11 'Some attach this passage to the previous one and insert the connector and between them, others detach and separate this passage and drop the "and" so that this passage begins as follows: "we know what these kinds of drugs consist of".' (Vagelpohl 2016, pp. 457–459).

12 On the different meanings of τρόπος, see Kühn et al. (1986–1989, s.v.).

13 'we know what these kinds of drugs consist of.' (Vagelpohl 2016, 459).

14 'what these kinds of drugs consist of, how and what they are' (Vagelpohl 2016, 457), which

ὧν γεγένηται, ὁκοῖα, ἅττα. The last of these interrogatives, ἅττα or ἅσσα (with rough breathing, the equivalent of ἅτινα) is also given by the majority of Hippocratic manuscripts (V I R).[15] The author of *Theriac to Piso*, however, adopts a different reading: in the same place he uses the indefinite ἄττα or ἄσσα (with soft breathing, equivalent of the enclitic τινά), which is given in only one of the Hippocratic manuscripts (R). The author of *Theriac to Piso* has understood, therefore, that thanks to Hippocrates we know 'from where they [the simple drugs] have come to be such things (ἐξ ὧν γεγένηται ὁκοῖα ἄττα)'. This is the third difference.

Another conundrum is the omission of ὁμοίως and whether to read σύγκειν-ται or εὖ κεῖνται in the subsequent phrase: οὐ γὰρ πάντες ὁμοίως, ἀλλ' ἄλλοι ἄλλως σύγκεινται. The masculine forms πάντες and ἄλλοι can only have τρόποι as their antecedent. One may notice that in both cases Galen and the author of *Theriac to Piso* read the same text: ὁμοίως (adopted by Littré and R. Alessi, but omitted in all the Hippocratic manuscripts) and σύγκεινται (instead of εὖ κεῖνται), a mistake which Robert Alessi suggests can be explained by an obvious error in capital letters (ΕΥΚΕΙΝΤΑΙ misread as ΣΥΓΚΕΙΝΤΑΙ). The reading σύγκειν-ται must be wrong. In the Hippocratic Corpus, as well the Galenic corpus, this verb does not refer to (ingredients) being mixed, but to (a whole) being composed (of parts): it is an anatomical term which describes the composition of the body in *Places in Man* (6.278.4 L.), or that of the parts of the body in *On Fractures* (3.348.13 L.), and that of the trachea in *Anatomy* (8.538.3 L. etc.). In the Galenic corpus, we do not find the verb σύγκειμαι used in reference to the composition of drugs, but συντίθημι.[16]

Galen and the author of *Theriac to Piso* must therefore have read the same Hippocratic text with the false reading of σύγκεινται, whose origin can probably be traced back to a same exemplar written in capital letters. Nevertheless, even here the two authors do not give similar interpretations. Galen understands σύγκεινται as a synonym of συντίθημι, referring to the mixing of drugs

means that Galen (as he explains this later on in his commentary) sees these as 1) of what the drugs consist, 2) the differences between the nature of the drugs, i.e. their properties, and 3) the individual substances of the simple drugs that are part of a compound drug. Galen remarks elsewhere that these three terms are listed by some in the order 1-3-2, which seems better to him because 'one should first know the substance of the compound drug, before knowing its properties.'

15 The abbreviations refer to the following manuscripts: V = Vaticanus gr. 276 (12th cent.); I = Parisinus gr. 2140 (13th cent.); R = Vaticanus gr. 277 (14th cent.).

16 Even if in other texts σύγκειμαι sometimes serves as the perfect passive of συντίθημι (see *LSJ Dictionary*).

('compound drugs differ from each other' according to the Arabic in his commentary),[17] which creates a syntactical difficulty, as the subject of σύγκεινται can only be τρόποι and not φάρμακα.

By contrast, the author of *Theriac to Piso* takes τρόποι as the subject of σύγκεινται, and, in accordance with the context of chapter 4—simple drugs can, depending on the case, produce different or even opposite effects—he understands that 'the effects of drugs (which he calls their "natures") appear (σύγκεινται) to be different from one another.'

Let us now turn to the question of how to interpret ληφθέντα. In his commentary, Galen considers ληφθέντα to relate to harvesting drugs, notably at the correct moment, for instance when they are very ripe, or when they are not yet ripe:[18]

أن الأدوية المركبة يخالف بعضها بعضا في طبائع الأدوية المفردة التي تركب منها وفي كيفياتها
وفي أوقات التقاطها، فإن منها ما يلتقط وقد نضج ثمره ومنها ما يلتقط وثمره فج.

> ... compound drugs differ from each other in the natures and qualities of the simple drugs from which they are composed and in the times at which they are picked, because some are collected when their fruit is ripe, and others when it is not ripe yet.

However, Galen also writes that some commentators thought that the participle related to drugs that must be taken (ληφθέντα) by the patient sooner or later during his disease.[19] Galen rejects this interpretation (which was adopted by Littré).[20] Like Galen, the author of *Theriac to Piso* understands the participle to relate to the moment at which simple drugs must be picked, as for example in the case of clover, about which Pseudo-Galen has previously written the following:[21]

---

17 See the quotation of Galen's explanation below.

18 Vagelpohl (2016), p. 458, lines 3–5 (text); p. 459, lines 3–5 (translation, with slight modifications).

19 Vagelpohl (2016), p. 460, lines 15–16 (text); p. 461, lines 16–17 (translation): 'لا أبدان المستعملين لها كما ظن قوم (... not the bodies of those who take them, as some people have thought.)'

20 'Il y a encore les différences qui résultent de l'administration anticipée ou tardive (There will also be differences depending on whether the drug is taken early or late).' (5.105 L.).

21 Pseudo-Galen, *Theriac to Piso* 4.7 (14.227 K.; Boudon-Millot 2016, p. 16, line 7). The Arabic translator (quoted above) read the same text, but understood the Greek ληφθέντα differently, namely as referring to the time when a drug is administered to the patient (*yusqāhu*) after production (*ba'da ṣan'atihī*).

> τὸ γοῦν τρίφυλλον, ἡ βοτάνη ἥτις τῷ ὑακίνθῳ ὡμοίωται, ὁπότε τοῦ ἔαρος ἐγκύμων γένεται καὶ τὸ σπέρμα ὅμοιον ἔχει τῇ ἀγρίᾳ κνίκῳ, ὅταν τις ἀφεψήσῃ πάνυ, εἶτα τῷ δήγματι τοῦ φαλαγγίου ἢ καὶ τοῦ ἔχεως τῷ ὕδατι ἐπαντλήσῃ, ἰᾶται αὐτὸ καὶ εὐθέως ἀνώδυνον ἐργάζεται.
>
> When one rightly boils clover, the plant which resembles hyacinth, when it matures in spring and releases seeds similar to that of wild safflower, and applies it with water on the bite of a spider or even a snake, it cures it and immediately alleviates the pain.

Likewise, the author of *Theriac to Piso* argues later on that the ideal time to hunt snakes (a principal ingredient of theriac) is 'not every season, but preferably at the beginning of spring (μὴ ἐν παντὶ καιρῷ τεθηραμένας, ἀλλὰ μάλιστα περὶ τὴν ἀρχὴν τοῦ ἔαρος).'[22]

Let us next look at the question of what καὶ τὰ τοιαῦτα refers to and how one should deal with the variant readings ἕως versus ἐῶ. These textual problems occur in the next passage, which discusses the different ways of preparation of simple drugs (whether one should dry, ground, or boil them). We find a number of significant difficulties as well as yet another difference of interpretation between Galen and the author of *Theriac to Piso*. A first difficulty relates to punctuation. When Galen cites the Hippocratic lemma in his commentary, he puts a full stop after 'καὶ τὰ τοιαῦτα (and other similar things.)', which he seems to interpret as 'καὶ τὰ λοιπά (and so on)'. In this way, 'καὶ τὰ τοιαῦτα' refers back to the previous list of 'manipulations' 'such as drying, crushing, boiling'. Littré, however, takes καὶ τὰ τοιαῦτα with what follows, namely to 'ἐῶ τὰ πλεῖστα', and translates the sentence as 'j' omets beaucoup d' autres remarques du même genre (I omit many other remarks of this kind).' If we rely on the punctuation of the oldest manuscript of *Theriac to Piso* (the *Laurentianus gr*. 74, 5), which places a period after καὶ τὰ τοιαῦτα, Pseudo-Galen seems to have understood the Hippocratic text similarly to Galen (or at least similarly to the Arabic translator of the lemma), but differently from Littré. The clear punctuation after the first καὶ τὰ τοιαῦτα actually establishes a parallel with the second καὶ τὰ τοιαῦτα where the quotation ends.

What did Galen read next? The manuscripts that can be directly traced back to Hippocrates read ἐῶ τὰ πλεῖστα. However, the Arabic expression '*mā huwa akṯaru min ḏālika* (more than that)' which translates the Hippocratic lemma

---

22 Ibid. 13.7 (14.264 K.; Boudon-Millot 2016, p. 65, line 3); the Arabic translator chose to understand like some commentators that the participle was related to drugs that must be taken (ληφθέντα) by the patient; see the discussion above.

quoted by Galen in his commentary seems to indicate that Galen did not read a superlative τὰ πλεῖστα but rather a comparative (πλείω *or* πλείονα): 'I shall not mention more of this.' In *Theriac to Piso*, we find an interesting variant reading in this place: 'καὶ τὰ τοιαῦτα ἕως τὰ πλεῖστα μειώσῃ πλείω'. In fact, the words μειώσῃ πλείω (added here to the Hippocratic text and with no equivalent in the Hippocratic manuscripts from the direct tradition) are likely to be a marginal gloss inserted into the text of *Theriac to Piso* by accident. '⟨Ση⟩μείωσαι πλείω (read "πλείω")' indicates an old variant reading πλείω for πλεῖστα, which was probably already known to Galen and which has only been preserved in *Theriac to Piso*.[23] The reading 'ἕως (until)' in *Theriac to Piso* instead of 'ἐῶ (I leave)' in the Hippocratic manuscripts likely results from the addition of a simple ς and a reconstruction which aimed to make the text readable after the incorrect insertion of the gloss ⟨ση⟩μείωσαι πλείω.

In conclusion, the oldest manuscript of *Theriac to Piso* (L) and its apographs have preserved an ancient gloss inserted by accident and unknown in other versions of the Hippocratic text, which proposes to read πλείω, a reading probably accepted and quoted by Galen in his *Commentary on the Epidemics*, instead of τὰ πλεῖστα, the only reading attested in the direct manuscripts of the Hippocratic text and also adopted by the author of *Theriac to Piso*.

The next textual difficulty regards ὁκοῖα versus ὁκόσα, about which Galen and Pseudo-Galen also differ. The author *Theriac to Piso* writes 'ὁκοῖα (which)' instead of 'ὁκόσα (how many)', which is given by the manuscripts of the Hippocratic text, thus substituting quality for quantity (or dose).[24] The author of *Theriac to Piso* wants to understand how a simple drug (or a particular part of a simple drug) can be a useful remedy for one person, but harmful for another. In this context, it is the quality (ὁκοῖα: which drugs for whom) which interests the author, and not that of the quantity or dose (ὁκόσα: how much for whom).

The subsequent part of the quotation contains several other textual problems. These include the use of ὁκοῖα before ἡ ὥρη as given by Pseudo-Galen instead of ὁκοίη given by the Hippocratic manuscripts but omitted by Galen in his quotation of the lemma; καὶ ἥτις καὶ in the Hippocratic manuscripts, rightly

---

23 I thank Ivan Garofalo, who suggested this solution to me after my talk on which this article is based.

24 In his commentary, Galen says that Hippocrates had the reading 'ὁκόσα' in the sense of 'how much'; to quote: 'وقال أولا: «وكم لكل واحد» يعني كم ينبغي أن يقدم لكل واحد من المرضى من الدواء الذي ألف (First he said: "how much for each one", that is, how much of the prepared drug should be given to each patient)' (Vagelpohl 2016, p. 462, lines 14–15 [text]; p. 463, lines 17–18 [translation]).

read by Galen but omitted by Pseudo-Galen; as well as ἀγομένη in the Hippocratic manuscripts, adopted by Galen but read as ἄγομεν by Pseudo-Galen. However, these differences are not so clear cut as to show different interpretations by the two authors regarding the end of this passage. I shall therefore not dwell on them, even though these questions must, naturally, be addressed by editors of Hippocrates, Galen, as well as Pseudo-Galen.

To conclude, in the Arabic translation of his commentary, Galen interprets the lemma from Hippocrates' *Epidemics* 2.3.2 as only relating to compound purgative drugs, as did Littré who knew Galen's interpretative decision largely through the fake Renaissance commentary. The author of *Theriac to Piso*, however, cites the same Hippocratic passage in support of an argument regarding simple drugs. He continues to say:[25]

> διὰ γὰρ τούτων, ὡς ὁρᾷς, καθολικώτερον ἡμᾶς διδάσκει, παραινῶν καὶ τὰς φύσεις τῶν φαρμάκων εἰδέναι, καὶ τὸν καιρὸν ἐξετάζειν, ἐν ᾧ τις τὸ φάρμακον μέλλει λαμβάνειν, καὶ τὰς κράσεις τῶν λαμβανόντων ἐπιβλέπειν. εἰσὶ γὰρ ὡς ἀληθῶς οἱ μὲν εὐκόλως λαμβάνειν δυνάμενοι, ὡς καὶ πέπτειν αὐτὰ πολλάκις, ἢ κατὰ μηδὲν ὑπ' αὐτῶν κακοῦσθαι, ἀλλ' ἐνίοτε καὶ τροφὴν αὐτοῖς γίγνεσθαι αὐτὸ τὸ φάρμακον. ἔνιοι δὲ ἀφυῶς οὕτως ἔχουσι πρὸς τὰς φαρμακείας ὡς μηδὲ τὴν ἀρχὴν αὐταῖς χρῆσθαι δύνασθαι, ἀποστρέφεσθαί τε αὐτοῖς τὸν στόμαχον καὶ πρὸ τῆς χρήσεως ἐκλύεσθαι ῥᾳδίως.
>
> Through these words, as you see, he teaches us most generally, advising us to get to know the natures of drugs, to examine closely the time at which someone should take it, and to observe the temperaments of the patients. For there are some who can truly take certain drugs so well that they even digest them often; or when they do not suffer any disease, the drug serves them as food. But some have a nature so disposed against the drugs that they are unable to use them at all, and the stomach returns them and quickly dissolves them before they can be of use.

Therefore, the context of the Hippocratic quotation in *Theriac to Piso* and the passage following it which we have just quoted revolves around drugs that a patient can or cannot digest, or may or may not take according to his mixture. This shows that Galen and Pseudo-Galen interpreted this passage fundamentally differently, and we have also seen that they have many divergent readings.

---

25 Pseudo-Galen, *Theriac to Piso* c. 4.15–16 (14.229 K.; Boudon-Millot 2016, p. 18, line 8–p. 19, line 6).

Yet, they also share the incorrect variant σύγκειντα instead of the correct reading εὖ κεῖνται of the Hippocratic manuscripts. Therefore during their age, the Hippocratic text was already in the process of becoming fixed.

Finally, Pseudo-Galen effectively divides the quotation from the *Epidemics* 2.3.2 in three large sections concerning 1) the preparation of drugs in general; 2) the time when to administer drugs; and 3) the mixture of the patient. Yet, he omits the end of the quotation and does not comment on it, as the passage quoted above shows. Pseudo-Galen's *Theriac to Piso* thus provides a witness that allows us to uncover a different reading and interpretation of this passage of the *Epidemics*, an interpretation which competes with, and sometimes diverges from, Galen's quotation of the passage as preserved in the Arabic translation of his commentary, which seems based on a different Hippocratic text.

2 *Aphorisms* 4.5

Theriac to Piso contains another quotation of Hippocrates, this time taken from the *Aphorisms*. It concerns *Aphorisms* 4.5. In this aphorism, the author first discusses the way in which one should purge the body, and argues in particular that one should purge from the top in summer and from below in winter. Then he declares: 'During and before a heatwave purging is dangerous (ὑπὸ κύνα καὶ πρὸ κυνὸς ἐργώδεες αἱ φαρμακεῖαι.)'[26]

Galen copies this passage in exactly the same form in his *Commentary on the Aphorisms* 3.14 (17b.664.2 K.), where he explains that summer heat (ἡ κατὰ τὸ θέρος θερμασία) makes purging dangerous because many patients suffer fevers when they are purged during this season (διὸ καὶ πυρέττουσι πολλοὶ τῶν ἐν τούτῳ τῷ καιρῷ καθαρθέντων). He also quotes this passage in exactly the same in his *Sects for Beginners* 8 (1.89.17 K.; Marquadt et al. 1884–1893, vol. 3, p. 20) and uses it to defend Empiricist medicine in the debate against Methodist medicine. He argues that 'similar symptoms in all patients do not always indicate a similar treatment (τῶν αὐτῶν κατὰ πάντα παθῶν οὐ πάντοτε τὴν αὐτὴν θεραπείαν ἐνδεικνυμένων)', but that rather the quantity of the remedy and the way it is administered change according to the age of the patient, the seasons, and the region in which he or she lives. Thus, no physician would risk bloodletting (διὰ

26 4.502 L. In his critical apparatus, Littré gives the variant reading πρὸ κυνὸς καὶ κατὰ κύνα, which he attributes to 'Magn. in marg.', meaning Paulus Magnolus' edition (Venice 1542). There he had found this variant reading in the margin. In fact, this reading can be traced back to the Latin translation of *Theriac to Piso* (the Aldine edition of Galen based on manuscript P, where this reading can be found).

φλεβὸς κενοῦν) someone very weak or a child. The context, both in Hippocrates and Galen, remains that of purging, and Hippocrates' passage is again understood as referring to purgative drugs.

The context in *Theriac to Piso* is considerably different. Pseudo-Galen cites this passage at the end of his treatise, as part of an argument where he advises against the using the theriac during summer, nor should it be taken by young people who are 'in the prime of life' and whose temperature is very warm. Pseudo-Galen explains that the theriac, a particularly heating drug, risks overheating the body during summer and thus causing dangerous fevers. The author adds the following:[27]

> καὶ τοῦτό γε συνιδὼν ὁ θαυμασιώτατος Ἱπποκράτης τὰς πρὸ κυνὸς καὶ μετὰ κύνα φαρμακείας ἐργώδεα εἶναι λέγει.
>
> The most wonderful Hippocrates was aware of this and therefore said that **before** the [rise of the] dog [star] and **after** the [rise of the] dog [star] purgatives are difficult.

This reading 'before the dog (πρὸ κυνὸς)' is found in a marginal note by J. Clementis who corrects the erroneous text of P 'πρὸς κυνὸς', also found in L; πρὸ κυνὸς is also adopted in the Aldine edition and underlies Niccolò da Reggio's Latin translation *ante canem* and the anonymous Arabic version as '*qabla ṭulūʿi l-šiʿrā al-ʿabūri* (before the rising of the Dog Star)'. Likewise, the reading 'after the dog (μετὰ κύνα)' occurs in the oldest manuscript L, and J. Clementis' marginal note, correcting the reading κατὰ κύνα found in P and adopted in the Aldine edition; Niccolò da Reggio's Latin translation *post canem* and the anonymous Arabic version ('and after its rising [*wa-baʿda ṭulūʿihā*]') support the reading μετὰ κύνα. I have adopted this text, as it must have been the reading of the archetype rather than the distorted text that appeared previously in the printed editions.

This is not the right place for us to deal with the textual problem of ὑπὸ κύνα καὶ πρὸ κυνὸς, which is found in the Hippocratic manuscript tradition, *Sects for Beginners*, and Galen's commentary, but which Pseudo-Galen quotes as 'πρὸ[ς] κυνὸς καὶ μετὰ κύνα'; nor that of ἐργώδεα, a neuter plural form found in the ancient manuscript of *Theriac to Piso* compared to ἐργώδεες, the feminine form found in the Hippocratic manuscripts. For this discussion, which relates to the editing of the text, I refer to apparatus and notes on this passage in my critical

27 Pseudo-Galen, *Theriac to Piso* 17.4 (14.285 K.; Boudon-Millot 2016, p. 85, line 17–p. 86, line 2).

edition of this text. What I am arguing here is that this passage is taken to refer to purgative drugs only in Hippocrates and Galen, whereas it is understood by Pseudo-Galen to refer to drugs in general and to the theriac in particular.

3 Conclusion

The author of *Theriac to Piso* reads and quotes a different text than that cited by Galen in the lemmas of his commentaries on the *Epidemics* and the *Aphorisms*. Several variant readings adopted by Pseudo-Galen were, however, also known to Galen, who discussed them in his commentary on *Epidemics* 2 before rejecting them. More importantly, unlike Galen, who in the two examples we have discussed understands φάρμακον and φαρμακεία to refer to simple purgative drugs in accordance with the Hippocratic tradition, the author of *Theriac* considers these two terms as referring to drugs in general, and in the second example to the theriac in particular.

Who could this physician be and from which school could he have taken his reading of Hippocrates? In *Sect for Beginners*, Galen uses his quotation from the *Aphorisms* to defend the Empiricist school. It is, however, impossible for the author of *Theriac to Piso* to have been one of the Empiricist physicians introduced by Galen. In fact, he is particularly critical of the members of this school of whom he spoke sarcastically.[28] This is another difference from Galen: although he did not claim to be an Empiricist, he still presented Empiricism, especially in *Sects for Beginners*, but also elsewhere, as coherent and convincing. Pseudo-Galen is equally harsh on the Methodist physicians. He himself championed reason and rational medicine.[29] Unlike Galen, however, he never refers to the rationalists as dogmatists, as their adversaries, the empiricists,

28 See *Theriac to Piso* 3a.3 (14.220 K.; Boudon-Millot 2016, p. 11, lines 6–11): 'For, unlike the Empiricist physicians who, without taking into account the natures of drugs, treat everyone without skill while shamefully pretending to hold the drugs useful for the art, some doing so inspired by dreams, and others by mere chance, unlike them, we deploy our zeal for medicine in this way, but etc. (οὐ γὰρ ὥσπερ οἱ ἀπὸ τῆς ἐμπειρίας ἰατροὶ ἄνευ λόγου τοῦ κατὰ τὰς φύσεις ἕκαστον ἀτέχνως ἰατρεύοντες, αἰσχρῶς τὰ μὲν ἐξ ὀνειράτων, τὰ δὲ καὶ παρ' αὐτῆς τῆς τύχης λαβεῖν φασιν εἰς τὴν τέχνην τὰ φάρμακα, οὕτως καὶ ἡμεῖς περὶ τὴν ἰατρικὴν σπουδάζομεν, ἀλλ' κτλ.)'. And also chapter 10.4 (14.245 K.; Boudon-Millot 2016, pp. 47–48): 'In fact, I do not approve of the Empiricist physicians themselves, because they behave like individuals who, because they only consider what they want, are surprised at what happens and ignore the cause of what happens (καὶ γὰρ αὐτοὺς τοὺς ἐμπειρικοὺς οὐκ ἀποδέχομαι, ὅτι καὶ αὐτοί, ὥσπερ ἰδιῶται μόνον ὁρῶντες τὸ βλεπόμενον, θαυμάζουσι μὲν τὸ γιγνόμενον, τοῦ δὲ γιγνομένου τὴν αἰτίαν ἀγνοοῦσιν.)'

29 See *Theriac to Piso* 10.7 (14.246 K.; Boudon-Millot 2016, p. 48, lines 16–17): τελείαν οὕτω καὶ

labelled them.[30] It would therefore be tempting to see the author of *Theriac to Piso* as one of the 'Hippocratics ('Ἱπποκράτειοι)' who were contemporaries of Galen; the latter violently inveighed against them in his commentaries and they seem to have been his most direct competitors.[31] If this hypothesis is correct, the quotations of Hippocrates in *Theriac to Piso* allow us to recover the activity of a 'Hippocratic' physician, a witness of a reading of the Hippocratic text that differs from that of Galen, almost completely and definitively overshadowed by the latter's fame and authority.

λογικὴν ἀναγκαίως ἔχομεν τὴν τέχνην; 16.4 (14.278 K.; Boudon-Millot 2016, p. 79, line 24): ὑπὸ δὲ τοῦ λογικοῦ ἰατροῦ; 16.6 (14.279 K.; Boudon-Millot 2016, p. 80, lines 7–8): διὰ τὴν τοῦ λογικοῦ ἰατροῦ τέχνην.

30 See, for example, Galen, *Method of Healing* (10.159.7 K.; Johnston, Horsley 2011, vol. 2, p. 244): εἰ δὲ διὰ λόγου τινὸς, ἢ μεθόδου, λογικός τε καὶ μεθοδικὸς καὶ δογματικός; and his *Commentary on Hippocrates' 'Nature of Man'* (15.60.9; Mewaldt 1914, p. 33) where Galen mentions dogmatists and speaks of 'logical' schools in the plural: Κατὰ πάντας ἰατρούς τε καὶ φιλοσόφους τοὺς τελείους δογματικοὺς ἡ συμμετρία τῶν στοιχείων ὑγείαν ἐργάζεται. διττῆς δ' οὔσης τῷ γένει τῆς ἐν ταῖς λογικαῖς αἱρέσεσι στοιχειώσεως, ἡ μὲν ἑτέρα ..., ἡ δὲ ἑτέρα ... See also *My Own Books* (Boudon-Millot 2007, p. 137): τὰ δὲ τῶν τριῶν αἱρέσεων ὀνόματα σχεδὸν ἅπαντες ἤδη γιγνώσκουσιν, τὴν μέν τινα δογματικήν τε καὶ λογικὴν ὀνομάζεσθαι, τὴν δὲ δευτέραν ἐμπειρικήν, τὴν τρίτην δὲ μεθοδικήν.

31 See Boudon-Millot (2015).

CHAPTER 13

Ancient Medicine in the Galenic Corpus: The Story of a Concealment

Sabrina Grimaudo

Alongside the commentaries on single works in the Hippocratic Corpus (a list of which we find in *My Own Books* 9),[1] the story of Galen's intense exegetic activity on the Hippocratic Corpus also includes some writings that, though not having the form of a commentary, are in fact almost entirely devoted to exposition of Hippocratic doctrines, as is the case for *Elements according to Hippocrates*, *The Soul's Dependence on the Body*, and, in some respects, *Doctrines of Hippocrates and Plato*.[2] There are also some doxographic sections scattered here and there in Galen's corpus and, conversely, we can also insert some significant silences on important Hippocratic texts that Galen actually shows he knew well.[3] Among these, first of all, there is *Ancient Medicine*, a work that represents an exemplary case of Hippocratic writing substantially devalued, in the wake of Galen, during the Middle Ages, but considered of capital importance in the modern period: exactly the opposite destiny to that which befell the treatise *Breaths*, as Jacques Jouanna (2003a, 7) observed.[4] Previous scholarship has accustomed us to considering the image of Hippocrates which emerges from this intense exegetic activity as a reconstruction that is also, to a great extent and especially in some strategic respects, a construction deeply conditioned by Galen's conception of medicine.[5]

---

1 The commentaries by Galen quoted there (17) relate to the following works by Hippocrates: *Aphorisms*; *Fractures* and *Joints*; *Prognostic*; *Regimen in Acute Diseases*; *Wounds*; *Wounds in the Head*; *Epidemics* 1, 2, 3, 6; *Humours*; *Nutriment*, *Prorrhetic* 1; *Nature of Man*; *Surgery*; and *Airs, Waters, Places*. To these there must also be added those mentioned at other points in the corpus (*Nature of the Child*; *Eight Months' Child*) and of course also the *Hippocratic Glossary*. For an up-to-date bibliography on Galen's commentaries, see Savino (2013).

2 For a more detailed discussion of this phenomenon, see the articles by Rosen and Singer above.

3 Among the most important texts in the Hippocratic Collection that Galen ignores, particular mention must be made of *Ancient Medicine* and *Sacred Disease*.

4 For the afterlife of the work in the modern period, see Schiefsky (2005), 66–71, who connects the rise of an interest in *Ancient Medicine*, in the Renaissance epoch, to the affirmation of a critical attitude towards Galen and his predilection for humoralism.

5 See Wesley D. Smith (1979/2002), Paola Manuli (1983), Armelle Debru (1987), Daniela Manetti

© SABRINA GRIMAUDO, 2021 | DOI:10.1163/9789004470200_015

Galen did not write a commentary on *Ancient Medicine*.[6] And, above all, he substantially ignored the existence of that significant work, thus in fact consigning it to oblivion that was to last throughout the Middle Ages, as Mark Schiefsky (2005, 66) has observed, 'by a determined policy of silence'. The present study aims to reconstruct in more depth than has been done until now the causes and consequences of this silence.

As far as I have been able to verify, no explicit reference to *Ancient Medicine* is contained in Galen's boundless work, with a single exception.[7] It is a well-known passage in the commentary on *Epidemics* 2, only extant in the Arabic translation produced by Ḥunayn ibn Isḥāq:[8]

فهذا هو معنى هذا القول الذي قصدنا لتفسيره ولا بأس عندي بأن أذكر أيضاً من فسر هذا القول على ضد معنى قول أبقراط. وذلك أنهم قالوا إن قول أبقراط في هذا الموضع إنما هو القول الذي يوجد في الكتاب الذي رسمه «في الطب القديم» وواضع ذلك الكتاب ينصره ويصححه وهو أنه لا ينبغي في قوله أن تُجعل الأغراض في مداواة الأمراض الحار والبارد والرطب واليابس — كأنا ليس نجد أبقراط في كتابه «في طبيعة الإنسان» يبين أن طبيعتنا إنما هي مركبة من هذه الأشياء وليس نجده في «كتاب الفصول» ولا في غيره[9] من كتبه الصحيحة قد ذكر هذه الأشياء مراراً كثيرةً ذكر ما ينتفع به في العلاج.

This is the meaning of the lemma we wanted to explain, and as far as I am concerned there is nothing wrong with also mentioning those who have explained this lemma in a way that is at odds with what Hippocrates meant. For they said that Hippocrates' observation here is (also) found in the book entitled *Ancient Medicine*, and the author of that book sup-

---

and Amneris Roselli (1994), Ineke Sluiter (1995), Heinrich von Staden (2002, 2009), Jacques Jouanna (2000, 2006), Véronique Boudon-Millot (2008), Rebecca Flemming (2008), and Philip J. van der Eijk (2012).

6 The fact that Galen did not consider the text authentic was not decisive in this connection, seeing that Galen's corpus also includes commentaries on some works in the Hippocratic Corpus explicitly declared to be spurious. This is the case, for example, of the commentary on *Prorrhetic* 1, on which see the recent essay by Roselli (2015).

7 Anastassiou and Irmer (1997), 455–457. Indirect references are contained, according to Anastassiou and Irmer (2001), 355 in: *Medical Definitions* 19.346.6–8 K. to *Ancient Medicine* 3; 1.578.9–10 L.; *Hippocrates' Regimen in Acute Diseases*, Westenberger (1914), p. 385, line 9–386, line 22 to *Ancient Medicine* 5; 1.582.13–14 L., and Westenberger (1914), p. 387, line 5–p. 390, line 5 to *Ancient Medicine* 16; 1.610.4–6 L.

8 Vagelpohl (2016), p. 299, lines 13–21.

9 *wa-lā fī ġayrihī* M : *om.* E1.

> ports and confirms it: there is, as he says, no need to make hot, cold, wet and dry the target in treating diseases—as if we do not find Hippocrates explaining in his book *Nature of Man* that our nature consists of these things or we do not find him mention these things in the *Aphorisms* or his other authentic books many times in a way that is useful for (medical) practice.

According to the interpretation by Smith (1979/2002, 209–210) and Schiefsky (2005, 65–66), the passage seems to constitute a clear example of that anti-empirical reading of *Epidemics* by Galen of which Philip van der Eijk (2012) has spoken in more general terms.

The passage concludes the long section devoted to the interpretation of a rather obscure point in *Epidemics* 2.2.12, a typical example of that elliptic and laconic character of this Hippocratic work, on which, among others, Volker Langholf has dwelt:[10]

> Ῥητέον ὅτι, αἵματος ῥυέντος, ἐκχλοιοῦνται καὶ ὅσα ἄλλα τοιαῦτα, ὅτι πρὸς τὸ ὑγραίνειν καὶ ξηραίνειν καὶ θερμαίνειν καὶ ψύχειν πολλὰ ἄν τις τοιαῦτα εἴποι.

> You must argue that when the blood flows, a person turns green and yellow, and other such things, and you can argue many such things with regard to moistening, drying, heating and cooling.

After having dwelt at length on a reading of the text consistent with the principles of Hippocratism outlined in *Elements according to Hippocrates* and in *Method of Healing*, and having maintained that the thought underlying it is that a person who has lost a lot of blood also loses bodily heat, Galen concludes by mentioning with some smugness the opinion of 'those who have explained this lemma in a way that is at odds with what Hippocrates meant (*man fassara hāḏā l-qawla ḍidda maʿnā Abuqrāṭa*)'. These commentators—resorting to the hermeneutic principle deriving from Homeric philology, consisting of 'explaining Hippocrates with Hippocrates',[11]—read the problematic reference to τὸ ὑγραίνειν, καὶ ξηραίνειν, καὶ θερμαίνειν, καὶ ψύχειν in *Epidemics* 2.2.12 as an

10 Langhoff (1977), (1990), 136–139 ('Lack of Explicitness in *Epidemics*'); Smith (1994), p. 34, lines 11–13; 5.88.18–20 L.

11 Which, however, is an exegetic principle employed by Galen himself. Cf. *About 'Coma' according to Hippocrates*, Mewaldt (1915), p. 182, line 23–p. 183, line 2. On the application of this exegetic principle in Galen cf. Manetti and Roselli (1994), 1564–1565.

allusion to and a summary of the positions expressed in *Ancient Medicine*,[12] whose author had denied that recourse to the concepts (the *hypothéseis*, to use the language proper to the work) of hot, cold, wet, and dry could present any utility for the treatment of diseases ('there is, as he says, no need to make hot, cold, wet and dry the target in treating diseases [*wa-huwa annahū lā yanbaġī fī qawlihī an yuǧʿala l-aġrāḍu fī mudāwāti l-amrāḍi l-ḥārra wa-l-bārida wa-l-raṭba wa-yābisa*]'): a position in stark contrast, according to Galen, with the theories repeatedly affirmed by Hippocrates in *Nature of Man*, in *Aphorisms*, 'or his other authentic books (*wa-lā fī ġayrihī min kutubihī l-ṣaḥīḥati*)'. The bad interpretation of the passage in *Epidemics*, as usual, is attributed to arrogant ignorance of the commentator, alleged not only not to have read those Hippocratic works, but also not to have correctly understood even the general meaning of *Epidemics* itself.

As we have said, both Wesley D. Smith and Mark Schiefsky—but not Jacques Jouanna in the previously mentioned edition for the Collection des Universités de France—see in the passage in Galen's commentary a reference to the Empiricists,[13] and cite it as proof of interest (in any case very probable, as we will see) of the exponents of that medical school in *Ancient Medicine*. But this interpretation, which does not seem to find any direct echo in the text, where there is a rather generic reference, creates some problems. And I say this, recognising that, as has been shown above all by Philip van der Eijk (2012), Galen's commentary on *Epidemics* 2 undoubtedly has an anti-empirical general approach and 'flavour'.

First of all, it is not clear how the obscure text of *Epidemics* 2, in which however it is said that 'you can argue many such things with regard to moistening, drying, heating and cooling (πρὸς τὸ ὑγραίνειν, καὶ ξηραίνειν, καὶ θερμαίνειν, καὶ ψύχειν, πολλὰ ἄν τις τοιαῦτα εἴποι)', could be set alongside that of *Ancient Medicine*, and specifically the chapters (15 and 16) in which it is expressly

12 See in particular *Ancient Medicine* 15.1 (Jouanna 2003a, p. 137, lines 11–17) and 16.1–2 (Jouanna 2003a, p. 139, lines 4–16).

13 On the question, no opinion is explicitly expressed in Anastassiou and Irmer (1997); they limit themselves to recalling (p. 456, note 1) Smith's opinion that the passage contains a reference to the exponents of the Empiric school. According to Smith (1979/2002), 210, '[Galen] gives us the information in one of his expansive moments in which he is apparently transmitting information given by Rufus of Ephesus.' Manetti and Roselli (1994), 1600, take a contrary position: 'Nel commento a *Epidemie II* Rufo è citato solo nell'ultima parte (sezione VI) ed è probabilmente utilizzato attraverso una fonte intermedia.' One should also consider that the quotation from an Empiric (Heraclides of Tarent) closest to the passage examined by us, in section 2.2 of Galen's *Commentary on Hippocrates' 'Epidemics' 2* occurs some ten pages earlier.

denied that the four elementary qualities, above all hot and cold, have a central role in the treatment of diseases. But this concerns the bad interpretation of the text that Galen here stigmatizes, criticizing it precisely on the basis of such incongruities.

On the other hand, the attribution of this bad interpretation to the Empiricists clearly seems in contrast with what Galen affirms in a well known passage in the preface to the commentary on *Epidemics* 3, when he observes that the Empiricists, at least before Lycus and Quintus (grouped among the Empiricists by Galen), correctly understood Hippocrates' humoralism in close connection with the theory of elements and qualities, and that in commenting on a Hippocratic text they attribute the cause of everything 'to the first principles (εἰς ταύτας τὰς ἀρχάς)', behaving like good actors, 'as in a play sticking to their own part of the character in question (καθάπερ ἐν δράματι φυλάττοντες … τὴν οἰκείαν ὑπόκρισιν τοῦ περικειμένου προσώπου)', that is to say adapting to the Hippocratic text, just as in commenting on a text by Herophilus, Erasitratus or Asclepiades they present themselves as Herophileans, Erasistrateans or Asclepiadeans.[14]

Apart from the issue of a correct identification of the polemic target it is addressed to,[15] one fact clearly emerges from the passage in the commentary on *Epidemics* 2: Galen did not consider *Ancient Medicine* authentic, as is shown by the contextual reference to *Nature of Man*, to *Aphorisms* and the 'other authentic books' in the Hippocratic Corpus.

We do not know if *Ancient Medicine* was quoted in the treatise that Galen devoted to the distinction between true Hippocratic and spurious works (*Περὶ τῶν γνησίων τε καὶ νόθων Ἱπποκράτους συγγραμμάτων*): this is a lost treatise, which is alluded to several times in the Corpus and an ample excerpt from which is given in the preface to the commentary on *Nature of Man*.[16] However, some lemmas in the *Hippocratic Glossary* (where actually *Ancient Medicine* is never explicitly

14 Galen, *Commentary on Hippocrates' 'Epidemics'* 3.1.4; Wenkebach (1936), p. 16, line 17–p. 17, line 7. On this passage see Manetti and Roselli (1994), 1593.

15 I would not rule out the possibility that Galen's criticism is addressed here to the Methodist physicians, who in Galen's *corpus* are frequently accused of not understanding the importance of hot, cold, dry and wet in the evaluation of the healthy state and the pathological one; see *Against Julian* 4 (Wenkebach 1951, p. 42, line 9–p. 43, line 3) as one example of many.

16 Galen, *Commentary on Hippocrates' 'Nature of Man'*, Mewaldt (1914), 7–8. The testimonies on this piece of writing were collected by Mewaldt (1909). For this work, and more in general for Galen's philological activity in relation to the 'Hippocratic question', the reader is referred to Boudon-Millot (2008) and, more recently, to the ample essay by Manetti (2015). Doubts on the existence of this Galenic work were advanced by Smith (1979/2002), 169–170, note 85 and Manetti and Roselli (1994), p. 1555, note 95.

mentioned) refer in all likelihood to this work, as Jacques Jouanna (2003a, 97–99) has shown. But also, over and above these precise textual echoes, other elements suggest that Galen was familiar with *Ancient Medicine*, and indeed he found in that work some orientations converging with his own vision of medicine, perhaps voluntarily ignored in the name of the evident incompatibility that he recognized between *Ancient Medicine* and *Nature of Man*. We will return to this later.

In the ancient world, before Galen, the Hippocratic paternity of *Ancient Medicine* had been affirmed by Erotian, who correctly inserted the work among those related to art (τῶν δ' εἰς τὸν περὶ τέχνης τεινόντων λόγον),[17] while doubt remains about whether a commentary on the text had been written by Rufus of Ephesus.[18] And also regardless of the possibility that the passage in the commentary on *Epidemics* 2 analysed above refers precisely to the Empiricists, it is entirely likely that the exponents of this medical school considered the work authentic, certainly having a particular liking for it. And this is because it contained a reconstruction of the history (or better of the *archaiología*) of medicine, and of its relations with dietetics, which, according to paragraphs 33–36 of the preface by Celsus, must have presented many points of contact with theirs. But above all because—as we know well—in the name precisely of an extreme empiricism,[19] the work radically rejected every *physiological* approach to medicine.[20] Finally, we cannot rule out the possibility that Celsus was referring precisely to *Ancient Medicine* when, in a famous passage in the preface, he affirmed that Hippocrates was the first to distinguish medicine 'from studying philosophy (*a studio sapientiae*)', implicitly recognizing the authenticity of the work.[21]

---

17 Nachmanson (1918), p. 9, lines 18–19. On the indirect tradition relating to *Ancient Medicine*, cf. Jouanna (2003a), 95–102: in addition to the glosses by Galen and Erotian, Jouanna refers to those contained in Hesychius' *Lexicon* and in the anonymous treatise *On Anger* (Diels 1918).

18 Cf. Anastassiou and Irmer (2006), 458, who recall the sceptical position of Sideras (1994), 1097–1098.

19 However, on the limits of a reading in a fully empirical key of *Ancient Medicine*, see Schiefsky (2005), 345–359 (Appendix 1, '*VM* and Medical Empiricism').

20 Another possible element of contact is the juxtaposition of *iatrikḗ* and *kybernētikḗ*: cf. *Ancient Medicine* 9 and, for empirical medicine, the passages cited by Deichgräber (1930), p. 92, line 23 (Celsus proem); p. 217, lines 15 and 21 (Sextus Empiricus). However, this aspect is already amply discussed in Plato and Aristotle.

21 Celsus, *On Medicine*, proem 8: [...] *Huius* [sc. Democriti] *autem, ut quidam crediderunt, discipulus Hippocrates Cous, primus ex omnibus memoria dignus, a studio sapientiae hanc disciplinam separavit, vir et arte et facundia insignis*. However, for a more problematic approach to the passage cf. Mudry (1977) and (1982), 63–65. In both works, Mudry

As for other writings in the Hippocratic Corpus, in the case of *Ancient Medicine* too—we see it clearly in the quoted passage in the commentary on *Epidemics* 2—the Hippocratic paternity of the text is denied by Galen not on the basis of historical-linguistic or stylistic parameters, but on the basis of the criterion that for him should weigh most heavily in this type of choice, and that is to say on a doctrinal basis. More exactly, on the basis of the lack of congruence with the theories expounded in *Nature of Man*, a text, however, that Galen explicitly recommended reading as preparatory to the reading of *Epidemics*.[22] This is a theme that is particularly dear to Galen, who, according to what he himself tells us in *My Own Books*, had written a work no longer extant in three books with the eloquent title *That in Other Works, Too, Hippocrates Proves to Have the Same Opinion as Expounded in 'Nature of Man'* (*Ὅτι καὶ κατ' ἄλλα συγγράμματα τὴν αὐτὴν δόξαν ἔχων ὁ Ἱπποκράτης φαίνεται τῇ κατὰ τὸ ⟨Περὶ⟩ φύσιος ἀνθρώπου*), for the purpose of dispelling the doubts on the authenticity of the treatise that continued to circulate even after the spread of his commentary.[23] Considering that *Elements according to Hippocrates* in actual fact also constitutes an analysis and a (re)reading of *Nature of Man*, we can conclude that the works devoted by Galen to this treatise were no fewer than three, proving the particular importance that he attributed to it.

On Galen's exegetic activity around *Nature of Man*, I do not need to dwell long. One only needs to turn to the essays that Jacques Jouanna has devoted to the theme, which also show the absolute centrality that this work occupies in the wholly Galenic characterization of the 'true' Hippocrates.[24] At the basis of this characterization was the translation of the theory of the four humours present in *Nature of Man* into elementary-quantitative terms: both in the commentary on *Nature of Man* and in *Elements according to Hippocrates* (which, as already mentioned, can to all intents and purposes be considered a further commentary on *Nature of Man*), the system of the four humours was presen-

also draws attention to paragraph 47 of the proem by Celsus, where Hippocrates and Erasistratus are recognised to have the merit of including *naturae rerum contemplatio* in the doctor's necessary preparation.

22 *Commentary on Hippocrates' 'Epidemics'* 1 proem, Wenkebach (1934), p. 6, lines 26–28.

23 *My Own Books* 9.12; Boudon-Millot (2007), p. 161, lines 14–20.

24 Cf. Jouanna (2000) and (2006). One should read in particular the famous passage in the preface to the commentary on *Nature of Man* in which Galen affirms that the first part of the work (chapters 1–8) is like the foundation of the whole Hippocratic theory (τὸ δὲ πρῶτον αὐτοῦ μέρος ἁπάσης τῆς Ἱπποκράτους τέχνης ἔχει τὴν *οἷον κρηπῖδα*), which Plato mentioned in *Phaedrus* 270c–d; see the articles by Hankinson and Singer in this volume for a more detailed discussion.

ted by Galen as exactly equivalent to that of the four elements (air, water, fire, earth) and of the four qualities (hot, cold, wet, dry).

Accordingly, the attitude taken by the author of *Ancient Medicine* with respect to the insignificance of elementary properties, of hot and cold particularly, from Galen's point of view must have been what mostly distanced the work from genuine Hippocratic spirit. In this way *Nature of Man* became the privileged canon on which to test out the authenticity of the other works in the Corpus. This is a situation that was to be literally turned upside-down by Émile Littré, for whom this canonical role was instead to be played precisely by *Ancient Medicine*: the work to which, in his opinion, Plato alluded in the famous passage in *Phaedrus* (270c–d), in which he attributed to Hippocrates a conception of medicine as a science that cannot be separated from analysis of nature as a whole. The work with which, and not by chance, he began his edition of Hippocrates' *Complete Works*.[25]

This is a particularly important point for Galen, who repeatedly in his vast corpus puts forward the idea of a Hippocratic-Platonic-Aristotelian-Stoic consensus on a theory of matter resulting from a composition and a mixture (κρᾶσις) of the four elements or of the corresponding qualities, against monist and atomistic-corpuscular theories.[26] Therefore, it is not difficult to understand how the polemic of the author of *Ancient Medicine* towards the employment in the medical sphere of *hypothéseis*,[27] alongside explicit identification of the latter with elementary properties like hot, cold, wet, and dry, must have appeared entirely incompatible to Galen with the image of Hippocrates as the first discoverer of the theory of the elements and qualities that he persistently proposes, particularly in *Elements according to Hippocrates*. At the same time, the negation of any physiological[28] characterization of medicine was in stark con-

25 1.557–637 L. Littré's choice is repeated in the editions by Kühlewein (1894, 1–30) and Jones (1923), 11–62.

26 I collected these passages in Grimaudo (2008), 35–54 See, just by way of example, *Constitution of the Art of Medicine* 8; Fortuna (1997a), p. 80, lines 20–23, where Galen attributes the theory according to which earth, water, air and fire are elements of what is born and perishes to 'all philosophers who do not fail to see the demonstration.'

27 A term dear to Galen, who employs it with great frequency (over 200 attestations in his extant works), though sometimes attributing a technical meaning to it that obviously it did not yet have in the fifth century BC. For this more technical use of *hypóthesis* in the description of the mechanisms of the hypothetical-deductive reasoning in Galen cf. above all Gourinat (2011). Among the passages that could instead be quoted for use of *hypóthesis* in a meaning close to that of *Ancient Medicine*, and that is to say with specific reference to the elementary theories, see for instance *Differences of Fevers* 1.3 (7.281.7–11 K.).

28 On the anachronistic reference of this term to texts preceding the Hellenistic age, in Galen, see Jouanna (2003b) and, in more general terms, Nutton (2012a).

trast with the ideal of a philosophical medicine, whose first founder and principal example Galen identified precisely with Hippocrates. This ideal amply runs through Galen's production, and is also clearly summed up in the title of one of the most successful works: *That the Best Physician is also a Philosopher*. This work was also known, as Galen himself informs us, as *Galen's Hippocrates* (*Γαληνοῦ Ἱπποκράτης*),[29] as has been confirmed by the discovery of a new manuscript, *Vlatadon* 14.

Various reasons therefore must have driven Galen to emphasize the points of contrast between *Ancient Medicine* and *Nature of Man*, and not to consider the existence of basic orientations substantially converging in the two works.[30] It is probably for the same reasons that Galen appears insensitive to the numerous consonances existing between *Ancient Medicine* and *Regimen in Acute Diseases*: he considered the latter an authentic work and wrote a long commentary on it.[31]

As I said at the start, Galen's condemnation of *Ancient Medicine* is essentially expressed through a strategy of silence. This is a silence that is all the more striking where one considers the numerous points of agreement that Galen could find between his own conception of medicine and that which emerges in the Hippocratic text. These points of agreement concern first and foremost Galen the hygienist. However, when in *Thrasyboulus* he sets about establishing a canon of Hippocratic treatises relating to protection of health, he quotes *Regimen* and *Airs, Waters, Places*,[32] significantly excluding the work in which with greatest depth and with most vivid historical and epistemological awareness the relationships between dietetics, medicine and gymnastics are investigated. Yet various and also very specific aspects of Galen's reflection relating to hygiene seem to be rooted precisely in *Ancient Medicine*.

One of these is consideration of the place that hygiene occupies in the history of medicine,[33] as well as reflection on its complex relationships with *gymnastiké̄*. In this connection, in the *archaiología* of hygiene that Galen works out in chapters 32–39 of *Thrasyboulus*, there very clearly emerges his awareness

29 *My Own Books* 9.14; Boudon-Millot (2007), p. 162, lines 7–11.

30 For an exhaustive examination of these convergences, see Jouanna (2002), 50–52, who stresses in particular the polemical attitude of both works towards a philosophical medicine.

31 Helmreich (1914). For an in-depth analysis of poins of contact between *Regimen in Acute Diseases* and *Ancient Medicine*, see Jouanna (2003a), 63–74.

32 *Thrasyboulus* 39; Helmreich (1893), p. 87, lines 6–11.

33 Though with some differences in the detail: according to Galen, therapeutics is more ancient than dietetics of the healthy, while for the author of *Ancient Medicine* the latter constituted the first stage of the development of the medical art.

of the 'hidden' character, so to speak, of this branch of medicine, which only developed in a subsequent phase of the history of medicine, originally having been identified with therapeutics.[34] For this reason—according to Galen's reconstruction—for a long time, and that is to say down to Erasistratus, hygiene seems not to have had a name of its own, and to have been variedly swallowed up in *gymnastikḗ* and sometimes confused with it. Besides, Plato, too, in the *Gorgias*, spoke of *gymnastikḗ* while really intending to refer to *hygieinḗ*, since this specific denomination was not yet in use in the fourth century BC.[35] These are words that immediately call to mind the reflection by the author of *Ancient Medicine*, who, going back to the dietetic origins of medicine (chapter 3), and noticing the identical nature of the lines of research followed by the one and by the other (chapter 4: κατὰ τὴν αὐτὴν ὁδὸν ζητέοντες), established a parallel between gymnastics and dietetics of the healthy; also showing the difficulty, for most people, of recognizing the latter as part of the medical art, it being instead unanimously identified with care for the sick (that is with therapeutics), which alone has a 'name and experts'.[36] In valorising perception (*aísthēsis*) and conjecture (*stochastikón*) in the sphere of hygiene, Galen appears particularly close to the positions of the author of *Ancient Medicine*.[37]

In this connection, to respond to the need to establish an epistemological criterion reflecting both the conjectural character of medicine, the inevitable corollary of its being knowledge of the particular, and its epistemic dimension, Galen works out an entirely new concept, that of 'conjecture founded upon art (*technikòs stochasmós*)'.[38] Galen's reflection on recourse to *technikòs stochasmós* in the sphere of hygiene very much recalls the positions of the author of *Ancient Medicine*. Among the many passages, one should read *Preservation of Health* 2.7 where, addressing the problem of determining the measure of exercises and massages to which to submit the patient to maintain him in good health, Galen presents attainment of an exact *métron* as the result of progressive stochastic refinement of the hygienist's knowledge:[39]

---

34 *Thrasyboulus* 26; Helmreich (1893), p. 67, lines 16–20.
35 Cf. Grimaudo (2008), 125–162.
36 Cf. *Ancient Medicine* 4,2; Jouanna (2003a), p. 123, lines 14–17, and above all 5.1; Jouanna (2003a), p. 123, line 18–p. 124, line 2.
37 As Schiefsky (2005), 66 observed: 'Galen's reluctance to mention *VM* is all the more striking given that he might have appealed to the use of the term στοχάζεσθαι in chapter 9 to gain Hippocratic authority for his notion that the practice of medicine requires a kind of rational conjecture or στοχασμός.'
38 On this concept, see in particular Boudon-Millot (2003b).
39 Koch (1923), p. 57, line 28–p. 58, line 2.

> ὁπόσον δ' ἐστὶ τὸ πλῆθος τῶν ἀνατρίψεων, οὐχ οἷόν τε λόγῳ δηλῶσαι, ἀλλὰ χρὴ τὸν ἐπιστατοῦντα, τρίβωνα τῶν τοιούτων ὑπάρχοντα, κατὰ μὲν τὴν πρώτην ἡμέραν οὐκ ἀκριβεῖ στοχασμῷ χρήσασθαι, κατὰ δὲ τὰς ἑξῆς ἐμπειρίαν ἤδη τινὰ τῆς τοῦ σώματος ἐκείνου φύσεως ἔχοντα τὸν στοχασμὸν ἀεὶ καὶ μᾶλλον ἐξακριβοῦν. καὶ μὲν δὴ καὶ κατὰ τὰ γυμνάσια τῇ μὲν πρώτῃ τῶν ἡμερῶν οὐ δυνατὸν ἀκριβῶσαι τὸ μέτρον, ἐν δὲ ταῖς μετὰ τήνδε καὶ πάνυ δυνατόν.
>
> One cannot show through theory what the quantity of massages should be; rather, the supervisor who is familiar with such matters ought to use imprecise conjecture on the first day, and on the following days when he already has a certain amount of experience with the nature of the [patient's] body, he ought to refine the conjecture constantly. This applies above all to exercises: on the first day it is not possible to specify the extent, whereas on the following days, this is quite possible.

And shortly after, speaking of the quantity of food to be administered, he adds:[40]

> εἰ γάρ τι καὶ παρέλαθεν κατὰ τὴν ἀρχήν, ἀκριβωθήσεται τοῦτο τῇ πείρᾳ διδαχθέν. οὕτως οὖν εἰς ἀκριβῆ στοχασμὸν ἔρχεται καὶ τὸ τῶν σιτίων μέτρον οὐδενὶ τρόπῳ κατ' ἀρχὰς γνωρισθῆναι δυνάμενον· ἀλλ' ἡ καθ' ἑκάστην ἡμέραν πεῖρα καὶ μνήμη τοῦ ποσοῦ τῶν σιτίων καὶ τῶν γυμνασίων, οὐδὲν ἀργῶς ὁρῶντος τοῦ προεστῶτος, ἀλλ' ἀεὶ μεμνημένου, ὅπως ἔπεψεν ἐπὶ τοσοῖσδε τοῖς γυμνασίοις τὰ τοσάδε σιτία, πλησίον ἀκριβοῦς ἐπιστήμης ἄγει τὴν διάγνωσιν ἐν τῷ χρόνῳ.
>
> If something has been missed at the beginning, experience will teach us how to improve it. In this way a precise conjecture is also attained about the quantity of food, which cannot in any way be known at the beginning. But daily experience and recollection of the quantity of food and exercises leads with time to a determination approximating certain knowledge, provided that the person responsible does not neglect anything, but always remembers how the patient digested a certain quantity of food after a certain quantity of exercises.

Here, as we can see, we are looking at an entirely original answer to the classical problem of how to establish the amount of food and exercises for a correct diet.

40 Koch (1923), p. 58, lines 24–31.

This problem already occurred in *Regimen* 1.2[41] and was, in more general terms, raised for the first time in *Ancient Medicine* 9;[42] this famous text clearly shares ideas with the passages in Galen quoted above. Besides, the great value of *aísthēsis*, which runs through the Galen's works and in particular the works on hygiene,[43] also tends in this direction, closely recalling the problematic affirmation in *Ancient Medicine* 9 that sense perception of the body (*aísthēsis toû sṓmatos*) is the most important criterion.

Yet, against so many points of contact, Galen's condemnation of *Ancient Medicine* is evident and takes on the characteristics of a genuine concealment. Evidently for Galen, the option for a model clearly privileging the humoralist-elementary approach remained dominant and hence proved stronger than all the other possible elements of congruence, however important, with *Ancient Medicine*. This option, as was said at the start, was for many centuries to condemn this work to oblivion. Only from the Renaissance onwards, when Galen and his predilection for humoralism was viewed with a more critical eye and later, as positivism exemplified by physicians such as Cabanis and Littré emerged, was there a complete change in the attitude towards *Ancient Medicine*, then considered one of the most significant writings in the Hippocratic Corpus. An extraordinarily advanced work, whose author, to quote once again Jacques Jouanna (2003a, 83–84), is 'a modern mind who dared to reject the excesses of modernity (un esprit moderne qui a eu le courage de refuser les excès de la modernité)'. It is a work that A.E. Taylor (1911) was to define as so important that anyone who had not studied it should not be deemed competent to speak or to write on the whole history of Greek philosophy: this is a further sign of the influence that Galen's exegetic activity, both positive and negative, exerted on the future destinies of the *Hippocratic Corpus*.

---

41 Joly (2003), p. 124, lines 21–26.

42 Jouanna (2003b), p. 127, line 15–p. 128, line 15.

43 On this aspect, see Boudon (2003b), who investigates in depth the question with specific reference to the concept of 'perceivable lesion of action (ἡ τῆς ἐνεργείας αἰσθητὴ βλάβη)'. More generally on *aísthēsis* in Galen, see Tieleman (2011).

CHAPTER 14

A New Anonymous Prologue to the Commentary on the Hippocratic Aphorisms in the *Harleianus* 6295

Giulia Ecca

The *Aphorisms* of Hippocrates are one of the most commented medical works from antiquity onwards.* If we consider the manuscript tradition of the various commentaries, we can find some Greek manuscripts that preserve so-called 'mixed commentaries', that is, exegetical works combining parts of commentaries by different authors (Galen, Stephen of Alexandria, and Theophilus).[1] In general, the parts of the different commentaries are simply juxtaposed one after the other without any gap. The manuscript London, British Library, MS Harley 6295 (*Londiniensis Harleianus* 6295, henceforth Hb; copied in the second half of fifteenth century) and its copy, Paris, Bibliothèque Nationale de France, MS 1884 fonds grec (*Parisinus graecus* 1884, henceforth R; copied in 1503), preserve a mixed commentary on the Hippocratic *Aphorisms*.[2] At Hb, fol. 157v, there is the short prologue to the *Commentary on Aphorisms* by Theophilus (Dietz 1834, vol. 2, p. 245, line 32–p. 246, line 7). Following it, we read the Hippocratic lemma, consisting in the first part of *Aphorism* 1.1, and the related commentary by Theophilus (Dietz 1834, vol. 2, p. 246, line 9–p. 248, line 4: in

* I wrote this paper during my postdoc at the University of Hamburg under the supervision of Christian Brockmann, whom I warmly thank for the support. I thank also the Department of Classics of the Humboldt University of Berlin and Philip van der Eijk for giving me the opportunity to work as visiting scholar in that Department, as well as Anna Motta for some remarks on the Neoplatonic schools. I am especially grateful to Peter E. Pormann and Peter N. Singer for the careful correction of this paper and their suggestions on the critical text and translation.

1 On the manuscripts containing mixed commentaries on *Aphorisms*, see Magdelaine (1994), vol. 1, pp. 275–279; cf. also Savino (2020b).

2 For Hb, see the catalogue by Nares, vol. III, pp. 354–355 and the website of the British library: http://www.bl.uk/manuscripts/FullDisplay.aspx?ref=Harley_MS_6295 [accessed 26 March 2020]; the project of the *Commentaria in Aristotelem Graeca et Byzantina* (CAGB) gives a detailed and updated description of this manuscript in its codicological and palaeographical aspects; see https://cagb-db.bbaw.de/vorhaben/index.xql?id=heuristik [accessed 26 March 2020]. For R, see the catalogue by Omont (1889), 2. 158. For a description of both these manuscripts with reference to Galen's *Commentary on Aphorisms*, see Magdelaine (1994), vol. 1, p. 226, notes 1–2 and Savino (2012), 34, 38.

© GIULIA ECCA, 2021 | DOI:10.1163/9789004470200_016

Hb, fols. 158r–158v). After this short part taken from Theophilus, we find Galen's *Commentary*, which runs from the second part of *Aphorism* 1.1 (17b.355.13 K.) to the end of book seven (from Hb, fol. 158v, line 18, to fol. 307v).

However, the peculiarity of this part of the manuscript tradition is not the mixed commentary itself. In fact, at Hb, fols. 157r–157v and at R, fols. 158r–159r, we find an anonymous and as yet unedited text that serves as prologue to this mixed commentary of Theophilus and Galen.[3] In the present contribution, I will focus my attention exclusively on the anonymous text: I will edit, translate and comment on it, trying to identify the cultural context in which it was composed. Instead of 'author', I will speak of 'compiler' of this anonymous text, since—as will become clear—he collected material from different sources and reorganized it according to his own purposes.

1 Edition and Translation

In the following edition of the text, I report the variants of both manuscripts in the footnotes (even the readings of R, although it is a copy of Hb). In some cases, it has been necessary to correct the transmitted text, which I have divided into seven paragraphs according to the content, in order to make the reading of my remarks easier.[4]

Ἀφορισμοὶ τοῦ Ἱπποκράτους

(1.) ἐπειδήπερ μέλλομεν συντόμως τε καὶ σαφῶς—χάριτι τοῦ ἐμοῦ Χριστοῦ καὶ Θεοῦ ἡμῶν τοῦ χορηγοῦ τῆς σοφίας καὶ πρώτου ἰατῆρος ψυχῶν τε καὶ σωμάτων τοῦ τὰς[5] ἀσθενείας ἡμῶν ἀναλαβόντος καὶ τὰς νόσους βαστάζοντος τε καὶ θεραπεύοντος—τοὺς Ἱπποκράτους Ἀφορισμοὺς ἐξηγήσασθαι, ἄξιον εἰπεῖν τε καὶ ἑρμηνεῦσαι πρῶτον τὸ ὄνομα τῆς ἐπιγραφῆς, εἶτα χεῖρα ἐπιβαλεῖν αὐτοῖς. **(2.)** ἔστι μὲν οὖν ἐπιγραφὴ αὕτη *Ἀφορισμοὶ Ἱπποκράτους* ἄλλως[6] ὅρος καὶ ἄλλως[7] ὁρισμός. ὁ μὲν οὖν ὅρος πολυσήμαντός ἐστι λέξις· σημαίνει γὰρ τὸ ὁροθέσιον, τὴν βασιλικὴν ἀπόφασιν, τὸν κατὰ φιλοσοφίαν[8] ὅρον εἰς ὃν ἀναλύ-

3 Magdelaine (1994, vol. 1, p. 226, note 1) already noticed the presence of the anonymous and unedited text in her dissertation; see also Ihm (2002), 229.

4 Hb, fols. 157r–157v; R, fols. 158r–159r.

5 τὰς Hb : *om.* R.

6 ἄλλως Hb : ἄλλον R.

7 ἄλλως *scripsi* : ἄλλον Hb R.

8 φιλοσοφίαν *scripsi* : φιλοσοφίας Hb R.

εται πᾶσα πρότασις συλλογιστική, καὶ τὸν ὁρισμὸν αὐτὸν τοῦ πράγματος. ὁ δὲ ὁρισμός (ταὐτὸν γὰρ ἐστὶν ἀφορισμὸς καὶ προδιορισμός) ὁρίζει καὶ διαφορίζει καὶ περιλαμβάνει καὶ ἀποχωρίζει τὰ προδιωρισμένα[9] ἀπ' ἀλλήλων, κἄν τε πράγματα εἶεν κἄν τε παθήματα καὶ νοσήματα [νοσήματος ἐστὶ λέξις].[10] ἀλλ' εἰ καὶ γραμματικῶν[11] παῖδες οὐκ ἔσχον κανόνα κανόνος ἀποδοῦναι, ἀλλ' οἱ τῆς[12] φιλοσοφίας ἀρχηγοὶ ὅρον ὁρισμοῦ ἀποδιδόασιν τῇ[13] δαψιλείᾳ τῆς γνώσεως· ἔστι μὲν οὖν[14] ὅρος ὁρισμοῦ· λόγος σύντομος δηλωτικὸς τῆς φύσεως τοῦ ὑποκειμένου πράγματος. (3.) ὅτι μὲν οὖν ὁ λόγος τετήρηται τῷ Ἱπποκράτει αὐτόθεν ἔχει τὸν ἔλεγχον καὶ οὐ χρείαν[15] ἑρμηνευμάτων. ὅτι δὲ ἀσαφεῖς ὑπάρχουσι,[16] τοῦτο μὲν ἅτε ποιητικώτερον[17] συντιθέμενοι τοῦτο δὲ καὶ[18] ὡς πολυλογώτερον παρὰ Γαληνοῦ ἐξηγησάμενοι καὶ ἀμφοτέρωθεν[19] πολλὴν τὴν ἀσάφειαν ἔχοντες, δῆλον τοῖς πᾶσι. ἑκατέρῳ οὖν ἀποσεισάμενος τοῦ μὲν Ἱπποκράτους περὶ τοὺς ἀφορισμοὺς ποιητικὴν ἀσάφειαν, μακρηγορίαν[20] δὲ τὴν περὶ αὐτούς—φησί τις τῶν καθ' ἡμᾶς προκρίτων θεοφόρων πατέρων· πολέμιος ἀκοαῖς κόρος λόγου[21] ὡς[22] ὑπερβάλλουσα τροφὴ σώμασιν[23]—εὐφραδέως[24] οὕτω καὶ συντόμως τὴν πραγματείαν ποιήσομαι. ἐπεὶ δὲ[25] περὶ ἰατρικῆς ἡμῖν ἐστιν ὁ λόγος, δέον αὐτόχρημα διορίσασθαι τί ἐστὶν ἰατρική· ἰατρική ἐστι τέχνη περὶ τὰ ἀνθρώπινα σώματα καταγινομένη ὑγείας περιποιητική.

(4.) Εἰδὼς[26] ὁ Ἱπποκράτης ὡς πᾶσα τέχνη καὶ ἐπιστήμη χρόνῳ μακρῷ ἀκριβῶς ἀσκεῖται καὶ εἰς ἄκρον κατορθοῦται—καὶ ἵν' εἴπω κατὰ τὸν θεῖον Ἰὼβ εἰς πίστωσιν ἄγω τὸν ἡμέτερον λόγον· ἐν πολλῷ χρόνῳ σοφία, ἐν δὲ πολλῷ βίῳ ἐπιστήμη—ἔφη περὶ τῆς ἰατρικῆς ὅτι ὁ βίος ἢ[27] ὁ χρόνος τῆς ζωῆς ἡμῶν ὀλιγοσ-

---

9 τὰ προδιωρισμένα *coniecit* Singer : τὰ πρὸς διορισμένα Hb R.
10 νοσήματος ἐστὶ λέξις *delevi* : *hab.* Hb R. These words are probably a gloss erroneously incorporated into the text: therefore I have deleted them.
11 γραμματικῶν *scripsi* : γράμματι τῶν Hb : γράμματα τῶν R.
12 τῆς Hb : τῶν R.
13 τῇ Hb : τῆς R.
14 οὖν Hb : *om.* R.
15 χρείαν *correxit* Pormann : χρείᾳ Hb R.
16 ὑπάρχουσι *correxit* Pormann : ὑπάρχωσι Hb R.
17 ποιητικώτερον Hb : ποιητικῶς τε R.
18 καὶ Hb : *om.* R.
19 ἀμφοτέρωθεν *scripsi* : ἀμφοτέροθεν Hb R.
20 μακρηγορίαν *scripsi* : μακρυγορίαν Hb R.
21 κόρος λόγου R : *om.* Hb.
22 ὡς R : ἡ Hb.
23 σώμασιν Hb : σώματος R.
24 εὐφραδέως Hb : εὐφραδῶς R.
25 ἐπεὶ δὲ Hb : ἐπειδὴ R.
26 Εἰδὼς *scripsi* : Ἰδώς Hb R.
27 ἢ *scripsi* : καὶ Hb R.

τός ἐστι πρὸς τὴν ἀκριβῆ κατάληψιν ταύτης· διὰ τοῦτο πολλὴ καὶ δυσκατάληπτός ἐστι καὶ χρόνου δεῖται πολλοῦ ὁ διαγνωσόμενος εἰς ἅπαν. (5.) 'ὁ δὲ καιρὸς ὀξὺς' ἤτοι ὁ τῶν πραττομένων στενότατος βραχύτατος συντομώτατος[28] ὑπάρχει διὰ τὸ τῆς ὕλης φθαρτὸν ἣν ἡ τέχνη μεταχειρίζεται[29] πρὸς ἐπικουρίαν τῶν καχεκτούντων. ἔστι δὲ καὶ ἄλλως εἰπεῖν καὶ διὰ τὸ εὐμετάβλητον τοῦ σώματος ἡμῶν· ὅπερ ἐν μιᾷ καιροῦ ῥοπῇ ῥᾳδίως πέφυκε ἀλλοιοῦσθαι καὶ μετατρέπεσθαι, μὴ μόνον ἐπὶ τῶν ἔξωθεν αἰτιαμάτων καὶ συμπτωμάτων, ἀλλὰ καὶ ὑπὸ τῆς ἐνούσης αὐτῷ φύσει φθορᾶς. (6.) 'ἡ δὲ πεῖρα σφαλερά' ἤτοι σαθρὰ καὶ κινδυνώδης καὶ εἰς ὄλεθρον ὅλου τοῦ ζῴου τελευτῶσα, διὰ τὸ δίχα τοῦ κατ' ἐπιστήμην[30] ὀρθοῦ λόγου προσάγειν[31] τὰ φάρμακα τοῖς νοσοῦσιν, ὑφ' ἧς συμβαίνει πολλάκις τὸ ἑτέρας νόσου ἴαμα ἄλλης γεννητικὸν[32] εἶναι προσενεχθέν.[33] (7.) 'ἡ δὲ κρίσις χαλεπή',[34] ἤγουν[35] ὁ ἐπιστημονικὸς[36] λόγος ὁ κρίνων καὶ διακρίνων τίνα δεῖ προσάγειν[37] τοῖς πάσχουσι καὶ τίνα οὐ δεῖ. χαλεπός τίς ἐστι καὶ δυσεύρετος ὡς[38] δηλοῖ καὶ τὸ πλῆθος τῶν κατὰ τὴν ἰατρικὴν τέχνην αἱρέσεων διαφόρων. οἱ δὲ τῆς πείρας μὴ δεχόμενοι ταύτην τὴν εἰσβολήν φασι κρίσει ἐνταῦθα λέγειν[39] τὴν ἐπίκρισιν τῶν βοηθημάτων τῶν διὰ τῆς πείρας εὑρεθέντων, δεινὴν οὖσαν καὶ οὐ ῥᾳδίαν εἰς τὸ εἰπεῖν ἐν τίνι τῶν γεγενημένων[40] ἰαμάτων συνέβη τῷ ἀσθενεῖ[41] ὠφεληθῆναι· ὅπερ ἐμοὶ μὲν δοκεῖ πιθανόν, οὐκ ἀληθὲς δέ.

Aphorisms of Hippocrates

(1.) Since we are going to explain in a concise and clear way the *Aphorisms* of Hippocrates—by the grace of my Christ and God, who dispenses wisdom and is the first doctor of souls and bodies, wins over our weaknesses, alleviates and heals our illnesses—it is appropriate first to state and to interpret the term used in the title, then to deal with them [the *Aphorisms*]. (2.) The same title *Aphorisms of Hippocrates* in some cases

28 συντομώτατος *scripsi* : συντομότατος Hb R.
29 μεταχειρίζεται *scripsi* : μετεριχειρίζεται Hb R.
30 κατ' ἐπιστήμην *scripsi* : κατ' ἐπιστήμης R: κατεπιστήμης Hb.
31 προσάγειν *scripsi* : προσάγ (*sic*) Hb R.
32 γεννητικὸν Hb : γενητικὸν R.
33 προσενεχθέν Hb : προσηνεχθέν R.
34 κρίσις χαλεπὴ Hb : κρίσεως χαλεπῆς R.
35 ἤγουν Hb : ἤτοι R.
36 ἐπιστημονικὸς *scripsi* : ἐπιστημονικῶς Hb R.
37 προσάγειν *scripsi* : προσάγει Hb R.
38 ὡς Hb : *om.* R.
39 φασι κρίσει ἐνταῦθα λέγειν *scripsi* : φησι κρίνει ἐνταῦθα λέγει Hb R.
40 γεγενημένων *scripsi* : γεγεννημένων Hb R.
41 ἀσθενεῖ *scripsi* : ἀσθενῆ Hb R.

means '*hóros*', in some others '*horismós*'. On the one hand, *hóros* is a word with many meanings: for it signifies the 'fixing of boundaries', the 'imperial judgement', the 'term' in philosophy, to which every syllogistic premise is reduced, and the very 'definition' of a thing. On the other hand, the *horismós* (for *aphorismós* and *prodihorismós* are one and the same thing) defines and distinguishes, includes and separates from each other objects previously distinguished, both if they are things and if they are affections and illnesses. Even if students of grammar are not able to explain a rule of a rule, nevertheless the masters of philosophy explain a definition of 'definition' [*horismós*] through the abundance of their knowledge. The definition of 'definition' [*horismós*] is then: 'a concise account, which explains the nature of the thing in question'. (3.) That this account was followed by Hippocrates himself has a clear evidence and does not need explanations. That [the *Aphorisms*] are unclear is evident to everybody, because they are composed in a more poetic way and also explained in a more long-winded way by Galen; for both these reasons, they have a lot of obscurity. After having shaken off both Hippocrates' poetic obscurity in the *Aphorisms* and [Galen's] long-winded account about them—one of our favourite fathers inspired by God says: 'a surfeit of words is adverse to the hearing of divine voices, as an excessive nourishment is for bodies'—I will put this treatise in a well-written and concise style. Since our account is about medicine, it is indeed necessary to define what medicine is: 'medicine is an art, which deals with human bodies and procures health.'

(4.) Since Hippocrates knew that every art and science has to be assiduously exercised for a long time and successfully accomplished to the utmost—and I confirm our account by saying, with the divine Job: 'wisdom [is acquired] in a long time, science in a long life'—he said of medicine that life, that is, the timespan of our existence, is too short to gain exact knowledge of it. For this reason [medicine] is long and difficult to apprehend and the one who wishes to make diagnoses in all contexts needs a long time. (5.) 'Opportunity is fleeting', that means, the opportunity for what is to be done is extremely brief, short and limited because matter, with which the art deals to help those who are ill, is perishable. One can say this in another way: [it is so] because our body changes easily, since at the only decisive moment of opportunity, [the body] is naturally predisposed to be readily altered and to change, not only moved by external causes and symptoms, but also by the deterioration intrinsic to its nature. (6.) 'Experiment is treacherous', that means, it is misleading and dangerous and brings about the death of the whole living being, because medicaments are administered to sick people without correct reasoning according to science: as a result of the [experiment], it often happens that the remedy for an illness generates another [illness], after it is administered. (7.) 'Judgment is difficult', that is to say, the scientific reasoning is what judges and discerns what one must administer to the patients and what not. It is somehow difficult and difficult to discover, as the great number of different sects in the medical art shows. The empiricists do not accept this onslaught and claim that by 'judgement (*krísis*)' Hippocrates means 'verification (*epíkrisis*)' of the remedies found through experiment; this verification represents a great task and it is not easy to say in which of the cures that have been brought about the patient happened to be helped. This seems to me plausible, but not true.

2 Remarks

The text is divided into two parts: in the first part (§§1–3), the compiler introduces the commentary on the *Aphorisms*, by explaining the title and offering a definition of medicine; in the second (§§4–7), he provides a word-by-word commentary on the text of the first part of *Aphorisms* 1.1. The only title present in both manuscripts (Hb and R) is 'Ἀφορισμοὶ τοῦ Ἱπποκράτους (Aphorisms of Hippocrates)', without any mention of a commentator, neither Galen nor Theophilus.

(§1) The Christian character of the text emerges from its very first lines: through an invocation, Jesus is defined as dispensor of wisdom, first doctor of souls and bodies, winner over human weaknesses, and physician who alleviates and heals human illnesses. It is well known that references to Jesus as physician, and in particular as physician of the soul, became widespread in Christian literature from the 3rd century.[42] At the end of Late Antiquity, which means more or less from the sixth century onwards, Christian features also started to appear in both philosophical and medical commentaries.[43]

The compiler claims that first of all it is necessary to explain the title (ἐπιγραφή) 'Aphorisms', which in some cases derives from the word ὅρος, and in

42 For a general overview on this topic, see Temkin (1991), 144–145, 157–158.

43 One of the first Christian philosophers in the Neoplatonic schools was John Philoponus. Among the medical commentators, it is not certain whether Stephen, the commentator on Hippocratic treatises, was also Christian. In the concluding words of his *Commentary on the Prognostic* (3. 32: Duffy 1983, p. 292, lines 31–32) we find an invocation to God, and

some others from the word ὁρισμός. The explanation of the title constituted one of the eight headings (κεφάλαια) of the so-called *schema isagogicum*, that is, the typical didactic list of topics to be addressed in the prologues of late antique commentaries.[44] As far as we know, among the commentators on the Hippocratic *Aphorisms*, only Stephen of Athens (sixth century) discussed the meaning of the title among the eight main points of the *schema isagogicum*, thus following the exegetical tradition of the Alexandrian Neoplatonists. Stephen argued that the title shows the way (τρόπος) in which Hippocrates taught medicine (Westerink 1985, p. 30, lines 18–19; cf. also p. 32, lines 7–9). The same interpretation is to be found in the Latin commentary attributed to Meletius, which almost exactly corresponds to the one by Stephen (Dietz 1834, vol. 2, p. 243, lines 12–14).

(§ 2) The compiler presents the definitions of ὅρος and ὁρισμός. The word ὅρος has four possible meanings: 1) the first one is concrete and indicates 'fixing the boundaries' (τὸ ὁροθέσιον); 2) the second one is political and means an 'imperial judgment' (ἡ βασιλικὴ ἀπόφασις); 3) the third one is philosophical and pertains to the field of logic: it means 'term' in a syllogistic sense (ὁ κατὰ φιλοσοφίαν ὅρος); 4) the fourth sense is more general and corresponds with the meaning of 'definition' (ὁρισμός). This is the first passage of our text which shows clear similarities with the *Introduction to Philosophy* (*Prolegomena philosophiae*) by David, a Neoplatonic commentator of the school of Olympiodorus,[45] who discusses and defines the notion of ὁρισμός (see especially πρᾶξις ε′: Busse 1904, p. 11, line 15–p. 15, line 9). Nevertheless, it is even more striking that the compiler of our text offers the same re-elaborated version of David's *Introduction* as is presented by John of Damascus (seventh to eighth century) in his *Dialectics*, and in particular in the eighth chapter, entitled Περὶ ὁρισμοῦ. Here John reports the following definitions of ὅρος and ὁρισμός (cf. also below):

similarly in the title of his *Commentary on Hippocrates' 'Aphorisms'* (Westerink 1985, p. 28, line 1). Nevertheless, as Temkin (1991), 236 suggests, 'such formulas may even be additions by Byzantine editors and scribes'.

44 See Mansfeld (1994), 10–11.

45 David's commentary also shows many affinities with Elias' *Prolegomena philosophiae*. On Elias and David, see Busse (1900) and (1904), respectively; cf. also Westerink (1962), pp. xx–xxiv and Westerink (1964). On the Neoplatonic *Prolegomena philosophiae* as introductions to the *Commentaries on the Isagoge* by Porphyrius, see Militello 2010, in particular pp. 53–73. The writings by Elias and David should not be confused with those of Pseudo-Elias (pseudo-David), edited by Westerink (1967).

> Ὁ μὲν γὰρ ὅρος δηλοῖ τὸ ὁροθέσιον, δηλοῖ δὲ καὶ τὴν ἀπόφασιν, ὥς φαμεν 'ὥρισεν ὁ βασιλεύς', δηλοῖ καὶ εἰς ὃν ἀναλύεται ἡ πρότασις, ὡς ἐν τοῖς ἑξῆς σὺν θεῷ μαθησόμεθα, δηλοῖ δὲ καὶ τὸν ὁρισμόν. Ὁ δὲ ὁρισμὸς μόνον δηλοῖ τὸν λόγον τὸν σύντομον, τὸν δηλωτικὸν τῆς φύσεως τοῦ ὑποκειμένου πράγματος (*rec. fus.* 8.83–88: Kotter 1968, 71–72).
>
> *Hóros* indicates the 'fixing of boundaries', and also the 'judgement', as in the expression 'the emperor judged'; it indicates also the 'term' to which a premise is reduced, as we shall learn later, God willing, and it indicates also the 'definition'. *Horismós*, however, only indicates a concise account which explains the nature of the thing in question.

It is certainly known that John used David's *Introduction to Philosophy* as one of the main sources for his *Dialectics*.[46] We must, however, emphasise that only John of Damascus presents the same structure, involving four definitions, that we find in our text: this could let us suppose that at least in this case the compiler used as his source John of Damascus, rather than David. On the other hand, the sentence 'εἰς ὃν ἀναλύεται πᾶσα πρότασις (to which every syllogistic premise is reduced)' often recurs in Neoplatonic texts, where it usually presents the form 'εἰς ὃν ἀναλύεται ἡ πρότασις' (with the article ἡ instead of the reading πᾶσα of our text): see, for example, John Philoponus' *Commentary on Aristotle's 'Analytics'* (Wallies, 1905, p. 11, lines 10–11 and p. 24, line 28) and David's *Introduction to Philosophy* (Busse 1904, p. 13, lines 18–20), as well as the above-mentioned passage of John of Damascus and his *Philosophical Fragments* (p. 9, lines 16–17 and p. 18, lines 39–40; Kotter 1968, 161 and 171).[47] This sentence clearly depends on Aristotle's *Prior Analytics* 24b16, where we find the philosophical definition of ὅρος: 'I call *hóros* that to which the syllogistic premise is reduced (Ὅρον δὲ καλῶ εἰς ὃν διαλύεται ἡ πρότασις).'

Whereas ὅρος encompasses a complex range of meanings, ὁρισμός bears the more specific meaning of 'distinguishing things from one another' and, in the medical field, 'distinguishing and defining illnesses'. Our compiler then draws a comparison between the young students of grammar (γραμματικῶν παῖδες), who only possess literary skills and cannot give a 'rule of a rule', and the mas-

---

46 See Richter (1964), 102–109 on chapter 8 of John of Damascus' *Dialectics* and its sources. The exact nature of the link between the late antique *Introduction to Philosophy* and the *Dialectics*, however, is not entirely clear. Roueché (1974) assumes that chapter 8 of the *Dialectics* as well as other parts of the text were composed from logical compendia circulating in the seventh century and not from complete lecture texts.

47 Cf. also pseudo-Zonaras' *Lexicon* (Tittmann 1808, p. 1463, lines 19–20).

ters of philosophy (οἱ τῆς φιλοσοφίας ἀρχηγοί), who, on the contrary, gave a 'definition of definition'. The name ἀρχηγός was used to define different philosophers, each of them considered the 'first' or the 'master' in his particular field or school.[48] Considering the similarities discussed above of our prologue with the Neoplatonic commentaries, it is immediately clear that the compiler refers to Plato and Aristotle with the expression οἱ τῆς φιλοσοφίας ἀρχηγοί. We have here another parallel to David's *Introduction to Porphyry's 'Isagoge'*, in which Plato and Aristotle are explicitly defined as masters of philosophy (Busse 1904, p. 105, lines 17–20).

Nevertheless, the definition of ὁρισμός that our text attributes to the masters of philosophy ('a concise account, which explains the nature of the thing in question') is not given by any work of Plato or Aristotle. Its earliest occurrence is to be found in pseudo-Galen's *Medical Definitions*, probably written in the first century AD:[49]

> Ὁρισμός ἐστι λόγος σύντομος δηλωτικὸς τῆς φύσεως τοῦ ὑποκειμένου πράγματος. ὁρισμὸς δὲ λέγεται ἀπὸ μεταφορᾶς τῶν ἐν τοῖς χωρίοις ὁροθεσίων.
>
> *Horismós* is a concise account which explains the nature of the thing in question. *Horismós* is used metaphorically in analogy with the 'fixing of boundaries' on land.

There are two possible explanations for this discrepancy: either the compiler quoted the definition of ὁρισμός from memory and generally attributed it to Plato and Aristotle without knowing the original source, or—and this option would be much more interesting—he considered Galen as one of the 'masters of philosophy', to whom the *Medical Definitions* were attributed. This last possibility is not to be excluded in the context of Neoplatonic schools, where medicine and philosophy were studied together.[50] This definition, in some cases referred to ὅρος and in others to ὁρισμός, became very widespread in Late Antiquity and Middle Byzantine Period: it often occurs in the introductions to different arts, in particular to philosophical, medical and rhetorical

48 For example, the founder of the natural philosophy is meant usually Thales of Miletus by Aristotle and the Aristotelian philosophers: See Aristotle, *Metaphysics* 983b20–21 and, for example, Alexander of Aphrodisias, *Commentary on Aristotle's 'Metaphysics'* (Hayduck 1891, p. 24, line 9).

49 The *Medical Definitions* are dated in the first century of our Era by Kollesch (1973), 60–66; the quotation is found at 19.349.6–8 K.

50 See Westerink (1964), Pormann (2010b) and Overwien (2018).

texts. Among the various introductory writings that use such a definition, it is worth mentioning, for example, the *Treatise on Definitions* (*Tractatus De definitionibus*) ascribed to Athanasius and dated to the seventh century (Migne 1856–1866, vol. 28, col. 533, lines 31–32), the seventh-century Berlin papyrus 11739A (it contains a Neoplatonic introduction to the Commentary on Galen's *On the Sects for Beginners*),[51] the *Introduction to Philosophy* by Elias (Busse 1904, p. 4, line 5), the *Introduction to Philosophy* by David (Busse 1904, p. 11, lines 17–18), chapter eight (Περὶ ὁρισμοῦ) of the *Dialectics* by John of Damascus (Kotter 1968, 69–72, in particular lines 83–88), and different Byzantine lexica.[52]

More generally, the use of definitions became very common from Late Antiquity onwards, especially in texts that served didactic purposes. The genre of the definitions (ὅροι) is similar to that of the ἐρωταποκρίσεις, and in many instances the definition is just presented as an answer to the question 'what is (τί ἐστιν)'.[53] Therefore the pseudo-Galenic *Medical Definitions* also became a very important source for the exegetical and didactic activity of that time.[54] Their use became instrumental in the transmission of philosophical learning (and in particular of Aristotelian logic) in the Middle Byzantine period.[55]

(§ 3) The compiler justifies the need to further explain the Hippocratic *Aphorisms* by emphasizing their obscurity: he argues that Hippocrates wrote the *Aphorisms* in a more poetic (ποιητικώτερον) but not clear way and that Galen explained them in a more long-winded (πολυλογώτερον), but also quite unclear way. The clarification of what is unclear was a fundamental exegetical principle since Galen's commentaries on Hippocrates,[56] and it became very common among Neoplatonists, too. Furthermore, we find in this paragraph another interesting parallel to the *Introduction to Porphyry's 'Isagoge'* by David, who mentions Galen as an example of obscurity because of his long-winded narrat-

51 See Manetti (1992).

52 For instance that by pseudo-Zonaras (Tittmann 1808, p. 1462, lines 13–15) and the *Etymologicum Magnum* (Gaisford 1848, p. 349, lines 24–25).

53 On the ἐρωταποκρίσεις see Garzya (1992) and Ieraci Bio (1995).

54 On the genre of the 'definitions' in antiquity, see Kollesch (1973), 35–38 with further bibliography.

55 See Roueché (1980) on the use of definitions in the Middle Byzantine period: he edits a Middle Byzantine text, which is a compendium of definitions pertaining to the *Isagoge* of Porphyry and the *Categories* of Aristotle and shows many similarities with the *Dialectis* by John of Damascus.

56 See Mansfeld (1994), 148–154.

ive (Busse 1904, p. 105, lines 13–16), and by Elias, who presents both Galen's prolixity and Hippocrates' brevity as examples of stylistic obscurity (Busse 1900, p. 41, line 30–p. 42, line 5).

In support of his aim to explain the Hippocratic text concisely and clearly, the compiler quotes a sentence from the treatise *On Holy Baptism* (*In sanctum baptisma*), written by the Cappadocian Father Gregory of Nazianzus (fourth century), who compares an excess of words, which is inimical to hearing the word of God, to an excess of food, which is bad for bodies: κόρος λόγου πολέμιος ἀκοαῖς, ὡς ὑπερβάλλουσα τροφὴ σώματι (*Orations* 40, Migne 1856–1866, vol. 36, p. 360, lines 24–25). It is rather significant that the only other quotation of this sentence is in John of Damascus' *Sacred Parallels* (Migne 1856–1866, vol. 95, col. 1345, lines 27–28). Moreover, from a philological point of view, it is noteworthy that this is the only case in which R, a copy of Hb, transmits a better text: the words κόρος λόγου are, in fact, missing in Hb. However, the fact that both Gregory of Nazianzus and John of Damascus put the words κόρος λόγου after πολέμιος ἀκοαῖς, whereas in R they occur before, seems to be a sign that the copyist of the manuscript R has intentionally added them, after having noticed their absence in the antigraph Hb.

By way of conclusion of the first section, the compiler uses the definition of medicine as 'an art which deals with the human bodies and procures health (ἰατρική ἐστι τέχνη περὶ τὰ ἀνθρώπινα σώματα καταγινομένη ὑγείας περιποιητική)', which has a clear original source in pseudo-Galen's *Medical Definitions* (19.350.17–18 K.). Exactly as was the case with the definition of ὁρισμός (see above), this definition of medicine, too, became very popular in the Neoplatonic schools: we find it in the *Commentary on Porphyry's 'Isagoge'* by Ammonius (Busse 1891, p. 2, lines 6–9), in that by Elias (Busse 1900, p. 5, line 34–p. 6, line 3) and in the *Introduction to Philosophy* by David (Busse 1904, p. 17, line 33–p. 18, line 6; p. 19, lines 3–4); it was also quoted in the same eighth chapter Περὶ ὁρισμοῦ of the *Dialectics* by John of Damascus (Kotter 1968, p. 70, lines 24–26). This definition contains—even if not explicitly—the clear Aristotelian distinction between the object (ὑποκείμενον) of the art, namely human bodies (περὶ τὰ ἀνθρώπινα σώματα καταγινομένη), and its purpose (τέλος), namely health (ὑγείας περιποιητική).[57]

The second section of the anonymous text offers a word-by-word exegesis of the first aphorism, or rather of its first part: 'Life is short, art long, opportunity

57 A very similar definition is also to be found in the scholia to Galen's *On the Sects for Beginners*, edited for the first time by Moraux in 1977: on this see Perilli (2000), 94–98.

fleeting, experiment treacherous, judgement difficult (ὁ βίος βραχύς, ἡ δὲ τέχνη μακρή, ὁ δὲ καιρὸς ὀξύς, ἡ δὲ πεῖρα σφαλερή, ἡ δὲ κρίσις χαλεπή).'[58]

(§ 4) The section immediately begins with the explanation of the words 'Ὁ βίος βραχύς, ἡ δὲ τέχνη μακρή' of the first Hippocratic aphorism. The expression εἰδὼς ὁ Ἱπποκράτης occurs only in late antique medical commentaries, and precisely in the *Commentary on Epidemics 6* by Palladius (Dietz 1834, vol. 2, p. 34, line 9 and p. 171, line 5) and in the *Commentary on Aphorisms* by Theophilus (Dietz 1834, vol. 2, p. 489, line 4).

The compiler incidentally quotes the words of the 'divine' Job, with the intention of confirming the dictum of Hippocrates through the Bible: ἐν πολλῷ χρόνῳ σοφία, ἐν δὲ πολλῷ βίῳ ἐπιστήμη (*Septuagint Job*, 12.12, translating the Hebrew בִּישִׁישִׁים חָכְמָה וְאֹרֶךְ יָמִים תְּבוּנָה). The same sentence from the *Book of Job* is often quoted by authors of the fourth to seventh centuries (one of the first occurrences is in John Chrysostom's *Fragments on Job*: Migne 1856–1866, vol. 64, col. 609, lines 12–13), and significantly twice by John of Damascus in his *Sacred Parallels* (Migne 1856–1866, vol. 95, col. 1308, lines 1–2 and vol. 96, col. 261, lines 21–22), where we have already found the sentence of Gregory of Nazianzus quoted in the third paragraph of our text (see above).

Turning his attention back to the Hippocratic words, the compiler specifies that life (βίος) is too short (ὀλιγοστός) for us to gain exact knowledge (πρὸς τὴν ἀκριβῆ κατάληψιν) of medicine, that is to reach perfection, which is not within the compass of human faculty. Moreover, one who wishes to make diagnoses needs a long time, since the science of medicine (ἐπιστήμη περὶ τῆς ἰατιρκῆς) is difficult to apprehend (δυσκατάληπτος). Galen uses the adjective δύσληπτος to explain the Hippocratic expression τέχνη μακρή, whereas both Stephen (Westerink 1985, p. 40, line 6) and Theophilus (Dietz 1834, vol. 2, p. 247, lines 34–35) use δυσκατάληπτος to explain the following κρίσις χαλεπή. It appears clear that here the compiler reworks Galen's text, as is also shown by the use of the participle διαγνωσόμενος used as a noun, which does not occur in any late antique commentary on the *Aphorisms*. The entire passage by Galen, which has been here reworked, reads (*Commentary on Hippocrates' 'Aphorisms'* 1.1 [17b.346.8–12 K.]):

> τὴν τέχνην δ' αὐτὴν διὰ τοῦτο ὑπολαμβάνω ἡγεῖσθαι μακράν, ὅτι τόν τε καιρὸν ὀλίγου δεῖν ἁπασῶν τῶν κατὰ μέρος ἐνεργειῶν ὀλιγοχρόνιον ἔχει καὶ κατὰ τοῦτο δύσληπτον, ὡς μακρᾶς δεῖσθαι τριβῆς τὸν διαγνωσόμενον.

58 Magdelaine 1994, 2. 375, 1–2 = 4. 458, 4–5 L.

> I presume that for this reason [Hippocrates] considered the art to be 'long', because the opportunity for almost all its individual activities is of short duration and therefore difficult to determine, so that someone who is going to diagnose needs a long practice.

(§5) The fifth paragraph explains the meaning of the words 'ὁ δὲ καιρὸς ὀξύς (opportunity is fleeting)'. The influence of Galen, already discussed in the previous paragraph, emerges again in the sentence '"Opportunity is fleeting", that means, the opportunity for what is to be done is extremely brief, short and limited (ὁ δὲ καιρὸς ὀξὺς ἤτοι ὁ τῶν πραττομένων στενότατος βραχύτατος συντομώτατος ὑπάρχει)', which defines better the meaning of the adjective ὀξύς; the correspondent passage in Galen's *Commentary on Aphorisms* reads: 'The opportunity for what is to be done is very fleeting in it [sc. the medical art], that is, extremely brief and of short duration (ὁ τῶν πραττομένων καιρὸς ἐν αὐτῇ ὀξύτατός ἐστι, τουτέστι στενότατός τε καὶ ὀλιγοχρονιώτατος)' (17b.353.4–6 K.).

The compiler then offers two different explanations of the Hippocratic expression. According to the first one, the opportunity is fleeting because the matter that medicine deals with (μεταχειρίζεται), that is to say the human body, is perishable (διὰ τὸ τῆς ὕλης φθαρτόν). Nevertheless, it is possible to explain it also in a different way (ἄλλως), namely through the expression 'because our body changes easily (διὰ τὸ εὐμετάβλητον τοῦ σώματος ἡμῶν)'. The correspondence with Galen's *Commentary* is evident also in this case, since Galen wrote (17b.346.16–18 K.):

> ὁ μὲν οὖν καιρός ἐστιν ὀξὺς διὰ τὸ τῆς ὕλης ῥευστόν, ἣν ἡ τέχνη μεταχειρίζεται· εὐμετάβλητον γὰρ ἡμῶν τὸ σῶμα καὶ ῥᾳδίως ἀλλοιούμενον.
>
> Opportunity is fleeting because the matter with which the art deals is in flux, for our body changes and alters easily.

This passage of Galen's *Commentary* was very popular in Late Antiquity: both Stephen in his commentaries on the *Aphorisms* (Westerink 1985, p. 38, lines 25–26) and *Prognostic* (Duffy 1983, p. 50, lines 6–7; Dietz 1834, vol. 1, p. 68, lines 7–8), and Theophilus in his commentary on the *Aphorisms* (Dietz 1834, vol. 2, p. 247, lines 20–21) used it, and it is also quoted or paraphrased in other anonymous texts which dealt with the first Hippocratic aphorism.[59] However, it is interesting to notice that neither Galen nor Stephen nor Theophilus used the adjective

59 See, for example, the anonymous text usually called *On Medicine* (*De medicina*; Kapetanaki–Sharples (2006), p. 88, line 13; Dietz 1834, vol. 2, p. 244, line 16: τῷ ἐν σώματι

φθαρτόν, but rather ῥευστόν. The adjective φθαρτός does not occur in any late antique or Byzantine commentary on the *Aphorisms*. I have found a similar expression only in a scholium to the Hippocratic treatise *Precepts*, based on Galen's *Commentary on Hippocrates' 'Aphorisms'* 1.1: in order to explain the sentence ὀξὺς ὁ καιρός διὰ τὸ ῥευστὸν δῆλον τῆς ὕλης καὶ εὐαλλοίωτον, taken from Galen,[60] the author of the anonymous scholium used the expression ἔμενον ἂν ἄφθαρτα with reference to the human bodies, which are necessarily subjected to the deterioration, since otherwise 'they would be imperishable'.

(§ 6) In his explanation of the expression 'experiment is treacherous (ἡ δὲ πεῖρα σφαλερή)', the compiler of our text mostly refers to Galen's *Commentary*, which says: 'to try something on a human body that has never before been attempted is extremely dangerous, as the bad experiment brings about the death of the whole living being (ἐπ' ἀνθρωπείου δὲ σώματος πειρᾶσθαι τῶν ἀπειράστων οὐκ ἀσφαλές, εἰς ὄλεθρον ὅλου τοῦ ζῴου τῆς κακῆς πείρας τελευτώσης)' (17b.354.2–4 K.). Nevertheless, he adds that experiment is dangerous, since medicaments can happen to have side effects: those medicines which can heal illnesses may also generate other diseases, if they have not been previously tested and verified.

(§ 7) 'ἡ δὲ κρίσις χαλεπή (judgment is difficult)', is explained once again through Galen's *Commentary*, which mentioned the large quantity of different medical schools as a sign that there was no consensus regarding medical theory: 'Also judgement—reasoning may be the judgement—is difficult and hard to obtain—especially correct [reasoning], as the great number of medical sects shows (καὶ μὴν καὶ ἡ κρίσις, ὁ λόγος δ' ἂν ἡ κρίσις εἴη, χαλεπὸς καὶ δυσθήρατός ἐστιν ὅ γε ἀληθής, ὡς δηλοῖ καὶ τὸ πλῆθος τῶν κατὰ τὴν ἰατρικὴν τέχνην αἱρέσεων)' (17b.354.6–7 K.). Nevertheless, in our text we find the couple of adjectives χαλεπός and δυσεύρετος, which have some parallels in late antique commentaries to Aristotle with reference to the θεωρία,[61] whereas Galen uses the couple χαλεπὸς and δυσθήρατος.

In particular, the school of Empiricists is taken into account: they did not accept the role of theory represented by the substantive κρίσις, and for this

ῥευστῷ μὲν διὰ τὴν ὕλην καὶ ἀβεβαίῳ). It is unclear whether this Galenic sentence has an Aristotelian origin, as Flashar (1962), p. 408, n. 3 noted.

60 For the edition of this text see Ecca (2016), 332–339; for a general interpretation of it see Ecca (2018).

61 Cf. Alexander of Aphrodisias, *Commentary on Aristotle's 'Metaphysics'* (Hayduck 1891, p. 139, lines 8–9 and p. 140, lines 14–15) and Asclepius, *Commentary on Aristotle's 'Metaphysics'* (Hayduck 1888, p. 116, line 9 and p. 117, line 1).

reason they introduced the substantive ἐπίκρισις, which refers to the practical 'verification' of the effects of a drug. Here the compiler uses the expression ἐνταῦθα λέγειν in order to attribute to Hippocrates, according to the Empiricists' interpretation, the use of ἐπίκρισις. We find an almost word-by-word quotation of Galen's *Commentary*, which reads (17b.354.10–15 K.):

> τοῖς δ' ἐμπειρικοῖς οὐχ ὁ λόγος εἰρῆσθαι δοκεῖ κρίσις, ἀλλ' ἡ τῶν διὰ τῆς πείρας εὑρισκομένων βοηθημάτων ἐπίκρισις. ὄντως γὰρ καὶ τοῦτο χαλεπὸν καὶ δυσθήρατον, ὅταν πολλῶν ἰαμάτων τῷ κάμνοντι γεγενημένων ἕν τι ἐξ αὐτῶν αἰτιᾶται τῆς ὠφελείας ἢ βλάβης.
>
> It seems that the Empiricists do not call the 'reason' 'judgement', but 'verification' of the remedies discovered through experiment. This is also really difficult and hard to grasp, when only one of the many cures that there are for a patient is alleged as the cause of benefit or harm.

The explanation of the first part of the first aphorism is followed by the prologue of the *Commentary* on the *Hippocratic Aphorisms* ascribed to Theophilus. In R, the division between the two sources was pointed out through a sign of *caesura*, which nevertheless was probably added by a later reader of the manuscript, who recognized the Theophilean prologue. I edit below the text of the prologue to Theophilus' *Commentary on Aphorisms*, as transmitted in our two manuscripts Hb and R. I will compare and, when necessary, correct it according to the text printed by Dietz:[62]

> τί ἐστιν ἀφορισμός;[63] λόγος σύντομος αὐτοτελῆ διάνοιαν[64] ἀπαρτίζων ἢ λόγος κατὰ μὲν τὴν προφορὰν ἤτοι τὴν φράσιν[65] πενόμενος,[66] πλουτῶν δὲ τοῖς ἐνθυμήμασιν. εἴρηται[67] ἀφορισμὸς διὰ τὸ περιορίζεσθαι ἐν αὐτῷ τὸ νόημα, ἀφορίζεσθαι δὲ καὶ ἀποδιΐστασθαι ἀπὸ τῶν πρὸ[68] αὐτοῦ καὶ τῶν μετ' αὐτόν.[69]

62 Unfortunately, there is no critical edition of Theophilus' *Commentary* yet.

63 τί ἐστιν ἀφορισμός Hb R] ἀφορισμός ἐστι Dietz. The interrogative form of the beginning of the prologue is to be found also in other manuscripts of the *Commentary* by Theophilus.

64 διάνοιαν Dietz : διανοίᾳ Hb R.

65 φράσιν Dietz Hb : φάσιν R.

66 πενόμενος Dietz : πενώμενος Hb R.

67 post εἴρηται *hab.* δὲ Dietz.

68 πρὸ Dietz : περὶ Hb R.

69 αὐτόν Dietz : αὐτοῦ Hb R.

> ἰστέον[70] ὅτι δύο προοίμια ἔχει ἡ παροῦσα πραγματεία· καὶ τὸ μὲν πρῶτον ἐστὶν ἀποφαντικὸν ἢ ἀποτρεπτικὸν κατὰ τρόπον,[71] ὡς τὸ[72] 'ὁ βίος βραχύς, ἡ δὲ τέχνη μακρά', τὸ δεύτερον συμβουλευτικόν, τὸ 'δεῖ δὲ οὐ μόνον ἑωϋτὸν[73] παρέχειν[74] τὰ δέοντα ποιέοντα καὶ τὰ ἑξῆς.'
>
> What is an aphorism? It is a concise account which determines a meaning that is complete in itself or an account which is poor in the utterance, that is, in the expression, but rich in meaning. It is called aphorism because it circumscribes in itself the thought, and at the same time it defines and distinguishes it from those that are before it and those that are after it.
>
> It should be known that the present treatise has two prologues: the first is declaratory or dissuasive in style, that is 'life is short, art is long …', the second is hortatory, that is '[scil. the physician] must be ready not only to do his duty himself' and so on.

Considering that the prologue by Theophilus partially corresponds in content to our anonymous text, one might think that our text represents just a longer version of Theophilus' prologue, which was not fully preserved in the rest of its manuscript tradition. This hypothesis, however, seems to be contradicted by that fact that the two texts often overlap with each other in their contents.

The prologue by Theophilus is divided into two parts. The first part (from τί ἐστιν ἀφορισμός up to τῶν μετ' αὐτόν) presents the definition of ἀφορισμός, which, exactly as in our anonymous text for the definition of ὁρισμός and medicine (see above §§ 2 and 3), shows a clear similarity with pseudo-Galen's *Medical Definitions* 19.349.14–17 K.):

> Ἀφορισμός ἐστι λόγος σύντομος αὐτοτελῆ διάνοιαν ἀπαρτίζων. ἢ οὕτως· ἀφορισμός ἐστι λόγος πενόμενος μὲν κατὰ τὴν προφορὰν ἤτοι τὴν λέξιν, πλουτῶν δὲ τοῖς ἐνθυμήμασιν.
>
> An aphorism is a concise account which determines a meaning that is complete in itself. Another definition is this: an aphorism is an account which is poor in the utterance, that is in the expression, but rich in meaning.

---

70 *post* ἰστέον *hab.* δὲ Dietz.

71 ἢ ἀποτρεπτικὸν κατὰ τρόπον *correxi* : ἢ ἀποτρεπτικὸν κατὰ τροπὴν Hb R : ἤγουν κατὰ προτροπὴν καὶ ἀποτροπὴν Dietz.

72 ὡς τὸ Dietz : τοῦ Hb R.

73 ἑωϋτὸν Dietz Hb : ἑωυτός R.

74 παρέχειν Dietz : παρέχει Hb R.

The commentaries by Stephen and Meletius on the Hippocratic *Aphorisms*[75] as well as the pre-Salernitan Latin commentary on the *Aphorisms*, known as 'Lat-A'[76] offer the same or a similar definition of aphorism at the end of the respective prologues. Nevertheless, it is significant that this definition, unlike the previous ones of ὁρισμός and medicine, has no parallel in David's *Introduction to Philosophy* nor in any other philosophical commentary of Late Antiquity, but is exclusively used by the medical commentators on the *Aphorisms*. This clearly indicates the difference in the use of sources between the compiler of our anonymous text, who mostly reworked philosophical material in the first part of the text, and Theophilus as author of the second prologue, who mostly used medical material.

The second section (from ἰστέον ὅτι up to the end) of Theophilus' prologue corresponds in content to Galen's *Commentary*, which divided the first aphorism into two parts with different introductory functions: a first declaratory part and a second hortative part (17b.347.9–14 K.):

> τὸ μὲν οὖν πρότερον αὐτοῦ μέρος τοῦ προοιμίου, κατὰ τουτὶ τελευτᾷ· τὸ δὲ δεύτερον οὐχ ὡς ἀποφαινόμενος, ἀλλ' ὡς συμβουλεύων γράφει. δεῖ δ' οὐ μόνον ἑαυτὸν παρέχειν τὰ δέοντα ποιέοντα, ἀλλὰ καὶ τὸν νοσέοντα καὶ τοὺς παρέοντας καὶ τὰ ἔξωθεν.
>
> The first part of the proem ends here. [Hippocrates] writes the second part not in a declaratory, but in a hortative way. The physician must be ready not only to do his duty himself, but also to secure the co-operation of the patient, of the attendants and of externals.

This distinction is important with regard to the exegetic activity on the text from Late Antiquity onwards, since both the *Commentary* by Stephen (which contains the same bipartition in the prologue)[77] and that by Theophilus comment on the two parts of the aphorism as if they were two separate aphorisms.

Finally, as we have seen above, after Theophilus' prologue the manuscripts Hb and R hand down the corresponding section of Theophilus' *Commentary* on the first part of *Aphorism* 1.1 (the 'declaratory' part), whereas they preserves Galen's *Commentary* from the second part of *Aphorism* 1.1 up to the end of the

75 Westerink (1985), p. 32, lines 14–17; cf. Meletius (Dietz 1834, vol. 2, p. 244; cf. Ihm 2002, 165–166).

76 Ed. Beccaria (1961), 41, 45–46: *Quid est aforismus? Sermo brevis, integrum sensum propositae rei scribens.*

77 Ed. Westerink (1985), p. 32, lines 26–27.

treatise. This means that the structure of our anonymous text, divided between prologue and commentary on the first part of *Aphorism* 1.1, exactly corresponds to the structure of Theophilus' *Commentary* as preserved in Hb and R. We must assume, therefore, that the juxtaposition of the Theophilean prologue is not due to the compiler of our text, but is the result of the later creation of the mixed commentary. For the compiler of our text would surely have noted the repetition of the contents in Theophilus' *Commentary* and would have had no reason to write the same things twice.

3 Conclusions

The analysis I have conducted so far offers some important considerations enabling us to infer the cultural and historical context to which this new prologue to the commentaries on the Hippocratic *Aphorisms* belongs. In the first part of our text, we found various elements derived from the tradition of the *Introductions to Philosophy* by David and Elias. These *Introductions* facilitated the study of the Porphyry's *Isagoge*, which was the first treatise to be read according to the philosophical curriculum of the Neoplatonic schools: the *Isagoge* was supposed to prepare the students for the reading of Aristotelian logic, since it is an introduction to the Aristotelian *Categories*.[78] Moreover, we detected an even more striking affinity of our text with the eighth chapter of the *Dialectics* of John of Damascus, who used David's *Introduction* as his main source. In this regard, the investigation on the transmission of logical handbooks between the end of the fifth and the middle of the eighth century in Byzantium is also important for the contextualization of our text. Roueché has pointed out that logical compendia, essentially those composed on the basis of the *Introductions to Philosophy* by David and Elias, 'undoubtedly played an important role in the transmission of the Aristotelian tradition during the 7th century: they form the likeliest bridge between the Alexandrian lectures on the one hand, and the Dialectica of John Damascene on the other'.[79] Among the medical commentaries, some scholia to Galen's *On Elements*, which presumably date back to Late Antiquity, also show similarities with the *Introductions to Philosophy* by David and Elias.[80] Our text certainly displays some features typical of a didactic-exegetical context (as, for example, the extensive use of

78 See Militello (2010).

79 So Roueché (1974), 67; see also Roueché (1980).

80 On this topic see Perilli (2000), which offers an important contribution to the investigation begun by Moraux (1977).

ἤτοι and ἤγουν in the sense of 'that means'). The compiler has tried to interpret the famous first Hippocratic aphorism through the reading of Aristotelian logic, which offered some important and basic definitions of ὅρος and ὁρισμός, useful for the explanation of the Hippocratic title.

In the second part of the text the presence of re-elaborated material taken from Galen's *Commentary on the Aphorisms* is evident, and this material is combined with elements revealing analogies with late antique medical commentaries. Unfortunately, these considerations do not enable us to identify the compiler, who was not necessarily a physician: in Late Antiquity and Middle Byzantine period, in fact, lectures on the first Hippocratic aphorism were probably common among philosophers too. One should not, then, be surprised that the compiler ended his text with the commentary on the first part of the first aphorism without commenting further on the Hippocratic text, since from the time of Galen onwards, it was considered a prologue somehow independent from the seven books of the *Aphorisms*. We find similar cases in other anonymous prologues, which reworked the famous first Hippocratic aphorism, and three are particularly worthy to be mentioned: first, the so-called prologue *On Medicine*, edited by Dietz and more recently by Kapetanaki–Sharples;[81] second, the anonymous text in the *Parisinus gr.* 2237 taken into account by Ieraci Bio;[82] and third, the scholium to the incipit of the Hippocratic *Precepts* transmitted in the *Vaticanus Urbinas graecus* 68, which I edited and commented on.[83]

The significant similarities with the *Introduction to Philosophy* and the *Dialectics* of John of Damascus, as well as the Christian character of the text, allow us to date our prologue no earlier than the sixth century. Beyond this, it is more difficult to establish a date for the composition of the text. Certainly, we can argue that the compiler studied the basic principles of Aristotelian logic derived from the late antique *Introductions* and commentaries on Porphyry's *Isagoge*. It is difficult to establish whether the compiler used the *Introduction* by David and the *Dialectics* by John of Damascus as direct sources or rather some logical compendia circulating in the Middle Byzantine period. The fact that, alongside the Christian invocation at the beginning, there are two further Christian quotations in the text (from Gregory of Nazianzus' *On Holy Baptism*

81 Dietz (1834), vol. 2, pp. 244–245, and Kapetanaki–Sharples (2006), 86–90. See also the studies by Flashar (1962) and Roselli (1998).

82 See Ieraci Bio (2006).

83 See Ecca (2016), 332–339 and (2018). It is worth to notice here that also in this scholium we find a quotation of a Cappadocian Father (Basil of Caesarea, *Sermon on the Holy Baptism*, Migne 1856–1866, vol. 31, col. 425), which was used also in John of Damascus' *Sacred Parallels* (Migne 1856–1866, vol. 95, col. 1273).

and from the *Book of Job*) is not decisive in excluding a Neoplatonic milieu. For it is certain that some Neoplatonic commentators of the sixth century were Christians, although we rarely find quotations from the Bible or the writings of the Church Fathers and other Christian authorities in their commentaries. The compiler probably wrote either around the seventh century—that is to say, in the same cultural milieu as John of Damascus—or he lived even later in the Middle Byzantine period and used compendia of Aristotelian logic for the composition of his prologue and his commentary on the famous first Hippocratic aphorism.

CHAPTER 15

On the Authorship of the Syriac *Prognostic*

Kamran I. Karimullah

It is well-known that Paris, Bibliothèque nationale de France, MS 6734 fonds arabe (hereafter referred to as P7) contains a portion of a translation of the Hippocratic *Prognostic*.[*,1] Jacques Jouanna (2013) has used the Arabic and the Syriac translations of the *Prognostic* in his recent edition of the Greek text. More than earlier editors of this text, Jouanna recognised that the Arabic and Syriac translations are valuable for reconstructing both the direct Hippocratic tradition and the indirect tradition from Galen.[2] He argues that the Arabic and Syriac translations were based on a lost Greek manuscript preserving the direct tradition that is 'three centuries earlier than the Greek manuscripts of Galen, the oldest of which dates from the thirteenth century' (Jouanna 2013, clxv). Based on Ḥunayn's remarks about his translation of Galen's *Prognostic* commentary and following a thorough comparision of the Arabic and Syriac versions of the *Prognostic* with the direct and indirect Greek tradition, Jouanna concludes that Ḥunayn took the indirect tradition of the *Prognostic* as the basis for his translation but used a manuscript preserving the direct tradition to fill in text in the Arabic and Syriac that are missing from the indirect tradition. From these considerations Jouanna concludes that the Arabic and Syriac translations provide crucial insight into the construction of the stemma of the Hippocratic *Prognostic*.

* I am extremely grateful to Peter E. Pormann for putting so much time and effort into editing this paper. My debt of gratitude grows daily. In preparing this paper I have also benefitted from Natalia Smelova's and Naima Afif's invaluable help, sage advice, and patience, which I gratefully acknowledge.

1 Degen (1981), 152; Grigory Kessel (2016) supplements Degen's work. The Arabic and Syriac *Prognostic* begins on P7, fol. 94[a] and ends on fol. 127[b]. The Syriac and Arabic texts terminate prematurely, the Arabic at '[...] وأصابه مكان وجع الفؤاد تمدد فيما <دون الشراسيف> ...', the Syriac at 'ܗܘ. ܣܠܩ ܚܒܫ ܠܒܐ ܕܗܡ' which corresponds to ἀντὶ δὲ τοῦ καρδιώσσειν, ἐν τῷ ὑποχονδρίῳ (Jouanna 2013, p. 74, lines 7–8; 2.184.15 L.) and Klamroth (1888), 231. Hence, Overwien's claim (2015, 164) that the manuscript contains the 'whole text of the Arabic and Syriac of the *Prognostic*' is incorrect.

2 Using Arabic translations in classical philology is an increasingly popular trend thanks, in large part, to the tireless efforts of Dimitri Gutas. See Gutas (2010, 2012), Gutas and Tarán (2012), and Ullmann and Schmidt (2012).

© KAMRAN I. KARIMULLAH, 2021 | DOI:10.1163/9789004470200_017

1 *The Hippocratic* Prognostic *in Ḥunayn's* Epistle to ʿAlī ibn Yaḥyā

In order to understand the text-critical relationship between the Arabic and Syriac *Prognostic* and the Greek text, Jouanna begins by consulting Ḥunayn's record of his Galen translations in the *Epistle to ʿAlī ibn Yaḥyā*.[3] There are in fact three different Arabic versions of the *Epistle* extant today. According to David Lamoreaux (2016, xxiii–xxvi) the recensions of the *Epistle* that Bergsträßer designated as 'A' and 'B' were written near the end of Ḥunayn's life and continued to be updated after his death. An edition of recension 'A', which Lamoreaux thinks represents a slightly later stage of the *Epistle* than 'B', was published by Bergsträßer in 1925. Following the discovery of a manuscript representing recension 'B' of the *Epistle* in 1929, Bergsträßer (1932) published the results of his collation of the two manuscripts as well as corrections to the 1925 edition. Bersträßer did not, however, prepare a new edition of the *Epistle*. In addition to listing eighteen notices that are not included in 'B', the information in recension 'A', which is the basis of Bergsträßer's 1925 edition used by Jouanna, often includes more information about the translations than recension 'B'. The third, highly abridged version of Ḥunayn's *Epistle*, edited by Fabian Käs (2010), is also extant, but does not concern us directly here.

At times the notices about the translation history of a single work as recorded in the two recensions are at odds.[4] We find this to be true in case of Ḥunayn's notice about the translation of Galen's commentary on the Hippocratic *Prognostic*. Here it is as it is recorded in recension A in Bergsträßer's edition:[5]

هذا الكتاب جعله في ثلاث مقالات. وقد كان ترجم هذا الكتاب سرجس إلى السريانية، ثم ترجمته أنا لسلمويه إلى السريانية، وترجمت فصّ كلامه إلى العربية لإبراهيم بن محمد بن موسى، وترجم التفسير عيسى بن يحيي إلى العربية.

Galen composed this work in three books. Sergius had translated this work into Syriac. Then I translated it into Syriac for Salmawayh. I trans-

3 Bergsträßer (1925). Lamoreaux (2016). On the latter see the reviews by Gutas (2018) and Karimullah (2018).

4 See Lamoreaux (2016), xxv. See for example the notice on his translation of Galen's *My Own Doctrines* (§ 113 Bergsträßer, § 123 Lamoreaux).

5 Bergsträsser (1925), 40–41.

> lated the lemmas (*faṣṣ*) of its [the book's] text into Arabic for Ibrāhīm ibn Muḥammad ibn Mūsā, while ʿIsā ibn Yaḥyā translated the commentary into Arabic.

Recension 'B', which is, in effect, what Lamoreaux's edition represents, records the following:[6]

> هذا الكتاب ألفه في ثلاث مقالات. وقد نقله سرجس الرأسي إلى السريانية. ثم نقلته أنا لسلمويه. ونقلته إلى العربية لإبراهيم بن محمد بن موسى.

> He [Galen] composed this work in three books. Sergius of Rēš ʿAynā had translated it into Syriac. Then I translated it [into Syriac] for Salmawayh, and I translated it into Arabic for Ibrāhīm ibn Muḥammad ibn Mūsā.

There are two details omitted from the earlier recension of Ḥunyan's letter that bear directly on Jouanna's argument and his understanding of the value that should be accorded to the Arabic and Syriac translations in reconstructing the direct and indirect traditions of the *Prognostic*. One is that unlike the later recension ('A'), the earlier recension of the *Epistle* ('B') does not explicitly refer to the fact that Ḥunayn made a seperate effort to translate the Hippocratic lemmas (*faṣṣ*) of the *Prognostic* into Arabic. Second, in the earlier recension ('B') Ḥunayn says that he himself translated Galen's commentary on the *Prognostic* into Arabic. In this recension, there is no allusion to the role that ʿĪsā ibn Yaḥyā played in translating Galen's commentary as recorded in the later recension of the *Epistle* ('A'). Lamoreaux observes that the differences between notices about the translation history of a single Galenic text as they are recorded in the earlier and later recensions of the *Epistle* often involve additional information that in many cases must have been supplied by Ḥunayn's colleagues shortly before or after his death.[7] Yet, the details contained in the two recensions about the translation Galen's commentary of the *Prognostic* are inconsistent. The earlier recension makes no mention of Ḥunayn's separate efforts to translate the Hippocratic lemmas apart from Galen's commentary, stating, rather, that Ḥunayn translated only Galen's *Prognostic* commentary.

6 Lamoreaux (2016), p. 97 (§ 97).

7 Lamoreaux (2016), xxi–xxvi.

2 On the Value of the Arabic and Syriac *Prognostic* for Reconstructing the Direct and Indirect Tradition of the Hippocratic *Prognostic*

This detail casts doubt on the evidence that Jouanna enlists for the claim that Ḥunayn made a deliberate effort to reconstruct the Hippocratic lemma of the *Prognostic* apart from Galen's commentary. Yet, it is difficult to deny Jouanna's conclusion that Ḥunayn must have had access to manuscripts from the direct tradition in some form, for how else could he have completed the portions of the Hippocratic text that Galen omitted from his commentaries as accurately as he did? For aside from Ḥunayn's efforts in the ninth century to reassemble the direct tradition on the basis of manuscripts from the direct and indirect tradition, Jouanna notes that, until the Aldine edition of Galen's commentary published in 1525, it was virtually unheard of for scribes to reintroduce the direct tradition of the *Prognostic* into the portions of Galen's commentary where it was omitted.[8]

Yet if we accept Jouanna's interpretation of Ḥunayn's report in recension A of the *Epistle*, namely that Ḥunayn used at least one manuscript from the direct tradition to reconstitute the direct Hippocratic tradition, we are faced with two serious objections. First, if Ḥunayn had manuscripts from the direct tradition at his disposal, why did he bother referring to the Greek text from the indirect Galenic tradition at all? Second, if the Arabic *Prognostic* is, as Jouanna claims, a mix of text from the direct and indirect tradition, is not Ḥunayn's translation of the *Prognostic* nothing more than a text 'disfigured by contamination', as Jouanna says of Kühn's 1830 edition? Jouanna's responses to both challenges are compelling. Ḥunayn's 'hybrid' direct tradition is not affected by a generalised contamination, counters Jouanna, for 'the Arabic translation generally goes along with Galen's lemmas when there is a divergence between the Hippocratic [that is, the direct] tradition and the Galenic [that is, the indirect] tradition'.[9] With regard to the second, Jouanna acknowledges that it would be strange for 'us moderns' to see that Ḥunayn took care to collect the lemmas separated by Galen in order to reconstruct the *Prognostic* while he had manuscripts containing the direct tradition at his disposal. Jouanna says:

> We must remember that Ḥunayn considered Galen an excellent philologist who guaranteed the validity of the Hippocratic text, whereas the text transmitted anonymously did not, for him, carry the same value. If, for

8 Jouanna (2013), clix.

9 Jouanna (2013), clxvii–clxviii.

> want of something better, Ḥunayn consulted the anonymous tradition in order to complete what Galen says he did not comment on (and did not recopy), it was in fact in order to recover as far as possible the authentic text of the *Prognostic* as Galen had established it.[10]

Hence the *Prognostic* that Ḥunayn appears to have reconstructed using manuscripts from the direct and indirect tradition should not, Jouanna believes, be classified as a 'contaminated' text, but as, in effect, a text that in most instances represents the Galenic indirect tradition, but gives insight into the direct tradition only in cases where Galen did not recopy the Hippocratic lemma.

In their translation of the Arabic *Prognostic*, Oliver Overwien and Uwe Vagelpohl come to a similar conclusion.[11] Having compared Klamroth's (1888) edition of the *Prognostic* with the Hippocratic lemmas quoted in the Arabic translation of Galen's commentary on the Hippocratic *Prognostic* preserved in manuscript (Oxford, Bodleian Library, Laud. Or. 139), Overwien and Vagelpohl observe that the two are 'identical', concluding that whenever there was a possibility of using the direct or indirect Galenic tradition, 'the Arabic translation going back to Ḥunayn was not created on the basis of manuscripts that preserve the direct tradition, but, above all, on the basis of the indirect tradition in Galen's commentary on the *Prognostic*'.[12] Yet, it seems that the Oxford manuscript used by Overwien and Vagelpohl might actually be a contaminated version of ʿĪsā ibn Yaḥyā's commentary. For we know that there was a Latin translation of an Arabic version of the *Prognostic* by Gerard of Cremona (d. 1187).[13] This version reconstructed the *Prognostic* in Latin on the basis of the incomplete lemmas quoted in ʿĪsā ibn Yaḥyā's Arabic translation of Galen's commentary. If it is true, as Overwien and Vagelpohl say, that Ḥunayn's hybrid *Prognostic* and the lemmas of the *Prognostic* in the Oxford manuscript are 'identical', we must conclude that it is likely that Ḥunayn's hybrid *Prognostic* was copied into an ancestor of Galen's commentary on the *Prognostic* contained in the Oxford manuscript.

In any event Jouanna sees the Syriac and Arabic translations as arising in the ninth century as part of a combined scholarly effort involving translators who were also medical professionals, as well as patrons such as Ibrāhīm ibn Muḥammad ibn Mūsā, who, though perhaps not professionally interested in

---

10 Jouanna (2013), clxix.

11 This translation is an appendix in Jouanna (2013), 273–298.

12 Jouanna (2013), 274.

13 Jouanna (2013), clxxix–clxxxiv.

Galen's lengthy commentary on the *Prognostic*, evidently wished to read Hippocrates' medical wisdom in Arabic. This effort culminated in a translation of Galen's commentary on the *Prognostic* into Arabic, a task which was eventually carried out by ʿIsā ibn Yaḥyā, a pupil of Ḥunayn.

3 The Syriac and Arabic *Prognostic* and the Direct Tradition

According to both recensions of the *Epistle* Ḥunayn produced his Syriac translation of the *Prognostic* for his patron Salmawayh. In neither recension of the notice on Galen's commentary is it made clear that there was a link between Ḥunayn's Syriac translation of Galen's commentary and the special effort he made to reconstruct the *Prognostic* at the behest of Ibrāhīm ibn Muḥammad ibn Mūsā. Nor is there any suggestion that ʿĪsā ibn Yaḥyā based his Arabic translation of Galen's commentary on Ḥunayn's earlier Syriac translation. Nevertheless, Jouanna's (2013, cxcvi) interpretation of the notice in the *Epistle* links the Syriac and Arabic *Prognostic* closely. He proposes that the Syriac translation for Salmawayh served as the preliminary model for the translation into Arabic that Ḥunayn agreed to do for Ibrāhīm ibn Muḥammad ibn Mūsā. In order to establish this model, Ḥunayn prepared, as it were, a hybrid Syriac *Prognostic*, which he completed by supplying in Syriac the lemmas that Galen did not recopy on the basis of manuscripts from the direct tradition of the *Prognostic*. The Arabic translation of Galen's *Prognostic* commentary by ʿIsā ibn Yaḥyā, on the other hand, was carried out based on the Syriac translation made earlier by Ḥunyan, which did not include the material from the direct tradition omitted by Galen's commentary.

The main evidence Jouanna's adduces in support of his hypothesis rests on the fact that, as he says (2013, clxxxix), the Syriac *Prognostic* and Ḥunayn's hybrid Arabic *Prognostic* edited by Klamroth 'behave' in the same way. Fundamentally, each provides a text from the indirect tradition, but is completed by making recourse to the direct tradition for the parts that Galen did not recopy into his commentary. One important way in which the Syriac and Arabic *Prognostic* behave similarly is in the fact that they share similar readings at key junctures. Ḥunayn's hybrid Arabic *Prognostic* and the Syriac *Prognostic* preserve readings, sometimes quite long stretches of text, from the direct tradition where the Arabic (and Latin) translations of the *Prognostic* that draw exclusively on the indirect tradition omit them.[14] The strongest evidence, therefore,

14 Jouanna (2013), cxc.

that the Syriac and Arabic versions rely on manuscripts from the direct tradition of the *Prognostic* comes from parallel passages in *Prognostic* 15 and 17 where the Arabic and Syriac *Prognostic* retain material from the direct tradition that is missing from the indirect tradition.[15] To get an idea of the strength of Jouanna's evidence, we may take a shorter example from *Prognostic* 1, where the indirect tradition omits the following sentence.[16]

> [1] Οὕτω γὰρ ἄν τις θαυμάζοιτό τε δικαίως [2] καὶ ἰητρὸς ἀγαθὸς ἂν εἴη· [3] καὶ γὰρ οὓς οἷόν τε περιγενέσθαι, ἔτι μᾶλλον ἂν δύναιτο διαφυλάσσειν [4] ἐκ πλείονος χρόνου προβουλευόμενος πρὸς ἕκαστα, [5] καὶ τοὺς ἀποθανουμένους τε καὶ σωθησομένους προγιγνώσκων τε καὶ προαγορεύων ἀναίτιος ἂν εἴη.

> [1] In this way anyone [able to use prognosis] would be rightly admired, [2] and would be a worthy physician. [3] For he would better be able to save those who can survive [4] by planning ahead for each eventuality. [5] Moreover, by recognising beforehand and predicting who will die and who will live, he would remain blameless.

Ḥunyan renders the Greek into Arabic as follows, according to the text in P7:[17]

> [1] فإنه إذا سلك هذا المسلك أعجب به الناس[18] وحق لهم أن يعجبون[19]، [2] وكان[20] طبيبا فاضلا. [3] وذلك أنه يقدر فيمن يمكن أن يسلم أن يكون أحرى أن يحفظه على ما ينبغي، [4] إذ كان يسبق قبل مدة طويلة فيروى[21] فيما يقابل به كل واحد من الأمور. [5] وإذا تقدم فعرف[22] وسبق فأنذر[23] بموت من يموت وسلامة من يسلم لم تلزمه[24] لا ئمة.[25]

---

15 Jouanna (2013), cxcii–cxcv.

16 2.113 L.; Jouanna (2013), 3.

17 P7, fols. 94ᵇ, line 2–95ᵃ, line 3. P7 is here compared to the edition of the Hippocratic *Prognostic* by Martin Klamroth (1888). The edition relied on three manuscripts in the Gotha library. The sigla are A = Gotha 2023, 3; B = Gotha 1900, C = Gotha 1899. Comparision reveals that P7 is, in general, an inferior copy of the text and and frequently contaminated by later scribes; though see Overwien's and Vagelpohl's comments in Jouanna (2013), 273–274.

18 أعجب به الناس] P7: عجب الناس به ABC.

19 يعجبون] P7: يعجبوا ABC.

20 وكان] P7: فكان ABC.

21 فيروى] P7, ABC: later hand modifies the diacritics of فيروى so that it becomes فيتروّى P7.

22 فعرف] P7: وعرف ABC.

23 فأنذر] conieci: post ف oblit. P7: وأنذر ABC.

24 تلزمه] P7: يلمه ABC.

25 لا ئمة] P7: لائم ABC.

> [1] If he [the physician] proceeds in this manner, people admire him and they would be right to have admiration, [2] so he would be an esteemed physician. [3] For in cases of those who can survive, he is better able to preserve them in the manner required, [4] since he would have looked a long time beforehand into each of the conditions with respect to what is opposed by it. [5] So when he recognises in advance (*iḏā taqaddama fa-ʿarafa*) and forewarns (*sabaqa fa-anḏara*) that those who will die will die, and those who will live will live, [6] no blame attaches to him.

And the parallel passage in Syriac in P7 runs as follows:[26]

> [1] ܗܟܢܐ ܒܢ̈ܝ ܡܬܕܡܪ̈ܝܢ ܒܗ ܐܝܟ ܙܕܩܐܝܬ: [2] ܘܐܣܝܐ ܡܝܬܪܐ ܗܘܐ ܐܝܬܘܗܝ. [3] ܐܦ ܒܢ̈ܝ ܠܗܠܝܢ ܕܡܨܝܐ ܕܢܬܦܪܩܘܢ: ܝܬܝܪ ܡܨܐ ܠܡܦܨܝܘ [4] ܟܕ ܡܩܕܡ ܒܙܒܢܐ ܕܣܓܝܐܐ ܡܬܚܫܒ ܥܠ ܟܠ ܚܕ ܚܕ. [5] ܘܟܕ ܩܕܡ ܝܕܥ ܕܐܝܠܝܢ ܥܬܝܕܝܢ ܕܢܡܘܬܘܢ: ܘܐܝܠܝܢ ܥܬܝܕܝܢ ܕܢܚܘܢ: ܘܩܕܡ ܡܘܕܥ ܥܠܝܗܘܢ [6] ܠܐ ܥܕܠܐ ܗܘܐ.

> [1] In this way people are rightly amazed with him, [2] and he will be an excellent physician. [3] And for those [patients] who can be rescued, he is more able to save [them], [4] by planning long before for each one. [5] When he knows in advance who is going to die and who is going to live, and informs about them in advance, [6] he is blameless.

By comparing the Arabic and Syriac with the Greek texts, we can certainly conclude that the translator or translators of the Syriac and Arabic must have had access to manuscripts from the direct tradition, for otherwise they could not supply the missing Hippocratic text. Moreover, in this instance at least the translations differ in style only slightly, the Arabic attempting to be more idiomatic than the Syriac. In an example that is typical in this text, the Syriac translator renders the Greek privative alpha adjective ἀναίτιος with the Syriac *lā ʿaḏīlā*, whereas the Arabic translator opts for the idiomatic *lam talzimhu lāʾimatun*. The translations are also characterised by some similarities. For example, there is the interesting use in both texts of combining two different verbs to render a single Greek verb. In the Arabic *Prognostic* preserved in P7, Ḥunayn uses a pair of conjoined perfect verbs to render a single Greek participle. Thus

26 P7, fol. 94[b], line 2–fol. 95[a], line 5.

taqaddama fa-ʿarafa is used to render the Greek προγιγνώσκων and *wa-sabaqa fa-anḏara* is used to render the Greek προαγορεύων. In similar fashion, the Syriac combines the present active participles *qāḏem* and *yāḏaʿ* to render προγιγνώσκων, and *qāḏem* with the infinitive *meḇdaq* to render προαγορεύων. Each translator also adopts a freer translation of clause 1, in which the Greek optative is rendered in Arabic through an indicative sentence adding the word 'people (*al-nās*)', '*people* are amazed by him (Ar. *uʿǧiba bihi l-nāsu*)', and the Syriac in similar fashion adds 'people (*nāš*)' to a nominal sentence, '*people* are righly amazed by him (*meṯdammar bēh nāš zāḏqāʾīṯ*).'

At first sight, then, the Syriac and Arabic translations would appear to support Jouanna's contention about Ḥunayn's authorship, both in the fact that each preserves the direct tradition of the Hippocratic text. But on the basis of such evidence Jouanna (2013, clxxxix) also concludes that the Syriac translation in P7 is by *Ḥunayn* not Sergius of Rēšʿaynā (d. 536). To my mind, however, we should not conclude that Ḥunayn is the translator of the Syriac *Prognostic* merely because the two texts each draw on the direct tradition, for this evidence does not exclude, for the sake of argument, the possibility that the Syriac was produced by a earlier scholar such as Sergius who may have had, like Ḥunayn, manuscripts from direct tradition available to him. Indeed, far from proving the point that Ḥunayn is the translator of the Syriac and Arabic *Prognostic*, the above example suggests that the translators were, in fact, different people.

Consider clause 4. The Arabic adds the apparently exegetical phrase 'with respect to what is opposed by it (*fīmā yuqābalu bihī*)', which is nowhere to be found in the Greek of the direct or indirect tradition.[27] This Arabic phrase appears to be an effort—by Ḥunayn or a later scribe whose manuscript is the ancestor of A,B,C, and P7—to explicate, by specifying more precisely, what 'planning ahead (*probouleuómenos*)' entails. This phrase in Arabic is not found in the Syriac *Prognostic*, which more accurately renders the Greek. There can be little doubt that Jouanna is right to conclude that the Arabic and Syriac *Prognostic* rely on manuscripts from the direct tradition. The evidence that proves this fact does not, however, provide unequivocal evidence for the authorship of the Syriac *Prognostic*. If clause 4 in the Arabic translation does in fact go back to Ḥunayn, the above example leads to the highly improbable conclusion that Ḥunayn based his earlier Syriac *Prognostic* on a correct, uncontaminated Greek manuscript, but then used a possibly contaminated Greek manuscript in his later Arabic translation.

27 Jouanna (2013), 3 (see apparatus).

4 Authorship of the Syriac *Prognostic*

It is not disputed that Ḥunayn produced an Arabic translation of the *Prognostic*, but the question of who translated the Syriac *Prognostic* has never been fully broached.[28] The debate surrounding the authorship of the Syriac *Aphorisms*, however, may be instructive in several respects. Henri Pognon edited the Syriac *Aphorisms* (1903) based on the Syriac text preserved in P7. He concluded that the Syriac *Aphorisms* preserved in P7 is not by Ḥunayn. Later, Degen (1978), Brock (1991), and Magdelaine (1994) discussed evidence in favour of Ḥunayn's authorship. Lately Oliver Overwien (2015) has forecefully asserted that the Syriac *Aphorisms* is by Ḥunayn. These studies tend to rely on shared readings between the Syriac and the Arabic translations of the *Aphorisms*. Recent studies by Mimura (2017a, 2017b) and Barry (2018), on the other hand, have focused on interpretive differences between the Ḥunayn's Arabic translation and the Syriac *Aphorisms*. They show how Ḥunayn and the author of the Syria *Aphorisms* interpreted the Greek text differently and must have used different Greek manuscripts as exemplars for their translations. Barry (2018) notes broad 'patterns' of lexicographical agreement between Ḥunayn's Arabic translation of the *Aphorisms* and the Syriac *Aphorisms*. He argues, however, that lexicographical similarities do not provide definitive evidence for Ḥunayn's authorship of the Syriac *Aphorisms* owing to the 'stronger pattern of divergent interpretations between the main Arabic and Syriac translations'.[29] Instead, Barry concludes that 'the terminological agreement between the two translations and the contrasting interpretive and stylistic modes they adopt point to their having been composed by two different authors within the same scholarly milieu'.[30] Hence, these studies show how Ḥunayn and the translator of the Syriac *Aphorisms* interpreted the Greek Hippocratic text in divergent ways—so divergent, in fact, that they cast serious doubt on Ḥunayn's authorship of the Syriac translation of the *Aphorisms*.

With regard to the Hippocratic *Prognostic*, it is tempting to use the fact of shared readings preserving the direct tradition against the indirect tradition as evidence for Ḥunayn's authorship of the Syriac translation. Overwien (2015, 165) has faulted Caroline Magdelaine for falling prey to misusing the evidence provided by shared readings in her pathbreaking edition of the Hippocratic

28 N. Peter Joosse (2013, 519) and Grigory Kessel (2016, 180) both lament the lack of scholarship on the Syriac *Prognostic*.

29 Barrry (2018), 173–174.

30 Barry (2018), 174.

Aphorisms. He argues that her argument rests entirely on the analysis of the 'Greek sources without taking into consideration the Syriac translator and his working methods'.[31] The fact that the Syriac and Arabic translations share readings that go back to the indirect tradition, Overwien avers, does not prove that the translators are the same person. Yet, in his own article, Overwien proceeds in the manner of Magdelaine. He compares the Arabic and Syriac with the Greek original, arriving at the conclusion that the Syriac and Ḥunayn's Arabic translation 'belong to the same textual tradition',[32] meaning that the Syriac and Arabic *Aphorisms* reflect the indirect tradition; and second, the fact that the same manuscript was used as the exemplar for each is proved by readings that they share but that go against the readings of the direct tradition.[33] Based on evidence from comparing the translation techniques in the Syriac and Arabic *Prognostic*, Overwien concludes that the translator of the Syriac *Aphorisms* is Ḥunayn because the amplifications of the Greek, which occur in both the Syriac and Arabic, are 'usually almost identical'.[34]

Yet, without the positive evidence supplied by so-called indicative 'errors' or 'variants', there is no way to judge whether the variants between the Syriac and Arabic translations are *peculiar* errors of the Syriac and Arabic manuscripts individually or *genealogical* errors inherited from the Greek exemplar or exemplars used for the translations.[35]

The need for data based on indicative errors rather than shared readings is especially urgent in the case of a textual tradition such as the *Prognostic*, where the likelihood of *contamination* is high, whether owing to contamination between the direct and indirect traditions, or to scribal interventions. We see the process of contamination unfold in P7 itself. For example, there are numerous instances of contamination, in which the scribe has altered Ḥunayn's Arabic translation of the *Aphorisms* based on the Syriac text. Taro Mimura (2017a, 2017b) has shown how P7's scribe Bahnām ibn al-Ḥaddād (manuscript dated AD 1205) modified Ḥunayn's Arabic translation of the *Aphorisms* on the basis of the parallel Syriac *Aphorisms*. A similar process of contamination may be observed in the *Prognostic*. For example, in *Prognostic* 1, the author speaks in a general way about the benefits and difficulties of prognosis. He says that while it is impossible to restore all patients to perfect health, it is nevertheless highly

31 Overwien (2015), 165.

32 Overwien (2015), 174.

33 Ibid.

34 Ibid.

35 See Maas (1952), 8–9. On the central role played by 'indicative errors' in textual criticism, see Mass (1952), 42–49.

desirable to know how the patient's disease will end. To assist the physician in making accurate prognoses about how individual diseases will terminate, the author says:

> … γνόντα οὖν χρὴ τῶν παθέων τῶν τοιουτέων τὰς φύσιας ὁκόσον ὑπὲρ τὴν δύναμίν εἰσι τῶν σωμάτων, ἅμα δὲ καὶ εἴ τι θεῖον ἔνεστιν ἐν τῇσι νούσοισι, καὶ τουτέων τὴν πρόνοιαν ἐκμανθάνειν.[36]

> Having known, then, to what extent the natures of these diseases exceed the strength of bodies, and, at the same time, if there should be something divine in the illnesses, it is also necessary thoroughly to master the foreknowledge that results from it.[37]

The Arabic in P7 reads as follows:[38]

> ينبغي[39] أن يعرف[40] الطبيب[41] طبائع تلك الأمراض التي هي مجاوزة لقوة[42] الأبدان. وإن كان أيضا[43] مع ذلك في الأمراض شيء[44] إلهي[45]، فقد ينبغى أن يكون الطبيب[46] سابق النظر فيه خبيرا.

> The physician ought to know the natures of these diseases that overcome the strength of bodies. If there is also something divine in the diseases, the physician must, therefore, have foreknowledge of, and be expert about, it.

It is evident from the different inks used by Bahnām and the later annotators that Bahnām had originally written 'divine (*ilāhī*)' in the text rather than 'heavenly (*samāwī*)', the latter of which is the text attested to in the hybrid direct

36 Jouanna (2013), 3.
37 For the translation of the Greek in this way see Jouanna (2013), 3 and 88.
38 P7, fol. 94[a], line 7–fol. 94[b], line 1.
39 ينبغي] ante correctionem P7: وينبغي P7: فقد ينبغي ABCBaġd et supra lin. P7.
40 يعرف] P7: تعرف ABCBaġd.
41 الطبيب] P7: om. ABCBaġd.
42 add. تلك A.
43 أيضا] BCP7Baġd: om. A.
44 add. آخر A.
45 إلهي] P7, in marg. AB: سماوى ABCBaġd., سماوي خ in marg. P7.
46 الطبيب] conieci: الطبيب ABCBaġd: oblit. P7.

tradition of the *Prognostic* created by Ḥunayn as well as in the indirect tradition in Baġdādī's *Prognostic* commentary.[47] Bahnām appears to have altered Ḥunayn's translation so that it would correspond to the Syriac which has *ilāhāyyā*. A later annotator added a correction in the margins of the Arabic to the effect that *samāwī* is the correct reading. As a justification, the same annotator provides a note that draws on the Arabic translation of Galen's commentary on the *Prognostic* to justify why 'heavenly' is the correct reading. For, as Jouanna has noted, Galen interprets 'divine' in this passage to refer to atmospheric factors that Hippocratic medicine holds responsible for causing disease.[48] In fact, it is likely that Galen's commentary prompted Ḥunayn to opt for the less literal 'heavenly' over the more literal 'divine'. In support of his correction in the margins, the annotator, drawing on Galen's commentary, writes:

يريد به حال الهواء المحيط بالأبدان، وقيل الاتصالات الكوكبية وأحوال القمر. وقيل يريد به المرض الذي يسميها بالأمراض الوافدة الحاصلة عن[49] فساد الهواء.[50] وغلط من ظنه أنه يريد الصرع أو العشق فإنهما يسمي[51] مرضهما إلهيا.

> By ['heavenly'] he means the condition of the air that surrounds bodies. It is said that [it means] planetary conjunctions and the conditions of the moon; it is said that he means diseases which he calls 'epidemic (*al-amrāḍ al-wāfida*)', and are caused by corrupt air. It is wrong to assume that he meant epilepsy or lovesickness because he [Hippocrates] calls both these diseases 'divine' (*fa-innahumā yusammī maraḍahumā ilāhīyan*).

In this example contamination of the Arabic text undermines the value of the Arabic *Prognostic* in P7 from a text critical perspective. Which is the correct reading, 'heavenly' or 'divine', is difficult to say for the contamination makes it virtually impossible to distinguish a *peculiar* error or variant in the manuscript from a *transmitted* error or variant. Taken naively, *ilāhīyan* in P7 would appear to preserve Ḥunayn's original translation because it is closer to the Greek text than *samāwī*. But given Ḥunayn's well-known sensitivity to the theological sensibilities of his patrons,[52] and his tendency to let Galen's interpretation

47 Joosse, Pormann (2012), 274. Klamroth (1888), 205.
48 Jouanna (2013), lviii.
49 عن] conieci: illeg. P7.
50 الهواء] conieci: illeg. P7.
51 يسمي] correxi: يسميان P7.
52 For example, Strohmaier (2012).

guide his translation of the Hippocratic text, *samāwī* is likely to be the original reading. The appearance of *ilāhīyan* in P7 is probably precipitated by the fact that the scribe compared and 'corrected' the Arabic text with the Syriac.[53]

> ܙܕܩ ܠܗ ܠܡܕܥ ܟܝܢܐ ܕܟܘ̈ܪܗܢܐ ܕܐܝܟܢ ܡܠܝܢ: ܕܚܠܨܝܢ ܠܚܝܠܗ ܕܦܓܪܐ.
> ܐܟܘܬܗ ܕܝܢ: ܐܦ ܡܕܡ ܐܠܗܝܐ ܐܝܬ ܒܟܘܪ̈ܗܢܐ ܐܦ ܠܡܩܕܡܘܬ
> ܡܬܝܕܥܘܬܐ ܕܟܠ ܗܘܐ ܙܕܩ ܠܡܐܠܦ.

> It is necessary for him to know the nature of the diseases, the extent of which they overcome the power of the body; and likewise even if there is also something divine in the diseases, and it is necessary to be skilled in apprehending beforehand.

Hence, the contamination in the Arabic *Prognostic* in P7 leads to a situation in which shared correct readings between the Arabic and Syriac are not necessarily because they were copied from the same Greek manuscript or from Greek manuscripts from the same branch of the stemma. The commonalities between the Arabic and Syriac in P7 may just as well be a result of the scribe altering the Arabic based on the Syriac, which is precisely what type of contamination appears in the Arabic *Aphorisms* and *Prognostic* in P7.

5 Limitations on the Method of Using Translation Style to Undermine Ḥunayn's Authorship

As was noted earlier, in order to prove that Ḥunayn is the translator of the Syriac *Prognostic* Jouanna relies on the fact that the Arabic and Syriac *Prognostic* consistently side on the same side of the *Prognostic*'s stemma, sometimes siding with the direct tradition and sometimes with the indirect tradition. Yet, contamination in P7 is not the only reason to be cautious about concluding that Ḥunayn is the author of the Syriac *Prognostic*. The above example from *Prognostic* 1.2 is a case in point. There are important similarities between the Arabic and the Syriac translations of the Greek that might lead us to venture that the translator or translators understood the text in similar ways. Notable for example is that in each the modal verbal phrase is repeated in Arabic (*yanbaġī an*) and in Syriac (*zādeq*). The translator or translators of the Arabic

53 P7, fol. 94[a], line 10–fol. 94[b], line 1.

and Syriac *Prognostic* adopt a similar strategy when they render the circumstantial participle clause beginning with γνόντα. In the Greek γνόντα begins the apodosis, marked by οὖν,[54] of a conditional sentence that began earlier with 'ἐπειδὴ …'.[55] Constructions like this have the force of subordinate clauses added to the main verb by conjunction and will agree in gender number and case.[56] There is evidence that Arabic translators of medieval medical texts used coordinated clauses connected by the conjunction 'wa- (and)', to render similar types of participle phrases.[57] In the above example, too, the Syriac and the Arabic translators use a similar technique, using '*zāḏeq leh l-maddaʿ … zāḏeq l-melap̄*' and '*yanbaġī an yaʿrifa … fa-qad yanbaġī an yakūna*', respectively, in coordination to render the participle phrase.

Moroever, it is possible that the Arabic and Syriac translators were also prompted to read the text in this way by Galen's remarks in the commentary on the Hippocratic *Prognostic*. Galen draws our attention to the fact that this text, located at the beginning of the *Prognostic*, is in effect restated at the end. Drawing a link between *Prognostic* 1.2 and *Prognostic* 25.2 (Jouanna 2013, 78), he records Hippocrates as saying:[58]

> χρὴ δὲ καὶ τὰς φορὰς τῶν νοσημάτων ἀεὶ τῶν ἐπιδημεύντων ταχέως ἐνθυμέεσθαι καὶ μὴ λανθάνειν τῆς ὥρης τὴν κατάστασιν.
>
> وقد ينبغي أن تتفطّن بسرعة دائما لحدوث الأمراض الوافدة ولا تفوتك حال الوقت الحاضر.
>
> It is also necessary always to consider promptly the course of the diseases that are present, and not to fail to observe the condition of the season.

To which Galen adds:[59]

> ὅτι μὲν οὖν χρὴ γινώσκειν τὸν ἰατρόν, εἴπερ τι καὶ ἄλλο τῶν εἰς τὰς προγνώσεις διαφερόντων, οὕτως καὶ τὸ περὶ τῆς τῶν ἐπιδημίων νοσημάτων γενέσεως ἐδήλωσεν, …

54 For οὖν used to mark the apodosis, see Denniston (1959), 428.

55 Jouanna (2013), 88.

56 Smyth (1920), 456–457.

57 Pormann (2004a).

58 Heeg (1915), p. 208, lines 23–25 (18b.21–22 K.), citing 2.188.12–14 L.; Klamroth (1888), 232. The text of P7 terminates before reaching this juncture in the *Prognostic*.

59 Heeg (1915), p. 208, line 25–p. 209, line 2 (18b.222 K.)

> The physician needs to know this, even if he [sc. Hippocrates] has also revealed other things that make a difference for the prognosis, and likewise what relates to the origin of epidemic diseases; …

In this way Galen emphasises the fact that, for Hippocrates, the physician must consider two things when treating a patient. He must consider the nature of the disease in relation to the patient, which Galen links to knowing differences between diseases. Second, he must apprehend well the elements that make up a prognosis, which Galen links to knowing the seasons of the year and the conditions in which the diseases is generated.

The Arabic and Syriac translations also reveal differences between the interpretation of the Greek source. The idea that what is known is the *extent* to which the natures of the diseases exceed the body's strength is conveyed in the Greek 'γνόντα … τὰς φύσιας ὁκόσον ὑπὲρ …'. This idea is also reflected in the Syriac with the phrase 'it is necessary to know the natures of the diseases, the extent they overwhelm the strength of the bodies (*zāḏeq leh l-madda' kyānē d-ḥaššē d-ḏāḵ hālēn d-'ālbēn l-ḥaylā d-pagrā*)', which follows the Greek syntax very closely in this regard. It is not, however, reflected in the Arabic, which says only that the *natures* of the diseases are what the physician should know (*yanbaġī an ya'rifa l-ṭabību ṭabā'i'a l-amrāḍi*).

These are not only differences in the interpretation of this brief text. They point to the possiblity that two different Greek manuscripts were used by the Arabic and the Syriac translators. To my mind, divergences like these reduce the value that Jouanna assigns to the readings that are shared by the Syriac and the Arabic *Prognostic* as evidence for Ḥunayn's authorship of the Syriac. In the following pages, I shall gather evidence to show that Ḥunayn's authorship of the Syriac *Prognostic* is unlikely. I shall approach this question by contrasting the translation styles of the Syriac and Arabic *Prognostic*, and contrasting how the translators interpret the Greek lemmas in different ways.

To put the point somewhat differently: in the following my conclusion that Ḥunayn is not the author of the Syriac *Prognostic* in P7 does not rest on the basis of slight differences in terminology or minor differences in interpretation. Differences such as these can easily be explained away as a consequence of Ḥunayn's having translated at two different, possibly quite remote, times in his life. Consider the following example of parallel texts from the Greek *Aphorisms* and *Prognostic*, which Ḥunayn translates into Arabic in different ways. Yet, no one seriously doubts Ḥunayn's authorship of either Arabic translation.

In the introduction to his edition of the Hippocratic *Prognostic*, Jouanna devotes several pages to comparing this passage from the *Prognostic* with a nearly identical passage in the Hippocratic *Aphorisms* vi.52. Jouanna includes

Ḥunayn's Arabic translation in the critical apparatus to this passage, but the Syriac is noticeably absent. In fact, the Syriac translation of the *Prognostic* differs noticeably from the Syriac translation of *Aphorisms* vi.52. First the Greek *Prognostic* (Jouanna 2013, p. 8, line 3–p. 9, line 1):

> Σκοπεῖν δὲ χρὴ καὶ τὰς ὑποφάσιας τῶν ὀφθαλμῶν ἐν τοῖσιν ὕπνοισιν· ἢν γάρ τι ὑποφαίνηται τοῦ λευκοῦ ξυμβαλλομένων τῶν βλεφάρων, μὴ ἐκ διαρροίης ἢ φαρμακοποσίης ἐόντι, ἢ μὴ εἰθισμένῳ οὕτω καθεύδειν, φλαῦρον τὸ σημεῖον καὶ θανατῶδες σφόδρα.
>
> It is necessary to examine what shows from the eyes during sleep, for if some of the white of the eyes appears whilst the lids are shut, but not because of diarrhoea, taking drugs, or because it is [the patient's] habit to sleep this way, it is a bad sign and extremely deadly.

Now the Greek of the *Aphorisms*, vi.52:

> Σκοπεῖν δὲ χρὴ καὶ τὰς ὑποφάσιας τῶν ὀφθαλμῶν ἐν τοῖσιν ὕπνοισιν· ἢν γάρ τι ὑποφαίνηται τοῦ λευκοῦ, συμβαλλομένων τῶν βλεφάρων, μὴ ἐκ διαρροίης ἐόντι ἢ φαρμακοποσίης, φλαῦρον τὸ σημεῖον καὶ θανατῶδες σφόδρα.
>
> It is necessary to examine what shows from the eyes during sleep, for if part of the whites of the eyes appears, whilst the lids are shut, without it being caused by diarrhoea or taking a drug, it is a bad sign and extremely deadly.

Arabic *Aphorisms*:

> قال أبقراط: قد ينبغي أن يتفقّد باطن العين[60] في وقت النوم فإن تبيّن شيء من بياض العين والجفن[61] مطبق وليس ذلك[62] بعقب اختلاف ولا شرب[63] دواء فتلك علامة رديئة[64] مهلكة جدًّا.[65]

---

60 العين ArMSS : العينين Tytler.
61 والجفن] Tytler: الجفن Mimura.
62 ذلك E5, E6, P1, Tytler : om. E7.
63 ولا شرب E5, E7, P1, Tytler : وشرب E6.
64 رديئة ArMSS : om. Tytler.
65 مهلكة جدا E5, E6, P1 : om. E7: مهلكة Tytler.

> Hippocrates said: it is necessary to examine the inside of the eye during sleep: if part of the white of the eye shows whilst the lid is shut and this is not following diarrhoea or taking a drug, this is a bad sign and is very deadly.

Arabic *Prognostic*:

> وقد ينبغى أن تتفقد ما يظهر من باطن[66] العينين في وقت النوم. فإنه إن ظهر شىء من بياضهما والجفنان منطبقان ثم لم يكن ذلك عن ذرب أو شرب دواء مسهل ولم يكن أيضا ممن[67] عادته أن ينام وعيناه بتلك الحال فإن ذلك[68] رديء قتال جدا.[69]

> It is necessary to examine what appears from the inside of the eyes during sleep. For, if part of the whites [of the eyes] appears whilst the eyelids are shut, and this is not because of diarrhoea or taking a purgative drug, nor is he [the patient] in the habit of sleeping with his eyes in this condition, this is a bad sign and is extremely deadly.

Many of the differences between the Arabic translations are, thus, not significant, relating mainly to word choice. For example, Ḥunayn uses *dalīl* and *ʿalāma* to render σημεῖον; he uses *qattāl* in one instance and *muhlik* in another to translate θανατῶδες; in the *Aphorisms*, Ḥunayn uses *tabayyana* to translate ὑποφαίνηται but uses *ẓahara* in the *Pronostic*; he uses *ʿayn* in the singular in the *Aphorisms*, but in the dual *ʿaynān* in the *Prognostic* for τῶν ὀφθαλμῶν, and likewise τῶν βλεφάρων in the Arabic *Aphorisms* is translated using the singular *ǧafn* 'eyelid' but the dual *ǧafnān* ('eyelids') in the Arabic *Prognostic*. Lastly, διαρροίης is translated in the *Aphorisms* as *iḫtilāf*, but in the *Prognostic* as *ḏarab*.

Yet other differences between the two translations are more substantial, with the Arabic *Prognostic* at times showing a slightly higher frequency of explication than Ḥunayn uses in the *Aphorisms*. For example, Ḥunayn twice translates φαρμακοποσίης using 'drinking of a drug (*šurb dawāʾ*)', but in the *Prognostic* Ḥunayn explicates further by adding 'drinking of a purging drug (*šurb dawāʾ mushil*)'. Ḥunayn's translations of the difficult word ὑποφάσιας are different in each text. In the *Aphorisms*, Ḥunayn translates this term slightly inaccurately as *the inside of the eye* (*bāṭin al-ʿayn*) whereas in the *Prognostic*

---

66 باطن ABCP7 : بياض خ in marg. P7.
67 ممن P7: فيمن ABC.
68 ذلك post add. دليل P7.
69 P7, fol. 97[a], line 8–fol. 97[b], line 1.

Ḥunyan uses a longer Arabic clause 'what appears from the inside of the eyes (*mā ẓahara min bāṭini l-ʿaynayni*)' to capture the meaning of the Greek term. In the *Aphorisms*, Ḥunayn interprets the ἐκ in 'μὴ ἐκ διαρροίης […]' as meaning that there is only prognostic value in observing the eyes during sleep if the observation is not *following in the wake of* diarrhoea (*laysa ḏālika bi-ʿaqibi ḫtilāfin*). On the other hand, in the *Prognostic*, Ḥunayn understands ἐκ to have a causative sense, so that the eyelids are not shut *because of* diarrhoea (*ṯumma lam yakun ḏālika ʿan ḏarabin*). Finally, Ḥunyan translates the genitive absolute συμβαλλομένων τῶν βλεφάρων differently in the *Aphorisms* and the *Prognostic*.

Likewise, the translation of the identical Greek phrase in the Syriac *Aphorisms* is different from the translation of the nearly identical phrase in the Syriac *Prognostic*.[70] The Syriac translator of the *Aphorisms* understood τὰς ὑποφάσιας to mean *the inside of the eyes*, just as the Arabic *Aphorisms* and *Prognostic* use *bāṭin* to render the Greek word. In the Syriac *Aphorisms*, then, we read:[71]

> ܘܙܕܩ ܕܝܢ ܕܬܬܒܥܐ ܒܓܘܝܬܗܘܢ ܕܥܝ̈ܢܐ ܒܙܒܢ ܫܢܬܐ. ܐܢܗܘ ܚܙܐ ܕܢܬܚܙܐ
> ܡܕܡ ܡܢ ܚܘܪܐ ܕܥܝ̈ܢܝܗܘܢ ܟܕ ܠܒܝܟܝܢ ܬܠܝ̈ܦܐ. ܟܕ ܠܐ ܗܘܬ ܠܕܪܝܗܐ
> ܡܪ̈ܕܝܬܐ ܕܟܪܣܐ ܐܘ ܐܫܬܝ, ܣܡܐ. ܐܝܬܐ ܗ̇ܝ ܒܝܫܬܐ ܡܡܝܬܢܝܬܐ[72] ܗ̇ܝ
> ܕܛܒ.[73]

> It is necessary to examine the inside of the eyes during sleep, whether something white appears from the eyes, whilst the eyelids are shut, without the flow from the stomach being caused by *diryāhā* or having taken a drug, it is bad and extremely deadly.

However, in the Syriac *Prognostic*, the Greek is rendered as follows:[74]

> ܘܙܕܩ ܕܝܢ ܠܡܚܙܐ ܘܠܐܘܦܘܦܐܣܝܣ ܐܘܟܝܬ ܡܬܚܙܝܢܘܬܐ ܕܡܢ ܠܓܘ ܕܥܝ̈ܢܐ.
> ܒܙܒܢ ܫܢܬܐ. ܐܢܗܘ ܚܙܐ ܕܡܕܡ ܡܢ ܚܘܪܗܘܢ ܡܬܚܙܐ ܟܕ ܠܒܝܟܝܢ ܬܠܝ̈ܦܐ:
> ܠܐ ܡܢ ܥܠܬ ܕܪܗܛܐ ܘܡܢ ܫܩܝܐ ܕܣܡܐ: ܘܡܐܟܘܠܬܐ ܕܠܐ ܡܕܡ ܗܘܝܐ
> ܠܡܕܡ̈ܝܢ. ܫܘܘܕܥܐ ܒܝܫܐ ܐܝܬ ܗ̇ܘ ܘܗܘܐ ܘܛܒ ܡܡܝܬܢܝܬܐ.

---

70 Overwien (2015, 166–167) analyses the same pair of texts but arrives at a different conclusion.

71 P7, fol. 84ᵃ, line 14–fol. 84ᵇ, line 6.

72 ܡܡܝܬܢܝܬܐ] P7: ܡܡܝܬܬܢܝܬܐ Pognon.

73 Pognon (1903), 27.

74 P7, fol. 97ᵃ, line 8–fol. 97ᵇ, line 1.

> It is necessary to look also at (*wa-ba-*) *ʾpwpsys*[75]—that is, the manifestation from the inside of the eyes—during sleep. If something from the whites appears while the eyelids are closed, if it is not caused by diarrhoea nor by taking a drug, and this [person] does not have the habit of sleeping this way, there is a bad sign there, and is extremely deadly.

Some of the differences between the two Syriac translations are evident but do not constitute evidence for or against single authorship.[76] For example, a minor difference is that the Greek ἐκ, which is used to convey a causal sense in these passages, is rendered in the Syriac *Aphorisms* with *l*(*a*)- and in the *Syriac Prognostic* with *men ʿellaṯ*. On the other hand, there are several noteworthy differences between the Syriac translations. The first is that the *Prognostic* opts to transliterate the Greek ὑποφάσιας and then to supply an explanatory gloss of the term, whereas the Syriac *Aphorisms* directly translates the phrase. Significantly, the translation in the *Prognostic* shows a different understanding of what ὑποφάσιας means in comparison with the Syriac *Aphorisms*. The latter somewhat problematically, translates the phrase as 'the inside of the eyes,' which resembles the slightly inaccurate translation of ὑποφάσιας in the Arabic *Aphorisms bāṭin al-ʿayn*. Though the *Prognostic* uses the technique of transliteration followed by explanation, the interpretation of ὑποφάσιας as 'the manifestation from the inside of the eyes,' is more accurate than the Syriac or Arabic *Aphorisms*. Thirdly, the translator (or translators) of the Syriac *Prognostic* and *Aphorisms* choose to translate διάρροια differently. The Syriac *Aphorisms* evinces a more literal understanding of the Greek text, which is closer to the lexical sense of 'flow from the belly'. The Syriac *Prognostic* shows greater appreciation for the Greek medical terminology, using the Syriac *dyālā* to translate the Greek term. Once again, the Syriac translator of the *Prognostic* transliterates the Greek διάρροια and then follows it with a brief explanation of its meaning.

Thus, we have before us four different renderings of nearly the same Greek text in Syriac and Arabic all of which have been ascribed to Ḥunayn. Yet, these translations differ not only in the literalness of the translation and word choice for translating technical terms into the target language. More importantly, all four translations show that the translator understood the Hippocratic text somewhat differently in each case. The Arabic *Aphorisms* and *Prognostic*

75 P7, fol. 97[a], line 11. Overwien (2015, 167) reads ܘܒܐܦܘܣܝܣ omitting the second *pē* in the manuscript.

76 Overwien (2015, 167) also observes that both 'Syriac translations are obviously not identical, but that was not necessarily to be expected as they were written independently of each other'.

show a greater degree of consistency in their lexical choices and in their interpretations of the two Greek texts. The Syriac *Aphorisms* and *Prognostic*, on the other hand, differ not only from the Arabic translations, but they differ from each other in terms of style and interpretation. This raises not only the question of whether the author of Arabic and the Syriac *Prognostic* are they same, but also of whether the author of the Syriac *Aphorisms* and *Prognostic* are the same. In the following section, I take up the first question only, providing evidence against Ḥunayn's authorhip of the Syriac *Prognostic* with examples from the Arabic and Syriac texts.

6 Evidence against Ḥunayn's Authorship

An instructive example appears in *Prognostic* 7, where Hippocrates speaks about a type of severe swelling affecting the entire area of the belly, or the 'hypochondrium (τὸ ὑποχόνδριον, *mā dūna l-šarāsīfi*)'.[77]

> Οἴδημα δὲ ἐν τῷ ὑποχονδρίῳ σκληρόν τε ἐὸν καὶ ἐπώδυνον, κάκιστον μέν, εἰ παρ' ἅπαν εἴη τὸ ὑποχόνδριον· εἰ δὲ εἴη ἐν τῷ ἑτέρῳ πλευρῷ, ἀκινδυνότερόν ἐστιν ἐν τῷ ἐπ' ἀριστερά.
>
> Swelling in the belly, being hard and painful, is worst when it is in the entire belly. If it is in one of the sides, it is less dangerous when it is to the left.
>
> وأما الورم[78] الحادث فيما دون الشراسيف إذا كان جاسيا مؤلما فأردأ ما يكون منه ما اشتمل على ذلك الموضع كله. فإن كان في أحد الجانبين فالأسلم منه ما كان في الجانب الأيسر.
>
> When a swelling occurring in the belly is hard and causes pain, it is very bad when it occupies this entire area. If it is on one side, it is safest when it is on the left.

The Syriac *Prognostic* reads as follows:[79]

77 Jouanna (2013), p. 18, lines 3–6; 2.126.7–9 L; P7 fol. 101^{b}, lines 7–13.

78 الورم ACP7 : التربل B : التربل *supra* lin. P7.

79 P7 fol. 101^{b}, lines 8–19.

ܪܘܒܠܐ ܕܐܝܬ ܕܗܘܐ ܒܐܘܦܘܟܘܢܕܪܝܘܢ[80] ܕܩܫܝܐ ܘܡܟܐܒ. ܐܦ ܗ̇ܘ ܒܝܫ
ܐܢܗܘ ܕܒܟܠܗ ܐܘܦܘܟܘܢܕܪܝܘܢ[81] ܢܗܘܐ. ܐܢܕܝܢ ܒܓܒܐ ܢܗܘܐ. ܐܝܬܘܗܝ
ܕܩܝܢܕܘܢܘܣ. ܕܐܢܗܘ [ܒ]ܓܒܐ ܕܣܡܠܐ [ܢ]ܗܘܐ.

> The swelling in the *hypochondrion*, which is hard and painful, is also bad, if [it is] in the entire *hypochondrion*. If it is on the side, it is dangerous when it is on the left side.

A comparison of the Greek, Arabic and Syriac texts yields two important results. First the Syriac and the Arabic translators adopt different translation techniques. In the Arabic, Ḥunayn uses the explicative translation *mā dūna l-šarāsīf* (literally 'what is below the rib-cartilage'), which captures the meaning and etymology of τὸ ὑποχόνδριον. In addition, in order to avoid repetition and perhaps to produce a more elegant translation, Ḥunyan replaces the second instance of τὸ ὑποχόνδριον in the passage with *fī ḏālika l-mawḍiʿ* (literally, 'in this place'). The Syriac translator on the other hand simply transcribes 'ὑποχόνδριον' twice, on both occasions without supplying a Syriac gloss of the term.

Finally, there is the problem of how the Greek privative comparative ἀκινδυνότερον ('less dangerous') is translated by the Arabic and Syriac translators. The Arabic translator uses the phrase *fa-aslamu minhu* ('it is sounder, safer …') in order to mimic the *morphology* of the Greek comparative. On the other hand, the Arabic translator makes use of a cognate of the verb *salima* (to be sound, free from) to render the *sense* of the Greek privative ἀκίνδυνος (lit. 'without danger'). Sadly, the Syriac portion of this text has been damaged by water so what Bahnām originally wrote in the manuscript has disappeared. A later scribe or annotator has overwritten portions of the Syriac text. It is unclear, however, whether this was done before or after the manuscript was affected by water damage or whether the later scribe was faithful to Bahnām's original. In the portion of the Syriac text in which the translation of ἀκινδυνότερον should appear, this later hand has written '(…) which is dangerous (*'īṯaw(h)ī d-qīndūnōs*).' This appears to be the opposite of the sense conveyed by the Greek text, and, to that extent, unlikely to have been originally copied by Bahnām. For in other passages of the *Prognostic* in P7 we notice that the antonym of ἀκίνδυνος, namely ἐπικίνδυνος, meaning *in danger, precarious*, is translated as, for

80 ܒܐܘܦܘܟܘܢܕܪܝܘܢ] correxi: P7 ܒܐܘܦܘܟܘܢܪܕܝܘܢ.
81 ܐܘܦܘܟܘܢܕܪܝܘܢ] correxi: P7 ܐܘܦܘܟܘܕܪܝܘܢ.

example, 'this signals danger (ܥܠ ܩܝܢܕܘܢܘܣ ܡܫܘܕܥܐ ܗܕܐ)' (P7 105[a], line 14) for ἐπικινδυνότερον. In another passage ܕܩܝܢܕܘܢܘܣ (*d-qīndūnōs*) and ܐܝܬ (*'īṯ*) are used together. The Greek καὶ ἐπικινδύνοισι is rendered as 'in which there is great danger (ܘܕܩܝܢܕܘܢܘܣ ܐܝܬܝܗܘܢ)' (P7 118[b], line 18–19); and οἱ δὲ γαργαρεῶνες ἐπικίνδυνοι καὶ ἀποτάμνεσθαι καὶ ἀποσχάζεσθαι is rendered as 'the uvula is in danger of being cut and incised (ܠܚܠܚܬܐ ܕܝܢ܂ ܕܩܝܢܕܘܢܘܣ ܐܝܬܝܗ̇ ܕܬܬܦܣܩ ܘܕܬܬܓܙܪܐ)' (P7 125[a], line 21–22). Hence, *'īṯaw(h)ī d-qīndūnōs* should be understood as 'it is dangerous'. This evidence suggests that the later scribe who tried to restore the manuscript ended up corrupting it, as the 'correction' conveys the opposite sense of the Greek.

At any rate, based on a similar construction in the Syriac *Aphorisms*, however, we might speculate about how the above Syriac could be reconstructed. At *Aphorisms* iv.43 the Hippocratic authors says:

> Οἱ πυρετοὶ ὁκόσοι, μὴ διαλείποντες, διὰ τρίτης ἰσχυρότεροι γίνονται, *ἐπικίνδυνοι*· ὅτῳ δ' ἂν τρόπῳ διαλείπωσι, σημαίνει ὅτι *ἀκίνδυνοι*.
>
> Those fevers that are not intermittent, intensifying thereafter to tertian, are *dangerous*; in the case of those that are intermittent in any way, it indicates that they are *not dangerous*.

Which in P7 is rendered in Arabic as follows:[82]

> إذا كانت الحمى غير مفارقة ثم كانت تشتد غبًّا فهي أعظم خطرًا، وإذا كانت الحمى تفارق على أي وجه كانت فهي تدل على أنه لا خطر فيها.
>
> When the fever is not intermittent and then intensifies to tertian, *it is more dangerous*; and when the fever is intermittent in any manner, this indicates that *there is no danger in it*.

And in Syriac as follows:[83]

> ܐܫܬܘ̈ܬܐ ܐܝܠܝܢ ܕܠܐ ܫܒ̈ܩܢ ܦܘܫܐ: ܚܕܐ ܠܬܠܬܐ ܡܬܩ̈ܦܢ: ܘܝܬܝܪ ܥܫܝܢܐܝܬ ܗ̇ܘܝܢ: ܝܬܝܪ ܐܝܬܝܗܝܢ ܕܩܝܢܕܘܢܘܣ. ܐܝܠܝܢ ܕܒܟܠ ܐܦܐ ܕܗܘ ܫܒ̈ܩܢ ܦܘܫܐ: ܡܫܘ̈ܕܥܢ ܕܕܠܐ ܩܝܢܕܘܢܘܣ ܐܝܬܝܗܝܢ.

82 P7, fol. 58[b], lines 1–6.

83 Pognon (1903), 17; P7, 58[b], lines 1–6.

> Fevers that are not intermittent, then strengthen considerably to three-day [fever] *are more dangerous*. If, however, they are in some way intermittent, they indicate that they are *not dangerous*.

From this example we see that the Greek *akíndunoi* ('they are without danger') is rendered into Syriac with a negation *d-lā qīndūnōs 'īṯēhēn* ('are not dangerous'). Based on this analysis I suggest that before it was erased the space before ܐܝܬܝܗܝܢ had ܕܠܐ ܩܝܢܕܘܢܘܣ. Following damage to the codex or erasure the space was incorrectly amended by a later annotator with ܕܩܝܢܕܘܢܘܣ.[84] Whatever the case may be, it is clear that the Syriac does not attempt, as Ḥunayn's Arabic does, to mimic the Greek morphology by using a comparative. Whilst Ḥunayn's Arabic translation dispenses with the privative morphology and follows the Greek comparative, the Syriac uses a privative construction but dispenses with the Greek comparative.

The next example comes from *Prognostic* 11 (a), where the Hippocratic author speaks about the qualities of faeces and the regular times and frequencies for defecating during the day and night:[85]

> Ἀλλὰ χρὴ κατὰ τὸ πλῆθος τῶν ἐσιόντων ὑποχωρέειν δὶς ἢ τρὶς τῆς ἡμέρης, καὶ τῆς νυκτὸς ἅπαξ, πλέον δὲ ὑπίτω τὸ πρωΐ, ὥσπερ ξύνηθες ἦν τῷ ἀνθρώπῳ.

> But it is necessary to evacuate in proportion to the quantity of nourishment given, either two or three times during the day, and once at night; let more be evacuated in the morning, as was the person's habit.

In the Greek, the final statement 'as was the person's habit' is vague. Jouanna supplies the gloss that the larger quantity of faeces is expelled in the morning as is the person's habit when he is healthy.[86] The Arabic translation explicates the Greek:[87]

> لكنه ينبغي أن يكون البراز بحسب ما يرد البدن مرتين أو ثلاث مرات بالنهار ومرة بالليل،
> ويكون أكثره نحو السحر أو كما[88] من عادة ذلك الإنسان أن يقوم.

84 Pormann (2012b), 159.

85 Jouanna (2013), p. 28, line 6–p. 29, line 1; 2.136.3–5 L.

86 Jouanna (2013), 28: 'Mais il faut évacuer proportionnellement à la quantité d'aliments ingérés, deux ou trois fois le jour, et la nuit une seule fois; qu'une plus grande quantité sort le matin, comme c'était habituel chez l'individu (quand il était en bonne santé)'.

87 P7 fol. 107[a], lines 6–10.

88 أو كما] P7: وكما ABC.

> But it is necessary for the faeces to be according to amount that enters the body, twice or three times during the day and once during the night, and most of it [namely, faeces, sc. *birāz*] at dawn or whenever one usually gets up.

The Arabic translation adds the phrase '... gets up (... *an yaqūma*)' to clarify that the habit (*ʿāda*) the Hippocratic author refers to is the time of the day that the person (*ḏālika l-insāni*) normally gets out of bed. By contrast the Syriac *Prognostic* renders the Greek in the following way.

> ܐܠܐ ܙܕܩ ܕܠܦܘܬ ܡܫܘܚܬܐ ܕܥܐܠܝܢ ܕܒܥܐܠ̈ ܬܬܦܢܩ ܒܡܒܥܘܬܗ: ܬܪ̈ܬܝܢ
> ܙܒ̈ܢܝܢ ܒܝܘܡܐ. ܐܘ ܬܠ̈ܬܐ ܐܘ ܚܕܐ ܙܒܢ ܒܠܠܝܐ ܐܝܟ ܕܒܨܦܪܐ
> ܕܢ ܬܬܦܢܩ ܣܓܝ̈ܐܐ. ܐܘ ܐܝܟ ܕܐܝܬ ܠܗ ܥܝܕܐ ܠܒܪܢܫܐ.

> But it is necessary that, of what comes in, the amount in proportion (*dalpūṯ* = κατὰ) is evacuated, two times a day, or three, or once in the night, as it is expelled in a large quantity in the morning, or as is the person's habit.

It is noteworthy that the Syriac here sticks closer to Greek than the Arabic does. In particular the Syriac translator does not add the clarification that the Arabic translator supplies. Possibly recognising that two translations are at odds, the Arabic annotators in P7 attempt to supply explanations that harmonise the translations, and to provide further details drawing on Galen's commentary.[89] One annotator says that in this passage 'habit (*ʿāda*)' means 'his [the patient's] habit of getting up when in good health (*ʿādatuhū fī ṣiḥḥatihī an yaqūma*).' Another annotator adds a legnthier note:

> الظاهر أنه ينبغي أن يكون أكثر من الوارد إذا كان (...) لأنه يكثر بالمادة المرضية وإنما يكون
> بالليل مرة لأن الطبيعة تغور لإنضاج المادة[90] واستمداد القوة و (...) عند القيام.[91]

> The purport [*al-ẓāhir*, of this passage] is that it is necessary that [what is expelled] be more than the nourishment given if (...), because [the faeces] is increased through the disease matter. It [expulsion] is only once (*mar-*

89 Heeg (1915), 272–273.
90 [المادة] conieci: الما P7.
91 In marg. P7, fol. 107ª.

ratan) during the night because the nature descends in order to concoct the matter and to nourish the faculty, and (…) at the time of rising [from sleep].

The above example is an example of explicitation by the Arabic translator which is not mirrored in the Syriac. The understandings of the passages differ, suggesting that the Arabic and Syriac translators are not the same person.

The next example concerns tapeworms:[92]

> Ἐπιτήδειον δὲ καὶ *ἕλμινθας στρογγύλας* διεξιέναι μετὰ τοῦ διαχωρήματος, πρὸς τὴν κρίσιν ἰούσης τῆς νούσου.
>
> It is advantageous when round worms are expelled along with excrement as the disease proceeds toward the crisis.

Ḥunyan translates the text into Arabic as follows:[93]

> ومما يحمد[94] أيضا أن تخرج مع البراز حيات إذا أمعن المريض[95] نحو البحران.[96]
>
> What is praiseworthy also is that intestinal worms are expelled with the excrement, if the patient proceeds toward the crisis.

And in Syriac it runs as follows:[97]

> ܥܘܕܪܢ ܕܝܢ ܘܐܦ ܕܚܘܪ̈ܩܐ ܚܠܩܠܐ ܬܬܦܠܛܘܢ ܥܡ ܡܦܩܬܐ܆ ܡܐ ܕܐܙܠܐ ܟܘܪܗܢܐ ܢܬܩܪܒ ܠܦܘܪܫܢܐ.
>
> It is also advantageous that round tapeworms are expelled with the excrement as the disease advances towards the crisis.

Two aspects of this set of texts merit our attention. In his edition of the Arabic *Prognostic*, Martin Klamroth ventures that Ḥunyan omitted στρογγύλας from his Arabic translation, simply translating ἕλμινθας στρογγύλας with a single

92 Jouanna (2013), p. 29, lines 3–5; 2.136.7–9 L.
93 P7 fol. 107ª, line 15–107ᵇ, line 2.
94 يحمد ABC: vacat P7.
95 المريض ABC P7 ante correctionem: corr. المرض P7.
96 P7 fol. 107ª, line 15–fol. 107ᵇ, line 2.
97 P7, fol. 107ª, line 19–107ᵇ, line 4.

Arabic word *ḥayyāt*.[98] We learn from Manfred Ullmann (2002, 235), however, that *ḥayyāt* was, in fact, a word frequently used to translate words referring to parasitic worms in the intestines as well as to refer to poisonous animals. Ḥunayn adopts the same translation in the Hippocratic *Aphorisms* 3.26, where he translates 'ἕλμινθες στογγύλαι' as '*ḥayyāt*'.[99] In other words, we have another case here of Ḥunayn opting for a less literal translation that seems to have accorded with lexical Arabic usage.[100] On the other hand, the translator of the Syriac *Prognostic* once again renders the Greek literally with 'ܥܘܪ̈ܠܐ ܓܠܠܝ̈ܬܐ' literally, 'round tapeworms', and an identical translation is adopted in the Hippocratic *Aphorisms* iii.26: 'ܥܘ̈ܪܠܐ ܓܠܠܝ̈ܬܐ'.[101] Such a literal translation is inconsistent with Ḥunayn's well-known tendency to avoid rendering the Greek literally.

The second point is the following. If the three manuscripts used by Klamroth, which I have collated with P7, are correct, Ḥunayn chooses to translate τῆς νούσου 'the disease,' which is the unanimous reading of the direct and indirect Greek traditions, with 'the patient (*al-marīḍ*)'. This should not be taken to imply, however, that Ḥunayn's manuscript had τοῦ νοσέοντος 'the sick person' rather than τῆς νούσου 'the disease', since, as we have seen, modifications such as these were relatively common in Ḥunayn's translation practice. The translator of the Syriac *Prognostic* opts for a more literal translation of the Greek τῆς νούσου, however, using ܟܘܪܗܢܐ 'disease, illness' to render the Greek. Recognising that the Arabic contains a different reading, a later annotator appears to have corrected the Arabic in P7 based on the Syriac translation. It is important to recognise that both Bahnām and later annotators tended to correct the Arabic based on the Syriac, not necessarily because they were able to compare each translation with the Greek original, but because these scholars appeared to assign greater weight to the testimony of the Syriac than the Arabic.[102] Given the disparity in the approaches to the translation, this example suggests that Ḥunayn was not the translator of this passage of the Syriac *Prognostic*.

A few lines after the lemma presented in the previous example, Hippocrates turns to discuss the colour and texture of faeces that indicate a bad outcome for the disease.[103]

98 Klamroth (1888), p. 222, n. 104, for Klamorth's comparison between the Arabic and the Greek texts where he indicates an omission.
99 P7, fol. 48b, line 4.
100 See for example Dozy (1881), 343, الحيات في الأمعاء.
101 P7, fol. 48b, line 6.
102 Mimura (2015).
103 Jouanna (2013), p. 29, line 6–p. 30, line 1; 2.136.10–12 L.

Ὑδαρὲς δὲ κάρτα ἢ λευκὸν ἢ χλωρὸν ἰσχυρῶς ἢ ἀφρῶδες διαχωρέειν, πονηρὰ ταῦτα πάντα.

Discharging what is extremely watery, white, strongly green or frothy is all bad.

وأما البراز المائي الرقيق جدا والأبيض والأصفر الشديد الصفرة والزبدي فكل ذلك رديء.[104]

Watery and extremely fine faeces; white [faeces]; intensely yellow [faeces]; and frothy [faeces] are all bad.

ܬܒܬܐ[105] ܕܝܢ ܕܗܘܝܢ ܡܝܢܝܐ. ܐܘ ܚܘܪܐ ܐܘ ܝܘܪܩܐ ܒܝܬܝܪܐܝܬ ܟܠܗܘܢ ܗܠܝܢ ܒܝܫܝܢ.

Faeces that are very watery, white, or green—all these are bad.

Here is another example in which the translation style adopted by Ḥunayn and the Syriac translator differ noticeably. Ḥunayn's translation endeavours to capture the Greek in a precise manner. Ḥunayn also uses the Arabic *zabadī* ('foamy', 'frothy', 'having drosses') to render the Greek ἀφρῶδες accurately. The Syriac translation on the other hand does not attempt to capture the sense of the Greek as accurately as Ḥunayn as he assigns a single Syriac word *mayyānāyā* (moist, watery) to capture the Greek ὑδαρές. Finally, it is noteworthy that the appropriate Syriac word corresponding to the Greek ἀφρῶδες is absent. In the Hippocratic *Aphorisms* 7.27 (ed. Pognon 1903, 30) we have the following:

ܠܐܝܠܝܢ ܕܪܘܥܬܢܝܐ ܬܒܬܗܘܢ ܒܪܗܛܐ ܡܢ ܪܝܫܐ ܢܚܬ ܠܗܘܢ ܡܕܡ.

Those whose faeces are frothy (*rūʿtanāyā*) in cases of diarrhoea, something of these descends from the head.

This is a translation of the Greek Hippocratic *Aphorisms* 7.30:[106]

104 P7 fol. 107[b], line 5.
105 ܬܒܬܐ conieci : ܬܐ(…) P7.
106 Magdelaine (1988), vol. 2, p. 64.

Ὁκόσοισιν ἀφρώδεα τὰ διαχωρήματα ἐν τῇσι διαρροίῃσι, τούτοισιν ἀπὸ τῆς κεφαλῆς καταρρέει.

In those who in cases of diarrhoea have frothy discharges, these descend from the head.

Given this, we would expect to encounter the Syriac word *rūʿtanāyā* in this portion of the Syriac *Prognostic*. It would be a mistake, however, to make too much of this omission, since its absence is most likely due to scribal omission.

Finally there is the following example from *Prognostic*, where Hippocrates speaks again about making medical predictions based on the colour of the urine.[107]

Ἔστ' ἂν δὲ πυρρόν τε ᾖ τὸ οὖρον καὶ λεπτόν, ἄπεπτον σημαίνει τὸ νόσημα εἶναι· εἰ δὲ καὶ πολυχρόνιον εἴη τοιοῦτον ἐόν, κίνδυνος μὴ οὐ δυνήσεται ὁ ἄνθρωπος διαρκέσαι, ἔστ' ἂν πεπανθῇ ἡ νοῦσος.

As long as the urine is flame-coloured and fine, [this condition] indicates that the disease is not concocted. If, in addition, it lasts a long time in such a state, there is a danger that the individual will not have the strength to last until the disease is concocted.

Ḥunayn translates the Greek into Arabic as follows:[108]

وما دام البول أصفر رقيق القوام فإنه يدل على أن المرض لم ينضج بعد. فإن كان مع ذلك في المدة طول فليس يؤمن أن يبقى المريض إلى أن ينضج مرضه.[109]

As long as the urine is yellow and its consistency is fine, it indicates that the disease has not yet been concocted. If, in addition to that, its duration is long, there is no assurance that the patient will last until his disease is concocted.

The Greek is translated into Syriac as follows:[110]

107 Jouanna (2013), p. 34, lines 1–6; 2.140.10–13 L.

108 P7, fol. 109ᵇ, lines 4–9.

109 P7, fol. 109ᵇ, lines 4–9.

110 P7, fol. 109ᵇ, lines 5–13. (Syriac). I am grateful to Naima Afif for greatly improving my original transcription of the Syriac text.

[ܟܠ ܙܒܢܐ] ܕܐܝܟ ܕܬܗܘܐ ܬܫܦܘ[ܪܬܐ] ܢܘܪܢܝܐ [ܠܓ]ܘܢܗ.[111] ܘܡܛܠܝܢܐ
ܫܘܐܝܬ܁ ܡܫܘܕܥܐ ܕܠܐ ܒܫܝܠ ܟܘܪܗܢܐ. ܐܢܕܝܢ [ܢ]ܘ[ܓ]ܪܐ[112] ܕܙܒܢܐ
ܬܦܘܫ [ܗܟܢ]ܐ.[113] ܡܣܬܟܢܘܬܗ ܐܝܬ܁ ܕܠܐ [ܢ]ܡܨܐ ܟܪܝܗܐ ܕܢܓܪܐ
[ܥܕ]ܡܐ ܕܢܒܫܠ[114] ܟܘܪܗܢܐ.

As long as the urine is fire-coloured, and equally fine, it indicates that the illness is not concocted. If the duration of time persists in this way, there is danger lest the patient [...] to last until the disease concocts.

The differences between the way the Syriac translator and the Arabic translator of the *Aphorisms* render the phrase 'in very old men (τοῖσι σφόδρα πρεσβύτῃσιν)' are noteworthy.[115] The Syriac translator stays quite close to the Greek, opting for a plural *aylēn*, where the Arabic uses a singular 'the elderly man (*al-šayḫ al-fānī*)'. Moreover, the Greek adverb *sphódra* is not directly mirrored in the Arabic. Ḥunayn uses the phrase '*al-fānī*' to emphasise that the man is elderly, already implied in the word *al-šayḫ*. The Syriac simply uses *d-saggī sāḇ*[*ū*] ('who are very elderly') to render the Greek.

These differences in the Arabic and Syriac *Aphorisms* punctuate the differences in the passage of the *Prognostic*, which we return to now. A few observations are in order. First, in Arabic Ḥunayn simply translates πυρρόν as 'yellow (*aṣfar*)', although the Greek literally means 'flame-coloured.' Ḥunayn's choice seems to be based on how Galen understood the Hippocratic lemma. In his commentary on the *Prognostic*, Galen understands Hippocrates to be speaking about urine that is yellowish-red, not about urine that causes a burning sensation upon exiting the body:[116]

Τὸ κατὰ φύσιν οὖρον μετρίως ἐστὶν ὠχρὸν ὡς ἂν ἐκ τοῦ πεφθέντος ὑγροῦ γεγονὸς ὀλίγον τε τῆς ξανθῆς χολῆς προσειληφός, ὅταν δὲ ἤτοι πλείων [ἢ] αὕτη τοῦ δέοντος ἢ ἄκρατος ἰσχυρῶς οὖσα προσαναμιχθῇ τῷ οὔρῳ, πυρρὸν φαίνεται.

111 The ܠ renders an accusative of relation. Compare Ὑπόπυρρον δὲ ἔστω which is translated by ܬܗܘܐ ܕܐܝܟ ܡܫܠܝܐ ܠܓܘܢܗ ܢܘܪܐ (fol. 107ᵃ, lines 17–18).

112 'Duration', cf. fol. 94ᵇ lines 9–10 where the Arabic has also في المدة طول.

113 τοιοῦτον is translated by ܗܟܢܐ elsewhere. Compare fols. 95ᵇ, l.ine 13, 96ᵃ, line 14, and 96ᵇ, line 5.

114 ܕܢܒܫܠ] correct: ܕܢܬܦܫܠ P7.

115 *Aphorisms* 2.40 (4.482.3–4 L.).

116 Heeg (1915), p. 284, line 26–p. 285, line 3; 18b.155 K.

> Natural urine is moderately yellow as if produced from the concocted moisture with the addition of a little bit of yellow bile. When the bile is either more plentiful than necessary or extremely pure and then mixed with the urine, it [the urine] appears to be flame-coloured.

The Syriac translates the Greek literally by using the word 'fiery (*nōrānāyā*),' which is not a Syriac word that is used to refer to colour but to heating and burning.

The Syriac strikes me as somewhat mysterious. As it stands, it appears to convey the opposite of the sense of the Greek phrase. The phrase ܡܣܟܢܘܬܗ ܐܝܬ ܕܡ properly conveys the sense of the Greek *kíndynos mḗ* ('there is a danger lest …'), but the Syriac text that corresponds to the Greek negative particle οὐ belonging to δυνήσεται appears to be missing from the text. In addition the imperfect verb ܕܢܩܒܠ seems out of place, although this is more likely because of textual corruption. Whatever the case may be, it is clear that Ḥunayn and the Syriac translator adopt two different approaches to the same Greek text.

7 Conclusion

In order to prove that Ḥunayn authored the Syriac text preserved in P7, Jacques Jouanna shows that the Syriac and Arabic *Prognostic* are textual hybrids constructed chiefly from the indirect tradition in Galen's commentary but supplemented from the direct tradition where the Hippocratic text was missing from the indirect tradition. Jouanna holds that Ḥunayn did not translate from a single Greek text, neither of the *Prognostic* nor of Galen's commentary. Rather, he sees Ḥunayn working with several Greek manuscripts, ultimately producing a hybrid Syriac and Arabic version of the *Prognostic* for which no single Greek archtype exists. As evidence for his hypothesis Jouanna cites numerous instances in which the Arabic and Syriac text share readings, sometimes both siding with the direct transmission other times both siding with one or the other Galenic recensions of the *Prognostic*. This signature editorial technique displayed by the text of the Arabic and Syriac *Prognostic*, a technique which is peculiar to Ḥunayn in Jouanna's eyes, leads Jouanna to conclude that both translations are Ḥunayn's.

My argument does not deal with the question of whether Ḥunayn actually constructed his Arabic translation in the way proposed by Jouanna (2013). It is aimed, rather, at the corollary that the Syriac translation is Ḥunayn's. The evidence reviewed above suggests that this conclusion needs to be reassessed. First, I have highlighted inconsistencies between the earlier and later recensions of Ḥunayn's *Epistle to ʿAlī ibn Yaḥyā*. I have pointed out that Jouanna's (2013, cxcvi) claim that the Syriac *Prognostic* preserved in P7 is Ḥunayn's preliminary Syriac translation that he produced before the Arabic version is not supported by explicit evidence from the *Epistle*. Second, I have examined the question of Ḥunayn's authorship of the Syriac *Prognostic* from the perspective of the author's translation technique and interpretation of the Greek text. I have drawn attention to the fact that this method has limitations, such as the problem of evident textual contamination in the Arabic translation preserved in P7. Moreover, I discussed an important instance in which Ḥunayn's Arabic translations of similar Greek texts in the *Prognostic* and the *Aphorisms* differ slightly in terminology and interpretation. Of course these minor differences do not lead one to conclude that the Arabic *Prognostic* and *Aphorisms* are not by Ḥunayn. This example shows that care must be taken when relying on evidence from translation technique and interpretation to prove or disprove Ḥunayn's authorship. With these caveats in mind I have nevertheless identified a number of stylistic and interpretive divergences between the Syriac and Arabic translations that are difficult to account for if we assume that Ḥunayn is responsible for both texts. Finally, I have highlighted several instances in which Ḥunayn's interpretation of the Greek is at odds with how the Syriac translator understood the text. Taken together, these examples speak against Ḥunayn's authorship of the Syriac *Prognostic*.

If Ḥunayn did not write the Syriac *Prognostic*, who did? Sergius immediately comes to mind, as he is the only other person said in the *Epistle to ʿAlī ibn Yaḥyā* to have produced a translation of Galen's commentary on the *Prognostic*. With such reasoning in mind Barry (2018: 174) proposes Job of Edessa or Ǧibrīl ibn Buḫtīšūʿ as the authors of the Syriac *Aphorisms*, since they are mentioend by Ḥunayn as having translated Galen's commentary on the *Aphorisms*. I am unconvinced by such arguments. Certainly, there is little if any positive evidence, textual or otherwise, to support the claim that Sergius translated the *Prognostic*. For the moment, we lack parallel passages in the Syriac *Prognostic* and in other texts ascribed with confidence to Sergius to verify this hypothesis. The time for thoroughly carrying out this task is drawing nearer as the research team led by Peter E. Pormann has recently made available a considerable amount of the Syriac translation of Galen's *On Simple Drugs*, which they attribute to Sergius rather than Ḥunayn.[117] While the question of who authored the Syriac *Prognostic* may never be adequately answered, I think the above evidence disproves the possibility of Ḥunayn's authorship. Sergius' and

117 Bhayro et al. (2013), 132; Afif et al., (2020).

Ḥunayn's authorship will probably not be definitively resolved until corpus-based techniques are developed to analyse Syriac translation techniques for different translators. Fortunately, preliminary steps are being taken in this direction.[118]

Whatever the case may be, these results confirm those arrived at earlier by Taro Mimura. With Mimura, I conclude that P7 contains contaminated versions of Ḥunyan's Arabic translations of the *Aphorisms* and the *Prognostic*. These texts have been altered to various degrees by Bahnām, P7's scribe, and by later annotators seeking to repair the damaged text on the basis of the parallel Syriac text. The scribe and the annotators worked in a scholarly environment in which Arabic was the language of science. P7 is heavily annotated, but entirely in Arabic, whereas there are no corrections or notes in Syriac in the margins. Yet, it is clear that for Bahnām and the annotators, the Syriac translation, preserved in the right column of P7, possessed a textual authority that was not shared in their eyes by Ḥunayn's Arabic translation. Mimura has shown how Bahnām altered phrases in the Arabic *Aphorisms* when the Arabic and Syriac *Aphorisms* disagreed on a reading. He has also shown that Bahnām rearranged or omitted aphorisms according to the structure and contents of the Syriac *Aphorisms*. Mimura suggests that Bahnām and the annotators made these changes not necessarily because they recognised that the Syriac was more consistent with the Greek than the Arabic, but out of deference to the Syriac text. In like manner, I have shown how Bahnām replaced Ḥunayn's 'heavenly' with 'divine' based on the Syriac parallel. I have also pointed to places where annotators recognised the differences between the Arabic and Syriac, sometimes correcting the Arabic text, and at other times making notes in the margins that attempt to harmonise the translations.

118 In addition to Peter E. Pormann's Syriac Galen Palimpsest project, Grigory Kessel leads a project at the Austrian Academy of Sciences (Österreichische Akademie der Wissenschaften) and funded by the European Research Council, called *HunaynNET: Transmission Of Classical Scientific And Philosophical Literature From Greek Into Syriac And Arabic*; see https://hunaynnet.oeaw.ac.at [accessed 11 March 2021].

CHAPTER 16

The Latin Commentary by Pedro Jaime Esteve on the Second Book of the Hippocratic *Epidemics* (Valencia, 1551)

María Teresa Santamaría Hernández

In 1551 the Valencian physician, Latinist and Hellenist scholar, Pedro Jaime Esteve (ca. 1500–1556),*[1] published in Valencia by Juan Mey his Latin commentary with translation of the second book of the Hippocratic *Epidemics*: *Hippocratis Coi medicorum omnium principis EpidemiΩn* (sic) *liber secundus a Petro Iacobo Steue medico Latinitate donatus, et fusissimis commentariis illustratus, adiecta et singulis sententiis graeca ueritate*.[2] Esteve, who was a Professor of Medicine at the University of Valencia, where he had also briefly been a professor of Greek, is one of the most outstanding figures of Spanish Medical Humanism, because he combines the qualities of philologist and physician, which are so characteristic of the most important European representative of this pedagogical and intellectual line of thought. The year after the publication of this commentary, he also brought out his translation in Latin hexameters of the *Theriaca* of Nicander of Colophon.[3] Nicander was the principal source in Renaissance toxicology, together with the apocryphal books of Pseudo-Dioscorides on the subject.[4] This translation by Esteve was also accompanied by Latin commentary, similar to that on the Hippocratic *Epidemics*. Both works were accompanied by the Greek text that he obtained from the Aldine edition (Venice 1499) in the first case, and, as we will see below, from the Venetian (1526) and Basel (1538) ones, in the second case.

* This article is part of the research project FFI2016–77240-P and of the Excellence Network *Opera Medica* (FFI2016-81769-REDT, Ministerio de Economía y Competividad).

1 The biographical repertories indicate he was born in Morella or San Mateo: Nicolás Antonio (1788), 203; Chinchilla (1967), 449; Hernández Morejón (1967), 365; López Piñero (1983), 312; Santander (1971), 85.

2 All references will be to this edition, which is foliated rather than paginated. I have modernized spelling and punctuation marks.

3 Esteve (1552). On this work see Santamaría (2002), (2004a), (2004b); and Radici (2012), 41–43. The information offered by Floris Overduin (2014, 136) that Esteve translated *Theriaca* into Spanish is not accurate, because it is a translation into Latin.

4 Sprengel (1830).

© MARÍA TERESA SANTAMARÍA HERNÁNDEZ, 2021 | DOI:10.1163/9789004470200_018

Especially from the 1520s onwards, the University of Valencia stood out within Spain as the principal promotor of humanistic thought, together with the University of Alcalá de Henares. In the case of Valencia, the reach of Humanism was particularly intense in the field of medicine. Indeed, besides the importance given to a new philological perspective, which can be exemplified by the creation of the chair in Greek in 1524, there was also a group of university physicians who represented the most modern understanding of medicine, which brought together Hippocratic Galenism from a doctrinal point of view, with the philological, linguistic and literary interests from a formal point of view. Members of this group were Miguel Jerónimo Ledesma, a professor of Greek and physician, and Esteve himself, who briefly replaced Ledesma as professor of Greek after his death (1547), as well as the Anatomists Pedro Jimeno and Luis Collado.[5]

In the first half of the sixteenth century, the Hippocratic *Epidemics* had not received much attention from European Medical Humanism, and Book 2 in particular even less. Besides the two complete editions of the Greek text published in Venice (1526) and Basel (1538), and the complete Latin translations by Fabius Calvus and Janus Cornarius published in the editions of the Latin *Opera* of 1525 and 1546, only Books 1, 3 and 6 had been subjects of special attention.[6] The First Book, in fact, appeared in Latin with the corresponding Galenic commentaries in 1531, translated by Hermann Cruser (1510–1574).[7] In this volume, however, his interest centred mostly on the three medical commentaries about it, as demonstrated by the titles and colophons of each of the three parts, in which the Hippocratic text is only a necessary complement for the corresponding explanations.[8] This remained the same in the 1550 edition in which Jan Was translated Galenic commentaries on Books 1, 3, and 6 of the Hippocratic *Epidemics*,[9] with the different sections focused once again on Galen.[10]

5 A philological study of the writtings of these physicians in Santamaría (2003). Biographical data in Nicolás Antonio (1783–1788); Chinchilla (1967); Hernández Morejón (1967); López Piñero (1979) and (1983); and Santamaría (2012a).

6 Calvo (1525); on this translator, see Witt (2018). Cornarius (1546).

7 Cruser (1531).

8 Fol. 1r *Claudii Galeni in primum Hippocratis librum de morbis popularibus, Commentarius Primus*; fol. 21r *Finis commentarii primi Galeni*; fol. 21v *Galeni in librum primum Hippocratis de morbis popularibus commentarius secundus*; etc.

9 Vassès (1550).

10 P. 43 *Galeni in primum Epidemorum Hippocratis commentarius primus*; p. 232 *Finis Commentarii Tertii in Primum Epidemiorum*; p. 233 *Galeni in tertium Epidemiorum commentarius primus*. etc.

Two common elements characterize these editions: first of all, as we have seen, the interest centred on Galen, as we can deduce from the titles and colophons of each section. Secondly, there is no sign of a 'modern' commentary, that is to say, a commentary by the author of the translation or by another humanistic physician.

The translation of Book 6 of the Hippocratic *Epidemics* published by Leonhart Fuchs in 1537 differs from these editions, as he included his own *expositio*, that is to say, his commentaries in Latin. This is precisely the fundamental characteristic that will mark modern works about the *Epidemics* (and about other Hippocratic writings), that centred not only on the translation of the Hippocratic text, but also on offering commentary on it with the modern perspective of Medical Humanism.

Moreover, this is also the characteristic that defines Esteve's commentary on Book 2, which made him a pioneer, as Fuchs had been for Book 6.[11] In reality, Esteve's commentary shares elements with Fuchs', and probably imitated him consciously. In fact, both editions have similar characteristics in form and content, from the use of the Omega in the genitive of the title, to the treatment of contextual matters of authorship (which had already been dealt with by Galen in his commentaries on the Hippocratic writing) and the assessment of earlier translations and editions, including the presentation of the Greek text and of the fragments from Galen duly translated into Latin by the respective authors.[12] All of this gives both works a very similar feel that makes it possible to situate the two writings on the same ideological level.

1 Esteve's Edition

Esteve's *Epidemics*, preceded by an epistle dedicated to Bernardo Simon,[13] another to the reader (*ad lectorem*) and a *praefatio* (the same, in fact, as Fuchs'), are organised following the scheme of the Hippocratic work on which they are based, in six *sectiones*. Of these, the fourth and the fifth are also presented with their prefaces. The Hippocratic text is divided into lemmas, combining in each case the Greek version—because it had to be offered for the reader to

11 In Spain, only the commentaries of Vallés (1577) were late published. See Martín Ferreira (1995), Ángel Espinós (2011), and Santander (1971).

12 Fuchs (1537), title: *Adiecta sunt ad calcem operis graeca, ut diligens lector haec ipsa cum latinis conferre possit*; Esteve (1551), title: *Adiecta Graeca veritate*.

13 Among other positions, he held that of *jurado* of Valencia, thereby forming part of the city government. See Expósito Navarro (2004).

understand the corresponding explanations—, Esteve's Latin translation, and the commentary on each of them.

To present the Greek text that serves as the basis of the translation and commentaries, Esteve followed, as would be expected, the Venetian edition of the *Opera omnia* (1526), that had appeared one year after the Latin translations by Fabius Calvus (1525). He also drew on the Latin version published by Janus Cornarius in 1538 by Froben.[14] Esteve frequently although not always referred to these two versions in his commentary as *exemplar Assulanum* and *Frobenianum*, or in a less precise manner with the term *exemplaria*, which was in fact common. His starting points was the Aldine edition, which he normally did not modify; but he compared it to the other Greek or Latin versions in order to correct the text, and was careful to document the variant readings and his emendations. However, Esteve's contribution to the Greek text is a subject that deserves further scrutiny.

As a result, then, of this practice of textual criticism, Esteve proposes emendations that are not found in any of the Greek or Latin editions. This is what he does for example when he amends the fragment in which Hippocrates exposes the signs that must be observed in the prognosis of diseases (2.1.6 [5.76 L.; Smith 1994, 22]). In this fragment Esteve proposes to correct 'βρωμάτων', the genitive plural of 'βρῶμα (food)', into 'χρώματα', the accusative plural of 'χρῶμα (colour)', and 'συμπτωσέων', the genitive plural of 'σύμπτωσις (collapse)', into 'συμπτώσιας', the accusative plural of the same word. He bases these corrections on a parallel passage in Book 6 (6.2.6 [5.280 L.; Smith 1994, 226]). In this way, and by adding a change in the segmentation of the text, the content of the fragment is made to coincide with what Hippocrates said in this book about the observation of colour and the pressure in the veins. This amendment was not found in the editions of the Greek text:[15]

> Caeterum cum tam praue nobiscum actum sit, ut nulla alia supersit spes, quam coniectura, Oedipum agere satius fuerit. Legebatur itaque in omnibus, quos hactenus uidere licuit codicibus, prima huius orationis pars in hunc modum: θεωρεῖν ἤ οὕτω δεῖ, βρωμάτων, συμπτωσέων. Φλεβῶν ὄγκοι ὑποχονδρίων. ἀναῤῥοπίων καταῤῥοπίων,[16] non inepte solum, uerum etiam

14 Hippocrates (1538).

15 Esteve (1552), fol. 33^{r}, lines 14–22.

16 Really, the editions of 1526 and 1538 offer the fragment with slight variants with respect to that of Esteve: θεωρεῖν δὲ οὕτω δεῖ. βρωμάτων συμπτωσέων. φλεβῶν ὄγκοι. ὑποχονδρίων. ἀναῤῥοπίων. καταῤῥοπίων (Hippocrates [1526], fol. 134, lines 38–39; Hippocrates [1538], p. 311, lines 47–48).

> indistincte, citraque ordinem, ut tanto uiro indigna penitus sententia censeretur. At nos ita restituimus, idque non absque ratione: θεωρεῖν δὲ οὕτω δεῖ, χρώματα, συμπ[π]τώσιας φλεβῶν, ὄγκους ὑποχονδρίων, ἀναῤῥοπίων, καταῤῥοπίων. Nam in libro *uulgarium morborum* sexto, sectione secunda, talis sententia legitur: φλέβες κροτάφων οὔχ ἱδρύμεναι, οὐδὲ χλώρασμα λαμπρὸν, ἢν πνεῦμα ἐγκαταλείπηται, ἢ βὴξ ξηρή, μὴ θηριώδης, ἐς ἄρθρα στήριξιν προσδέχεσθαι δεῖ.
>
> Since the remaining part has reached us in such a bad state that there is no other hope than conjecture, it would be better to take on the role of Oedipus.[17] So, in all the manuscripts that we were able to see to date, the first part of this sentence reads as follows: 'One should observe in this way: food (*brōmátōn*), collapse (*symptōséōn*). Swelling of the blood vessels of hypochondria (*phlebôn ónkoi hypochondríōn*). Upward tendencies, downward tendencies.' This is not just absurd, but also confused and not properly arranged. This sentence cannot, therefore, have been written by such a [distinguished] man [as Hippocrates]. We have restored it with good reason in the following way: 'One should observe in this way: colours (*chrṓmata*), collapse of blood vessels (*symptṓsias phlebôn*), swelling of the hypochondria (*ónkous hypochondríōn*). Upward tendencies, downward tendencies.'.[18] Because in book 6, section 2 of the *Epidemics*, this phrase reads: 'Blood vessels in the temples unstable, colour bad; if there be breathing trouble or a dry cough [not too violent], you must expect a deposit on the joints'.[19]

In the assessment of the versions of the text, Esteve frequently consults the earlier translations of Fabius Calvus, Cornarius and even Fuchs' of book 6. In this regard, for example, he rejects the versions of the Hippocratic fragments by Calvus and Cornarius based on erroneous readings and interpretations of the Greek text. He does so in the case of the commentary on *Epidemics* 2.1.1, where Hippocrates treated the appearance of anthrax in the summer: 'In Crannon in summer: anthrax. During the hot weather there was continuous violent rain. It occurred more with wind from the south ("Ανθρακες ἐν Κρανῶνι οἱ θερινοί. ὗεν ἐν καύμασιν ὕδατι λαύρῳ, δι' ὅλου ἐγένετο, καὶ μᾶλλον νότῳ [5.72 L.; Smith 1994, 18–

---

17 Oedipus solved the riddle of the sphinx; 'take on the role of Oedipus' means 'to find a solution to a difficult riddle'.

18 Trans. Smith (1994), 23.

19 Trans. Smith (1994), 227.

19])'. Esteve offers the text of the Aldine and Frobenian editions, and shows how Fabius Calvus mistook '*nótos* (south wind)' for '*nôtos* (back)':[20]

> Fabius Caluus, qui omnia Hippocratis opera Latio donauit sermone, in hac parte turpissime lapsus est. 'Carbones (inquiens) aestiui Cranone uiguerunt: sub aestu ualde pluit: qui per totum corpus, sed *in tergo* magis fiebant'. Quod enim Hippocrates καὶ μᾶλλον νότῳ scripsit, καὶ μᾶλλον νώτῳ legere uisus est, nominum similitudine deceptus. Nam Graece, νότος, per ο Austrum significat, per ω mega uero dorsum seu tergum.

> Fabius Calvus, who translated the complete works of Hippocrates into Latin, made a clumsy mistake in this part, saying: 'In Cranon there were summer carbuncles. In hot weather it rained a lot. These appeared all over the body, but especially *on the back* (*in tergo*)'. Although Hippocrates wrote καὶ μᾶλλον νότῳ, he apparently read καὶ μᾶλλον νώτῳ, because he was deceived by the fact that [both] words are similar. In Greek *nótos* with omicron means 'south wind', but with omega, it means 'back'.

Another example occurs at *Epidemics* 2.1.2: '*In hot weather when it is dry* fevers are mostly free from sweat (*'Ev καύμασιν ἀνυδρίης*, οἱ πυρετοὶ, ἀνίδρωτες τὰ πλεῖστα [5.72 L.; Smith 1994, 18–19])'. The question here is whether to take 'In hot weather when it is dry' with the preceding or the following sentence. Cornarius had taken in with the preceding sentence, but this is clearly wrong according to Esteve:[21]

> Caeterum admonendi in hac parte sumus, Cornarium, medicum alioqui doctissimum, oscitanter admodum, ne dicam inepte, hunc locum interpretatum fuisse, quoniam initium propositae orationis ἐν καύμασιν ἀνυδρίης, id est, in aestibus squaloris, cum praecedente, nulla prorsus seruata sententiae consecutione, copulasse uidetur hunc in modum: 'Deinde pustulae, uelut ab igne inustae, excitabantur et sub cutem uri sibi videbantur *in ardoribus siccitatis*'.[22] Cuius sane lapsus occasionem sibi praebuerunt Graeca propemodum omnia exemplaria uitiata. Nec mirum profecto est uirum uertentem solum, non tamen penitius scrutantem autoris sensa, interdum delinquere.

20 Esteve (1551), fol. 15^{v}, lines 2–7.

21 Esteve (1551), fol. 16^{r}, lines 26–35.

22 Cornarius (1546), 410.

> Moreover, we have to be warned here that Cornarius, otherwise an extremely learned physician, translated this passage carelessly, not to say, inappropriately. For he seems to join the beginning of the sentence in question, 'ἐν καύμασιν ἀνυδρίης', meaning 'in foul hot weather', with the preceding one, so that the sense of the arrangement is lost. This is his translation: 'then small blisters as though from burns rose up and seemed like burns on the skin beneath in the dry heat.' This error is undoubtedly due to the Greek manuscripts, which are all full of mistakes. It is, therefore, not surprising that someone who translates only without delving deep into the author's meaning sometimes makes mistakes.

Esteve thus explained Cornarius' error in terms of corruption of the Greek manuscript tradition. In Cornarius' own 1538 edition of the Greek text (p. 311, lines 18–20), the two sentences are linked to each other and not separated. Esteve's solution certainly has a lot of merit, and Littré (5.72 L.) adopted it some three centuries later.

Esteve thus wrote a critical commentary on *Epidemics* 2, and Fuchs' Latin translation on book 6 was of much help, for there are many parallel passages between books 2 and 6. This can best be illustrated with an example from *Epidemics* 2.3.7. There we have the mysterious sentence: 'Cure for continuous yawning, long breather; for inability to drink and difficulty drinking, short breather. ('Ιητήριον συνεχέων χασμέων, μακρόπνους, τοῖσιν ἀπότοισι καὶ μόγις πίνουσι, βραχύπνους)' [5.110 L.; Smith 1994, 54–55]. In he Greek printed editions available to Esteve, however, the second part of this phrase was corrupted to '... τοῖσιν ἀπότοισι καὶ μόγις μακρόπνους',[23] which is very difficult to translate, but could be rendered as 'for inability to drink also long breather with difficulty.' Yet, Galen's explanation of a similar passage in book 6 (6.2.4 [5.278 L])[24] allowed Esteve to restore the text:[25]

> Sed postquam expositionem omnem absoluimus, operae pretium erit quod in Hippocratico codice deprauatum admodum mendosumque est, impraesentiarum adnotare, ne loci corruptela facessere negotium cuiquam possit. Primumque studiosos commonemus, in secunda huius orationis parte, deesse uocem alteram πίνουσιν, atque in hunc modum legen-

23 Hippocrates (1538), p. 315, lines 27–28; and Littré (5.110 L.) adopted the reading 'μικρόπνους'.

24 Galen, *Commentary on Hippocrates' 'Epidemics'* 6.2.12–13 (17a.919 K.; Wenkebach, Pfaff 1956, 74); the commentary on book 2 has recently been edited by Vagelpohl (2016), 493–506.

25 Esteve (1551), fol. 109^{v}, lines 14–24.

> dum esse locum: τοῖσιν ἀπότοισιν, καὶ μόγις πίνουσιν, quod est in emaculatis Hippo[cratis] codicibus recte habetur. Quin, et ultima dictio plane est mendosa, cum habeat, μακρόπνους, atque legendum pro ea sit βραχύπνους, quod facile ex sexto libro *de morbis uulgaribus*, sectione secunda, restitui potest, in qua eadem prorsus oratio legitur. Quare doctam Leonardi Fuchsii expositionem non contemnas, quin potius ad eam te conuertito si quid compendiosius a nobis dictum, non plane tibi satisfaciat.
>
> After finishing the commentary, however, it will now be useful to indicate the places where the Hippocratic manuscript contains mistakes and errors, so that the corrupt passage does not cause difficulty to anyone. First of all, scholars should be aware that in the second part of this sentence the second word 'πίνουσιν' is missing and that it should read as follows: 'to those who cannot drink or drink with difficulty'. This text is preserved in the pure copies of Hippocrates' text. Moreover, the last word is also corrupt, as the text has 'long breather (μακρόπνους)', for which one should read 'short breather (βραχύπνους)'. This correction is easily made on the basis of book 6, section 2 of the *Epidemics*. There the text is very similar. Therefore, you should not neglect Leonard Fuchs' explanation, but consult it, if the rather brief explanation that I have given is not entirely satisfactory for you.

In this way, Esteve defends the addition of a term πίνουσιν and the correction of 'μακρόπνους' (offered by the Aldus's and Froben's editions) into 'βραχύπνους', which we find in Galen's commentary. Esteve also shows his admiration for Fuchs and sends his readers to him.

In addition to textual criticism, Esteve's commentary also contains exegesis of various aspects, from medical terminology to style, as well as medical doctrine. His explanations are notably varied and show great attention to detail. The preface already discusses the problem of who authored the different books of the *Epidemics*, the usefulness of translating it into Latin, the need to restore the Greek text, and the value of astronomy to physicians.

Esteve therefore pursued exegetical and didactic aims in this commentary by using resources such as glosses and definitions. In this, he followed trends in Renaissance commentaries on medical and other technical subjects. Esteve employed a characteristically humanistic medical Latin, from which medieval vocabulary and syntaxe are notably absent. This 'new' Latin contained a renewed medical terminology drawn from the principal sources of Renaissance medicine, Pliny the Elder and Celsus.[26]

---

26 See Santamaría (2004c), 353–373.

2 Esteve's Medical Humanism

In his commentary, but most particularly in the two prefatory epistles and the preface, Esteve detailed the programmatic principles that characterised his work, through which he expressed his humanist mentality and his assessment of the Hippocratic writings. He thus emerges as a physician-philologist who aims at restoring text of *Epidemics* 2 and thus the truth of Hippocrates' doctrine (the *Hippocratica ueritas*).

Esteve wants to restore both the text and the context so as to get at the exact text and its correct interpretation. Like many notable physicians representing Medical Humanism who outlined their objectives in the prefaces, prologues and epistles of their editions and translations, Esteve wanted to revive ancient medicine by searching for the correct Greek texts (*Graeca ueritas*) and their true meaning (*sensus* and *auctoris mens*). Declaring this overall objective became almost a cliché in editions, translations and commentaries on ancient Greek and Latin medical authors, in particular on Hippocrates and Galen.[27] It also affected other illustrious representatives of ancient medicine, such as Nicander of Colophon,[28] and even the Latinized works of the Arabs, frequently considered to be transmitters of Greek medical doctrine.[29]

Esteve is clearly aware of the internal problems posed by the work of Hippocrates, the differences in style, the disparate information, and the brevity of expression, which are aggravated by the passage of time. In the face of these, he declares his objectives of restoring the text 'into its original form (*in pristinum statum*)', and of searching for the 'author's intention (*scopus hominis*)' and the 'Hippocratic truth (*Hippocratica ueritas*)'. In this Esteve differs from Cornarius: the former criticises the latter for clinging too closely to the text as it is transmitted, and not using critical judgement to improve it:[30]

27 As we can see, for example, in Serveto (1537), a Galenist author: fol. 2, lines 7–8: 'The right defense of the Galen's doctrine (*Galenici dogmatis iusta defensio*)'. Critical edition in Santamaría (2011).

28 For example, in his Latin translation of *Theriaca*, Esteve explained his intention to discover the meaning of Nicander's verses: Esteve (1552), fol. 2ᵛ, lines 29–30; fol. 3ʳ, lines 1–3. See Santamaría (2018b), 56–57.

29 For instance, the Valencian physician and Hellenist Miguel Jerónimo Ledesma (1547, fol. 2ᵛ, line 24) says himself that he wants to restore the 'Arabic truth (*Arabica ueritas*) when translating the first part of the Avicenna's *Canon* into Latin.

30 Esteve (1552), fol. 3ʳ, lines 27–29; and fol. 97ᵛ, lines 35–38.

> Quod autem prae ceteris magis exoptabam, id quidem erat, ut in Galeni commentarios inciderem, quibus maximam huius libri partem in pristinum statum restituere possem.
>
> But what I wanted most of all was to consult Galen's comments in order to restore most of this book into its original form.
>
> Nos vero, in hunc modum, hanc Hippocratis partem conuertimus, longe quidem aliter quam aut Cornarius fecerit, aut alius quispiam, quoniam ad Hippocratis mentem magis accedere ita videremur.
>
> But we translated this section of Hippocrates in this way, quite differently from what Cornarius or others have done, in order to be seen to be closer to Hippocrates' thinking.

Esteve also pitched himself against medical 'barbarism', the perceived impure Latin and the corrupt doctrines of the Middle Ages.[31] This occurred in the wider context of a controversy that raged through Renaissance medical humanism, with the 'new' Latin replacing the 'corrupt' expressions of medieval medical authors, often translated from Arabic and seen to have distorted the Greek medical doctrine. This controversy brought together specifically medical aspects with others of a philological nature. There is no Latin work by any self-respecting medical humanist who does not declare his opposition to medieval Latin transmitter of medical errors in a programmatic way or as a central theme in a commentary or translation. This opposition, however, was projected especially against the scholastic Latin developed in particular since the twelfth century in commentaries and translations, and against its authors, starting with Gerard of Cremona (d. 1187) and his Latin version of the Avicenna's *Canon*, followed by the Italian commentators. On the whole, however, the Arabs were not automatically included, or at least some of them such as Rhazes were valued as transmitters of Greek medical doctrine, although they received the rejection of the staunch opponents of Arabs, such as Fuchs.[32]

In any case, this programmatic positioning against the formal and conceptual barbarism of medical scholasticism also informed the works of Esteve, and particularly his writing on *Epidemics* 2. In fact, as early as in his 'Letter to the Reader (*epistula ad lectorem*)' he attacks the *Pandects of Medicine* (*Pandectae*

31 See Santamaría (2018a).

32 See Pormann (2011b), Hasse (2016).

medicinae) by Mattheus Sylvaticus (ca. 1280–1342), the *Antidotarium Nicolai* (a famous manual on compound drugs) and Avicenna's *Canon of Medicine*. He attacks the *Pandects of Medicine*, the *Antidotarium Nicolai* and Avicenna (that is to say, his *Canon* translated into Latin) as the origin of the lack of knowledge of medicine and of professional malpractice, and, what turns out to be truly relevant for understanding the linguistic nature of this controversy, he pitches the exponents of this barbarism against 'those who favour good literature (*bonarum literarum professores*)':[33]

> … qualem, aliquando nos uidimus, qui eo venerat inscitiae, ne insipientiam dixerim, ut qua passim utimur theriacam, non ex Andromachi scriptura esse confingendam assereret, sed potius ex suo medicamentorum luco, nimirum aut Pandectario, aut tenebricoso luminari, aut maxime deprauato Nicolao, qui utique chaos est, ac rerum male conditarum congeries. Vides quo tandem hominum indignatio aduersus bonarum literarum professores procedat, ut dum animo suo faciant satis, non dubitent, et suorum etiam praeceptorum dogmata subuertere? Nam quod Auicenna, quem ipsi ut Deum colunt, Andromachi potissimum praeparationem in usus redigendam esse censeat, aut plane non norunt, aut dum nobis contendant inficiari non uerentur.

> I once met such a man [sc. such an intemperate physician]. He reached such a point of ignorance, not to say stupidity, that he claimed that the theriac that we use should not be made according to Andromachus' recipe, but rather from the grove (*lucus*) of his own drugs, or surely from the *Pandects*, or from the dark light (*tenebricosus luminaris*),[34] or indeed from the totally corrupt Nicholas, who is a total mess and a collection of badly conceived things. Do you not see how far the contempt of these people for those who favour good literature goes? In order to indulge themselves, they do not even hesitate to falsify the doctrines of their own teachers. For Avicenna, whom they adore like God, thought that one should mostly employ Andromachus' composition. Yet, they either simply do not know this, or they are not afraid to deny it in order to attack us.

33 Esteve (1552), sig. a3 v, line 30–sig. a4 r, line 2.

34 There is a Latin wordplay here, with 'grove (*lucus*)' being linked to 'light (*lux*)'.

This last idea is repeated later, when Esteve attributes medical malpractice to the lack of knowledge and engagement with the classical medical authors, using the significant terms '*classicus*' and '*barbarus*' to flag this opposition:[35]

> Nostri vero medici, suam temeritatem prodentes, medicamentorum multitudine naturam coeptum opus exequi non permittunt. Inter quos quidam eo temeritatis peruenerunt (dispeream si quenquam falso insimulauero) ut se nunquam decretorios dies expectasse arroganter, aut verius stulte ac insolenter asserant, neque expectaturos affirment. Quos (proh dolor) quantam aegrotantibus perniciem allaturos esse credendum est. Enimuero digni maxime sunt qui non minus quam homicidae ac totius reipublicae ἀλάστορες crucibus affigantur. Sed huius rei non tam imperitia in causa est, quam indecens ambitio ac inanis quaedam singularis nominis gloria. Quae sane omnia hinc maxime proficiscuntur quod a veterum classicorum medicorum doctrina desciuerunt, atque in penitissimam Barbarorum Stigiam se praecipitarunt, in qua tam immensus viget undiquaque chaos, ut temere quisque caecorum ritu prout libet ultro citroque ferri possit.
>
> Our physicians, however, show their recklessness by using too many different drugs, so that they do not let nature complete the task that they began. I do not want to accuse anyone falsely, but among them are those who declare that they do not observe, and are not going to observe, the critical days. They do this out of arrogance, or rather out of stupidity and insolence. One surely has to believe that they cause grave harm to their patients. Indeed, they deserve no less than murderers and traitors to the state to be crucified. One should not attribute this to inexperience, but to an unbridled desire for fame and fortune. All these things stem from the fact that they have deserted the teachings of the ancient classical physicians and thrown themselves into the deepest waters of the Barbarian Styx, where the greatest disorder reigns everywhere, so that one can be tossed back and forth randomly like a blind man.

This quotation shows Esteve's humanist mindset. Medical ideas should be expressed in a new literary Latin; he dedicates his commentary to those who grew up 'in the lap of the Muses (*in Musarum sinu*), saying 'but we speak to the

35 Esteve (1552), fol. 45^r, lines 22–34.

learned ... to those who have long been nurtured in the lap of the Muses (*Sed doctis loquimur ... his qui in Musarum sinu fuerint diutius enutriti*)'.[36]

Esteve also tackles the problem of Hippocrates' notoriously brevity (*breuiloquentia*). He recognises that 'the truth is sometimes hidden under such a condensed sequence of words (*ueritas sub tam compendiosa uerborum serie interdum latet*)'.[37] Therefore, unraveling this brevity becomes a key element in interpreting the text. One can thus have access to Hippocrates' ideas, as Esteve explains:[38]

> Caeterum, cum Hippocrates in his ordini sermonisque consecutioni non studeret, quandoquidem non in hoc ipsa scribebat ut in lucem prodirent, sed dumtaxat ut ea quae tum ratione, tum experimento colligebat memoria seruaret. Haec perpetuo meminisse decet, ne quispiam ipsum calumniari propterea possit. Siquidem sermonis propositi in his libris ueritatem non docendi modum contemplari oportet, quemadmodum et in *Aphorismis*, et in aliis nonnullis ipsius commentariis.

> Moreover, in his text Hippocrates did not pay attention to word order and sequence, because he did not write for publication, but merely to keep a record of the things that he discovered through reason and experience. One should always bear this in mind, so that no one can rebuke him because of this. Therefore, one ought to look at the truth that is expressed in the text contained in these books and not the manner of exposition, as is also the case with the *Aphorisms* and some other works by him.

Fuchs (1537, p. 1, lines 30–31) had already remarked that 'Hippocrates ... talked extremely unintelligibly because of his old habit to endeavour to be brief. (Hippocrate ... qui ob antiquae breuitatis studium obscurissime locutus est)' and noted his 'typical expression and laconic brevity which he used everywhere (*singularem phrasim, et laconicam qua passim utitur* [sc. *Hippocrates*] *breuiloquentiam*)'. This shows yet again that Esteve approached Hippocrates in a similar way to Fuchs.

European medical humanism generated notable translators of the works of Hippocrates, and particularly of the *Epidemics*. Since the 1525 publication of Fabius Calvus' translations, several physician-philologists were interested in improving, completing and commenting on Calvus' work and on the new

36 Ibid., fol. 134^{r}, lines 11–22.
37 Ibid., fol. 23^{v}, line 27.
38 Ibid., fol. 23^{v}, lines 20–26.

versions that were progressively published; this interest animated Fuchs, Cornarius, Esteve and Vallés. In this list of authors, Esteve occupies a special place, because of his dedication to *Epidemics* 2: his commentary is the only one in European Renaissance, just as Fuchs' was the only on *Epidemics* 6. The formal elements of the Esteve's commentary, as well as the principles and procedures that guided him when accessing ancient medicine reveal a work and an author fully integrated in the medical humanist movement that prevailed in sixteenth-century Europe.

CHAPTER 17

The First Complete Renaissance Commentary on the Hippocratic *Epidemics*

Jesús Ángel y Espinós

The commentary on the Hippocratic *Epidemics* (1577) by the Spanish physician Francisco Vallés (1524–1592) belongs to a series of works that Vallés devoted to Hippocrates, such as his books on the *Aphorisms* (1561), the *Prognostic* (1567), and *Regime in Acute Diseases* (1569).[*,1] As a follower of Hippocratic Galenism, which dominated medical studies in the second half of sixteenth century Spain, Vallés also wrote several commentaries on Galen's works such as *Affected Parts* (1559), *Art of Medicine* and *Uneven Bad-Mixture* (1567), and *Distinct Types of Fevers* (1569). Furthermore, he devoted several books to translations and commentaries of the Aristotelian Corpus on natural and physical subjects, in which the author defends the necessity of studying Greek in order to re-establish the *studia litterarum* in Spain with the patronage of the King. Owing to his high regard for classical values and heritage, Vallés is a prime representative of humanist medicine in Renaissance Spain. Therefore, in the dedication letter to the King Philip II in his commentary on the *Physics* of Aristotle (1562), Vallés praises the monarch's efforts to stem the tide of decline that had befallen Classical Studies:[2]

> Per hanc regum [sc. Philippi II eiusque patris Caroli V] potentiam et virtutem, iustitia quae languebat antea, multum convaluit, et otium et libertas abunde suppetentia bonis omnibus, ad excolendum literarum [sic] studia converterunt multorum animos [...]. Omne etiam literaturae [sic] genus videtur iam ad antiquum nitorem redire [...]. Nam ob Graecae

* This paper is part of Research Project DGICYT (FFI-2012-36474), with the title of *Estudios sobre la lengua del Corpus Hippocraticum y su influencia*, with the direction of Ignacio Rodríguez Alfageme. This project has the financial support of the Spanish Ministry of Science and Technology.

1 For the full titles of Vallés' works, see the bibliography. On Francisco Vallés' life and works more generally, see Santander Rodríguez (1971), 29–33, 72–74, 92–100, 103–107; Granjel (1980), 30–32; Martín Ferreira (1995), 58–64, and Ángel y Espinós (2011).

2 See Vallés (1562), 2.

© JESÚS ÁNGEL Y ESPINÓS, 2021 | DOI:10.1163/9789004470200_019

> linguae ignorationem, et corruptionem latinae, sordebant hucusque disciplinae omnes. Nunc vero revocari coeptis his idiomatis videntur paulatim dignitatem recuperare. Qua in re ego, cum multis aliis qui huic labori incumbunt, ut siquid possum iuvem, inter multa medicinae opera, quae partim in lucem prodierunt, partim latent in scriniis, partim sunt in manibus, in ea parte philosophiae, quae ad naturam spectat, volui laborare. [...] Iuniorum enim vix unus aut alter potuit Graecos codices consulere, et quid autor [sic] dicat, aut neget ab ipso petere. Veteres non praeviderunt sophysmata [sic], quae tempus p⟨ro⟩duxit, et ego extirpo [...].
>
> Through this power and virtue of the Kings [Philip II and his father, Charles V] justice which had grown weak became strong again. Leisure and liberty which support all good things made the minds of many turn towards literary studies. [...] All genres of literature have returned to their previous splendour. [...] Since Greek remains unknown and Latin badly understood, all disciplines here are in dire straits. But now these have begun to come back and the language has regained some of its dignity. Therefore, together with many others who strive to accomplish this task, I help as much as possible. Of the many medical works, some have been published, some are still stored away in cupboards, and some circulate [in manuscript]. I therefore decided to work on natural philosophy. [...] Among the young, there is hardly anybody who can read a Greek manuscript or find out what its author affirms or denies. The ancients did not foresee the sophisms which time has produced and which I [now] eradicate. [...]

Vallés belonged to a brilliant generation of scholars which flourished during the reign of Philip II,[3] one of the most prominent and controversial figures of sixteenth-century Europe. Among his many titles, he was King of Spain from 1556 and of Portugal from 1580 until his death in 1598. He also occupied the throne of England and Ireland from 1556 to 1558, because he was married to Mary I of England, the maternal first cousin of his father, the emperor Charles V.[4] It could be suggested that, unfortunately, the most noteworthy feature of this generation was perhaps the fact that they faced a new and difficult cultural situation imposed by the King's foreign policy, forcing them to adapt to

3 See Subiza Martín (1954) and Granjel (1980), 30–38.

4 From the almost limitless bibliography about Philip II, see in English the standard works of the British historians Kamen (1997) and Parker (1998), (2014).

a Spain that was rapidly becoming ever more isolated from the rest of Europe. This fact was reflected in the distancing of Spain from the ideological and scientific evolution being followed by other European nations and in the return to a new version of dogmatism as an intellectual manifestation linked to the block imposed by the monarchy.

In large part, this isolationism was caused by the King's prohibition, in 1559, of foreign study to Spanish scholars.[5] A few years previously, reports by the Dominican Friar, Baltasar Pérez, to the Holy Inquisition concerning the possible heterodoxy of certain groups in the University of the Flemish city of Leuven had rung early alarm bells. It is known that, although the religious situation in Flanders was very delicate, in any other city of that problematic area, religious orthodoxy was as tightly supervised as in Leuven; Philip II even visited the University in order to try to calm inflamed attitudes and to stop any theological fickleness as soon as possible, particularly among the Spanish students. The declaration by Philip II, made 22 November 1559 in Aranjuez, a village near Madrid, had as its pretext the large number of students who, by leaving Spain to study abroad, were reducing enrolment in Spanish universities. However, there were clearly other economic and, more importantly, ideological reasons for the prohibition. For the economic reasons, the prohibition attempted to prevent the excess expenses incurred with travel, stays abroad and other related costs. Nevertheless, it is clear that this was not the true cause, since Phillip II did not specify these monetary restrictions for universities in Rome, Naples and Coimbra; a fact that suggests that the financial troubles were, in reality, a smokescreen. As may be expected from such a complex and religiously obsessed individual, what truly concerned the King were other issues, as openly confessed in a private letter, written in Brussels 21 June 1559, addressed to his sister, Joanna of Austria, who was at this moment the regent of Spain because of the long absences of her brother. The tenor of this letter can be seen in the following sentence:[6]

> Porque de salir a estudiar fuera de estos reynos se ha visto por la experiencia los daños que se han seguido y siguen en lo de la Religión y costumbres y conviene mucho remediallo y excusallo.

5 See Tellechea Idígoras (1965) and (2000), Gil Fernández (1997), 440–448, Crespo Solana-Herrero Sánchez (2002), and Cantarero de Salazar (2015), 551–552. On the isolationism prompted by the royal decisions, see Parker (2014), 132–133.

6 See Fernández Álvarez (1966), 237 and Gil Fernández (1997), 445.

> Because going abroad to study has been shown to damage religion and customs, it is necessary to remedy and prevent this.

As can be easily inferred from these words, it is evident that the main preoccupation of Philip II was to maintain the Catholic orthodoxy, free from external influences and heresy, according to the doctrines embodied by the Counter-Reformation movement.[7]

The 1559 proclamation urged Spanish students and teachers as subjects of the King to return to Spain within four months, on pain of being deprived of their possessions (in the case of lay people) or of their benefits (in the case of clergy); moreover, the degrees of those who wanted to remain abroad would not henceforth be valid in Spain. In short, the damage to their contemporaries and those who would come later, had already been done; a few years later, Benito Arias Montano, orientalist and editor of the Antwerp Polyglot Bible, wrote a letter to the Duke of Alba (1 March 1570), in which he exhorted the creation of a Spanish professorship in Flanders and the return of the educational exchanges, at least with Leuven. Unfortunately, the 1559 proclamation of Philip II made it impossible for the future physicians to the ancient Crown of Aragon to continue their studies in Montpellier, famous for its medical training, as they had done since the thirteenth century. For example, the physician Arnau de Vilanova (born in the Kingdom of Aragon, *c.* 1240) taught medicine in Montpellier from 1289 to 1299 and in fourteenth century Valencia graduates of the University of Montpellier exerted a great deal of influence on the establishment of medical schools in the town.[8] It is worth noting that, in 1767, more than two centuries after the 1559 prohibition, the Spanish historian and writer Gregorio Mayans y Siscar (1699–1781), was still complaining about this erroneous and disastrous decision:[9]

> Una de las causas porque han descaecido tanto las artes y las ciencias ha sido aquella ley que mandó promulgar Felipe Segundo, prohibiendo los estudios en las Universidades extranjeras.
>
> One of the reasons why the arts and sciences have declined so much was the law enacted by Philip II which prohibited to study at foreign universities.

7 Parker (2014), 92–93 observes that Philip II was extremely devout and had a messianic conviction about his destiny in history.

8 See Bartolomé Martínez (1985), 22–24, 32.

9 See Peset (1975), 309.

It was in this atmosphere of incipient isolation and Counter-Reformation dogmatism that Vallés wrote his significant commentary on the Hippocratic *Epidemics*. The first edition appeared in Madrid in 1577 (Royal Privilege, 1576) and placed him at the forefront of European Renaissance medical science. It is highly significant that a century and a half later, the renowned Dutch physician Herman Boerhaave, the founder of modern clinical teaching, considered Vallés to be one of the leading lights, because he possessed all the qualities of a true physician:[10]

> Hos [Galenum, Jacobum Hollerium, Franciscum Vallesium] ubi quis habebit facile et sine damno carebit reliquis. Nam recenciores [sic] omnes scribunt ex sua hypothesi; nos vero tantum laudamus eos, qui ex observatione ipsa explicant sensum auctoris [...].
>
> Once someone has mastered those [sc. Galen, Jacques Houllier, Francisco Vallés], he can easily and without any harm omit the others. For all recent authors write on the basis of their own arguments. We, however, only praise those who explain the meaning of an author through their own observation.

Vallés, the personal physician to the King Philip II, states in his dedication to him that writing this series of scholarly commentaries on the seven books of the *Epidemics* is a great task of unprecedented magnitude:[11]

> [...] scribere decrevi, ea praecipue causa, quod nullius neque veterum neque recentium, extent, aut (quod equidem sciam) extiterint unquam integra commentaria.
>
> I decided to write [the complete commentary on the *Epidemics*] primarily because no complete commentaries by any ancient or modern author (as far as I know) exist or have ever existed.

Immediately afterwards, Vallés created a succinct listing of the authors who preceded him in this task and who certainly served as models to his great and novel enterprise:[12]

---

10 See Boerhaave (1726), 429.

11 See Vallés (1577).

12 Ibid.

> Galeni enim extant adhuc in primum, tertium et sexti partem: scripsit vero, ut eiusdem constat testimonio, etiam in secundum: recentiores in minora frustra secant. Leonhartus Fuchsius scripsit in sextum. Petrus Iacobus Esteve in secundum. Quartum, quintum et septimum nullus attigit, ac proinde a plerisque (iniuria ut censeo) habentur despecti ii, quasi alieni et spurii.
>
> [Commentaries] by Galen on Books 1, 3, and parts of Book 6 survive; he also wrote one on Book 2, as he himself says. Modern authors have cut the subject matter annoyingly into smaller parts. Leonard Fuchs wrote one on Book 6, Pedro Jaime Esteve on Book 2. No one has touched Books 4, 5, and 7, and therefore these [books] are disregarded by most (wrongly, as I think), as if they were foreign and spurious.

We know that Galen of Pergamum, whose first Greek edition rolled off the Aldine Press in Venice in 1525, did not feel that the fourth, fifth and seventh books of *Epidemics* were worthy of his hermeneutic effort, believing the fifth and seventh books to be spurious:[13]

> ὥσπερ οὖν τοῦτο προεῖπον, οὕτω καὶ τόδε προειπεῖν ἀναγκαῖόν ἐστιν, ὡς τὸ τῆς ἑρμηνείας εἶδος ἐν τῷδε τῷ βιβλίῳ πάμπολυ διαλλάττει τοῦ κατὰ τὸ πρῶτον καὶ τρίτον τῶν Ἐπιδημιῶν, ἃ σχεδὸν ἅπαντες ἡγοῦνται γεγράφθαι πρὸς ἔκδοσιν ὑφ' Ἱπποκράτους μόνα, τῶν δ' ἄλλων πέντε τὸ μὲν πέμπτον τε καὶ ἕβδομον ἐναργῶς εἶναι νόθα, τὸ δ' ἕκτον τοῦτο καὶ πρὸ αὐτοῦ τὸ δεύτερον, ἐξ ὧν αὐτὸς ⟨ὁ⟩ Ἱπποκράτης ἑαυτῷ παρεσκευάσατο, φασὶν ὑπὸ Θεσσαλοῦ τοῦ υἱέος αὐτοῦ συντεθῆναι. καὶ τινὲς μὲν ἡγοῦνται καὶ αὐτόν τι παρεγγράψαι τὸν Θεσσαλόν, τινὲς δὲ ἄλλους τῶν μετ' αὐτόν.
>
> Just as I said this beforehand, so I need to say the following. The mode of explanation in this book is completely different from that in Book 1 and 3 of the *Epidemics*. Nearly everyone agrees that these two books are the only ones that Hippocrates wrote for publication. Of the remaining five, Books 5 and 7 are clearly spurious. Book 6 and before it Book 2, which Hippocrates himself used as preparation, were reportedly composed by his son Thessalus. Some think that Thessalus himself had interpolated some things, and others think that other later [authors] did so.

13 Galen, *Commentary on Hippocrates' 'Epidemics'*, Book 6 (17a.796 K.; Wenkebach, Pfaff, 1956, 5).

Moreover, and in addition to the commentaries by Galen, reference was also made to commentaries by the German Leonhart Fuchs (1501–1566), and the Spanish Pedro Jaime Esteve (d. 1566) in the quotation above. Fuchs (1532) published a translation with notes of the sixth book of *Epidemics* in the Alsatian city of Haguenau. The extensive dissemination of this work was evidenced by the appearance of a new and extended edition in Basel in 1537.[14] Meanwhile, the Spanish physician Esteve (1551) offered commentaries on the second book of *Epidemics* which were published in Valencia.[15] These commentaries were subsequently criticised by adversaries of Esteve who claimed that they were in fact the work of Galen. Esteve was a professor of Anatomy, Greek, Surgery and Mathematics at the University of Valencia. He was trained as a doctor at the universities of Paris and Montpellier, where he acquired a deep knowledge of Greek and a solid mastery of anatomy and natural history. This can be seen from his commentary on the *Theriaca* by Nicander of Colophon, in which the original Greek text appears with its Latin translation and with abundant notes, in which Esteve included the common names of many plants.[16] The work on *Theriaca* reveals the Esteve's profound interest in medical botany. This interest was probably piqued in Montpellier, where he attended the lectures of Guillaume Rondelet, a renowned anatomist and naturalist specialising in botany.

Apart from the commentaries used by Vallés other texts also commented on the Hippocratic *Epidemics*. For a variety of reasons, however, Vallés did not consult them when writing his commentary. Examples include Galen's commentary on *Epidemics*, Book 2; and Palladius' and John of Alexandria's commentaries on Book 6.

Nevertheless, before considering these works, let us note that in Spain the interest in the *Epidemics* increased considerably between Esteve (1551) and Vallés (1577). Works by Núñez de Coria and Francisco Franco which appeared in this period contain a large number of references to the *Epidemics*.[17] These works, despite being granted licences for publication, are not available to us, either because they were never printed or because they have been lost.

Little is known about Núñez de Coria (or de Oria). He was a doctor of medicine and a Latin poet of some renown: he published a long poem in hexameters, *Lyrae heroicae*, in Salamanca in 1581, which extols the exploits of the legendary

14 Fuchs (1537).

15 On Pedro Jaime Esteve, see Montero Cartelle (2001), 112–113, and Santamaría Hernández (2002), (2003), (2012a), and her contribution to this volume.

16 Esteve (1552); see Santamaría Hernández (2012b), 197, *pace* Overduin (2015), 136, who mistakenly thinks that this is a Spanish translation.

17 See Santander Rodríguez (1971), 42, 90–91, and Granjel (1980), 23, 206, 231–236, 261–263.

medieval hero Bernardo del Carpio. As a physician, he was the author of one of the most relevant books on hygiene and dietetics printed in Renaissance Spain: the treatise *Auiso de sanidad* (*Notice of Health*), published in Madrid in 1569, and reprinted in 1572 and 1586. The work offers precise information about the health effects of different foodstuffs and the best way to consume them. His *Tractado del uso de las mugeres* (*Treatise on the Use of Women*) is dedicated to sexual hygiene and gives advices on sex and relationships with women. This treatise was published in 1572 and 1586 together with the *Notice of Health*, but it soon became a rare book, because of the censure of the Inquisition. In 1580, in Alcalá de Henares, the *Libro intitulado del parto humano* (*Book with the Title 'On Human Childbirth'*) came to light, which deals with diverse aspects related to midwifery and gynaecology.

Francisco Franco, who was of Jewish descent, served as physician at the court of John III, King of Portugal, and taught at the University of Seville. In 1569, he published in Seville his *Tractado de la nieve y del uso della* (*Treatise on Snow and its Use*) and his *Libro de enfermedades contagiosas y de la preseruación dellas* (*Book of Contagious Diseases and their Prevention*). In the latter work, Franco gives a series of recommendations on the diagnosis, treatment and prevention of the 'plague', a term that refers generically to all kinds of infectious diseases. In the former work, a short booklet of 30 pages, the author explains the different ways to use snow to cool drinks, a common custom at this time, and analyses the convenience of drinking cold beverages from the dietetic point of view.

Let us now consider the texts Vallés did not use when writing his commentary. Galen's commentary on *Epidemics*, Book 2 survives in the Arabic translation by Ḥunayn ibn Isḥāq (d. ca. 873).[18] This translation is extant in four manuscripts, including one recently discovered by Peter Joosse.[19] The oldest Arabic manuscript (possibly the thirteenth century), Scorialensis 804, comprises Books 1–3 and appears to have been inventoried as item 35 in a bilingual Arabic-Spanish catalogue from the late sixteenth century.[20] This manuscript contains marginal notes in Hebrew and Judaeo-Arabic dating back to the fourteenth century and therefore probably was in Jewish ownership at least for a time. Another important manuscript is Ambrosianus B 135 sup., which was copied in 1624 by the Scottish Catholic monk, David Colville, during his 10 year stay in the Escorial and it comprises Book 2 and the last third of Book 6, both

18 Vagelpohl (2016).

19 See Hallum et al. (2012).

20 Morata (1934), 100–102, proposes Diego de Urrea to be the author of this catalogue; Rodríguez Mediano and García-Arenal (2002), 509, share this opinion.

not preserved in Greek.[21] As Peter E. Pormann (2008) stated and Ivan Garofalo (2010) confirmed, the Ambrosianus B 135 sup. has some correct variant readings not contained in the Scorialensis ar. 804, suggesting that Colville made use of some Arabic manuscripts that were later destroyed in the fire of the Escorial in 1671. Colville himself stated that he copied the commentary on Book 2 'from a number of manuscripts (a pluribus exemplaribus)'. Today, there is only one Arabic manuscript of this text in the Escorial (Scorialensis ar. 804). It therefore makes sense that Colville was referring to item 33 of the bilingual catalogue, which later went up in flames. Unfortunately, although these two Arabic manuscripts were probably already on the shelves of the nascent Escorial library when Vallés was compiling his commentary on the *Epidemics*, he did not make use of them, as he did not know Arabic. He did know, however, that Galen had written a commentary on Book 2, as we have already seen.

We shall now consider the two commentaries on *Epidemics*, Book 6 which Vallés failed to mention in his dedication, although they existed in Greek, a language that he understood perfectly; they are the commentaries by Palladius and John of Alexandria. These two texts were written in Alexandria and show the importance of Book 6 for medical teaching there.[22] Gesius, an iatrosophist who worked in Alexandria in the beginning of the sixth century, wrote a commentary on Book 6 of which we have no trace in the original Greek. Nevertheless, as Grigory Kessel (2012) has recently suggested, it has been partially preserved in a Syriac translation (Damascus, Syrian Orthodox Patriarchate, MS 12/25), adapted and with additions by the translator, who appears to be Sergius, a well-known scholar who died in 536. Kessel (2012, 120–121) has also concluded that the work of Gesius was one of the sources of John of Alexandria's commentary.

Palladius' commentary has been partly preserved in Greek, with larger gaps comprising sections 2 and 8 and other smaller omissions. Within the manuscripts from the work of Palladius, there is the codex Scorialensis y. I. 8, which formed part of the collection of Diego Hurtado de Mendoza (1503 or 1504 to 1575), a distinguished figure in Spanish diplomacy during the time of Charles V and Philip II.[23] The Scorialensis y. I. 8, described by Giovanni Baffioni (1963), is a miscellaneous paper codex from the sixteenth century that has two sections.

21 Pormann (2009), (2008), 265–266.

22 See Pormann (2010b).

23 On this important figure and his library, see Graux (1880), 163–273, Revilla (1936), lxxxv–cxi, and Hobson (2001). A brief description of this codex, included the characteristic bookbinding of the collection of Hurtado de Mendoza, can be found in De Andrés (1965), 186.

The first one, copied by a certain Νικόλαος,[24] contains short texts from the Hippocratic Corpus (*Testament*, *Law*, and *Oath*), the commentary of the Byzantine physician Theophilus Protospatarius on the *Aphorisms* and that of Palladius on the *Epidemics*, Book 6. The second contains an anthology of Aretaeus of Cappadocia and was written by Petrus Karnavaka, a regular copyist of Hurtado de Mendoza, who signed it with his monocondyle.[25]

When Hurtado de Mendoza died in 1575, he left his book collection to Philip II, who moved it into the Escorial from June 1576 onwards. Unfortunately, it was seriously damaged by the 1671 fire.[26] It comprised 256 Greek manuscripts which all ended up in the Escorial. Today 136 remain there, the other 120 having been lost in the fire.[27] Palladius's commentary arrived in the Escorial in the same year as Vallés received the Royal Licence to publish his commentary on the *Epidemics*, although he was unaware of this. Once again, as had occurred with the commentaries of Galen on the second book of *Epidemics*, the paths of Vallés and Palladius would not cross, even though Vallés was apparently commissioned by Philip II, along with Benito Arias Montano and Ambrosio de Morales, to supervise and create the monastery's library.

Finally, we shall look at the commentary by John of Alexandria. It first appeared in Latin translation in 1483 in Venice together with the second edition of the *Articella*. Pritchet (1979, ix), the editor of the text, believed Bartholomew of Messina to be the translator of the Latin version from the Greek source text; the latter worked at the court of Manfred, King of Sicily (1258–1266). Moreover, fragments of the original Greek text still exist. These fragments, some quite extensive, have been entered in the margins of the Vaticanus graecus 300, an

24 According to De Andrés (1965), 186, the copyist Νικόλαος has to be identified with Nicolas Nathanael from Crete, who was the possessor of the Scorialensis X. IV. 12, a manuscript dated either to the thirteenth or fourteenth centuries, as it is indicated in the codex X. IV. 12 itself (f. 3): κτῆμα Νικολάου Ναθαήλου τοῦ Κρητός. Hobson (1999), 237 adopts De Andrés' proposal. On the Scorialensis X. IV. 12 see De Andrés (1965), 343–344.

25 Bravo (1982) lists and briefly analyses all the manuscripts of the Escorial library in which the handwriting of Petrus Karnavaka can be identified. All these manuscripts formed part of Hurtado de Mendoza's estate, which also contains works by other scholars, such as Valeriano Albini, Andronicus Nucius, Nicolas Marulus Gaitanus, Nicolas Murmuris, Joannes Mauromates and the Flemish Arnout van Eynthouts (Arnoldus Arlenius), the librarian of Hurtado de Mendoza.

26 According to De Andrés (1963), 240, the collection bequeathed to the King consisted of 853 manuscripts, the majority Latin (270), Arabic (268) and Greek (256).

27 Even what remains of Mendoza's Greek library constitutes the most important Spanish Renaissance collection of Greek secular texts; Caballero Sánchez (2014), 241, points out that Mendoza's wide-ranging interest in the Greek culture included scientific subjects such as geography.

Italo-Greek manuscript dating back to the twelfth century, and containing an Arabic medical handbook, Ibn al-Ǧazzār's *Sustenance of the Traveller and Provisions for the Sedentary Person* (*Zād al-musāfir wa-qūt al-ḥāḍir*), translated into Greek under the title *Ephódia toû apodēmoûntos*. Furthermore, as Duffy (1997) stated in the preface to his edition, there are a further 23 manuscripts containing the Greek translation of Ibn al-Ǧazzār's treatise, where fragments from John of Alexandria are inserted into the text rather than the margins. Likewise, Duffy (1997, 16) has also found pieces of a commentary on the sixth book of *Epidemics* that belongs neither to Palladius nor to John of Alexandria.

Unlike the two previous commentaries by Galen and Palladius, no manuscripts of the Latin version of the commentary by John of Alexandria existed in the Escorial library. Two manuscripts which also belonged to the library of Hurtado de Mendoza, Scorialensis X. II. 4 and Y. III. 5, contain the *Ephódia*, the work into which Greek fragments of John's commentary were interpolated.[28] Nevertheless, before the studies on Vaticanus graecus 300 by Cardinal Giovanni Mercati in the first decades of the twentieth century, it was not known that the *Ephódia* contained fragments of this commentary.[29] However, the fact that the work of John of Alexandria appears in Latin in printed editions of the *Articella* suggests that Vallés should have had access to this text, although this was apparently not the case.

In short, we have attempted to offer a brief statement on the vicissitudes faced by certain texts that comment on the Hippocratic *Epidemics* and which were in Spain, in the Escorial library, or were known by scholars or physicians during the sixteenth century. In the end, the fate of these texts resembles a story of missed opportunities: due to fate and other reasons, Vallés, despite his important position in the Escorial library, was unable to make use of these valuable manuscripts which, in some cases, were even within his grasp.

28 Cf. De Andrés (1965), 266–268 and 150–151.

29 See Duffy (1997), 13.

Bibliography

Adams, Francis (1849). *The Genuine Works of Hippocrates Translated from the Greek with a Preliminary Discourse and Annotation*, Vol. 1, London.

Adamson, P., R. Hansberger, and J. Wilberding, eds. (2014). *Philosophical Themes in Galen*. Bulletin of the Institute of Classical Studies Supplements, London.

Anastassiou, A. and D. Irmer (1997–2012). *Testimonien zum Corpus Hippocraticum*, Göttingen.

Andrés, G. de (1964). *Documentos para la historia del Monasterio de San Lorenzo el Real de El Escorial*, Vol. 7, Madrid.

Andrés, G. de (1965). *Catálogo de los códices griegos de la Real Biblioteca de El Escorial*, Vol. 2, Madrid.

Andrés, G. de (1987). 'El incendio del Monasterio de El Escorial en 1671 y sus consecuencias en las artes y las letras'. *Cuadernos de Investigación Histórica* 11, 247–263.

Ángel y Espinós, J. (2011). 'El comentario de Francisco Vallés *In libros Hippocratis de Morbis Popularibus*: Contexto histórico y antecedentes'. *Minerva* 24, 195–208.

Aselli, G. (1627). *De lactibus sive lacteis venis ... dissertatio*, Milan.

Asulanus, F. (1526). *Omnia opera Hippocratis*, Venice.

Baader, G., and R. Winau, eds. (1989). *Die hippokratischen Epidemien. Theorie—Praxis—Tradition. Verhandlungen des ve Colloque International Hippocratique (Berlin, 10.–15.9.1984)*, Stuttgart.

Baffioni, G. (1958). 'Scolii inediti di Palladio al "De sectis" di Galeno'. *Bollettino dei classici greci e latini* 6, 61–78.

Baffioni, G. (1963). 'Il *Codex Scorialensis* Y.I. 8'. *Bollettino del Comitato per la preparazione della Edizione nazionale dei classici greci e latini* n.s. 11, 25–32.

Bardong, K. (1942). 'Beiträge zur Hippokates- und Galensforschung'. *Nachrichten der Akademie der Wissenschaften in Göttingen, Phil.-Hist. Klasse* 7, 577–640.

Barnes, J. and J. Jouanna, eds. (2003). *Galien et la philosophie*, Entretiens Hardt 49, Geneva.

Barry, S.C. (2018). *Syriac Medicine and Ḥunayn ibn Isḥāq's Arabic Translation of the Hippocratic 'Aphorisms'*. Journal of Semitic Studies Supplement, Oxford.

Bartolomé Martínez, B. (1985). 'Estudiantes y profesores españoles en universidades extranjeras. Siglos xii–xvi'. *Revista Interuniversitaria de Historia de la Educación* 4, 7–35.

Batten, R. (2018). 'The Arabic Commentaries on the Hippocratic Aphorisms: Arabic Learned Medical Discourse on Women's Bodies (9th–15th cent.)'. PhD thesis, University of Manchester.

Beccaria, A. (1961). 'Sulle tracce di un antico canone latino di Ippocrate e di Galeno ii'. *Italia medievale e umanistica* 4, 1–75.

Bell, T.A. et al. (1997). *Ioannis Alexandrini In Hippocratis De natura pueri commentarium*, Corpus Medicorum Graecorum 11.1.4, Berlin, 130–175.

Bendz, G., ed. (1990). *Caelii Aureliani Celerum passionum libri iii, Tardarum passionum libri v*, Corpus Medicorum Latinorum 6.1, Berlin.

Bergsträßer, G. (1925). *Ḥunain ibn Isḥāq über die syrischen und arabischen Galen-Übersetzungen*, Abhandlungen für die Kunde des Morgenlandes 17.2, Leipzig.

Bergsträßer, G. (1932). *Neue Materialien zu Ḥunain Ibn Isḥāqs Galen-Bibliographie*, Abhandlungen für die Kunde des Morgenlandes 19.2, Leipzig.

Biagini, L. (2007). 'Il commento di Galeno alla peste di Atene', PhD thesis, Università di Bologna.

Biesterfeldt, H.H. (2007). 'Palladius on the Hippocratic *Aphorisms*'. In Cristina D'Ancona (ed.), *The Libraries of the Neoplatonists*, Leiden, 385–398.

Boerhaave, H. (1726). *Methodus discendi medicinam*, Amsterdam.

Börno, M. and S. Coughlin (2020). 'Galen on Bad Style (*kakozēlía*): Hippocratic Exegesis in Galen and Some Predecessors'. *Technai* 11, 145–175.

Boudon-Millot, V. (2003a). 'Aux marges de la médecine rationnelle: médecins et charlatans à Rome au temps de Galien (IIe s. de notre ère)'. *Revue des Études Grecques* 116, 109–131.

Boudon-Millot (2003b). 'Le rôle de la sensation dans la définiton galénique de la maladie'. In Isabelle Boehm and Pascal Luccioni (eds.), *Les cinq sens dans la medécine de l'époque impériale: sources et développements. Actes de la table ronde du 14 juin 2001*, Lyon, 21–30.

Boudon-Millot, ed. (2007). *Galien, Vol I. Introduction générale. Sur l'ordre de ses propres livres. Sur ses propres livres. Que l'excellent médecin est aussi philosophe*. Paris.

Boudon-Millot (2008). 'Galien commentateur d'Hippocrate: de l'authenticité des traités hippocratiques'. In Pascale Hummel (ed.), *Vérité(s) philologique(s). Études sur les notions de vérité et de fausseté en matière de philologie*, Paris, 75–92.

Boudon-Millot (2009). 'Galen's *bios* and *methodos*'. In Gill et al. (eds.), 175–189.

Boudon-Millot, V. (2011). 'L'ecdotique des textes médicaux grecs et l'apport des traductions orientales'. In R. Goulet and U. Rudolph (eds.), *Entre Orient et Occident. La philosophie et la science gréco-romaines dans le monde arabe*, Vandœuvres, Geneva, 321–387.

Boudon-Millot (2015). 'Ce qu'"hippocratique" (ἱπποκράτειος) veut dire: la réponse de Galien'. In Dean-Jones, Rosen (2015), 378–398.

Boudon-Millot (2016). *Galien. Vol. VI, Thériaque à Pison*, Paris.

Boudon-Millot (2021). 'Is the Theriac to Piso attributed to Galen authentic?', in Caroline Petit, Simon Swain, Klaus-Dietrich Fischer (eds.), *Pseudo-Galenica: The Formation of the Galenic Corpus from Antiquity to the Renaissance*, Warburg Institute Colloquia 34, London.

Boudon-Millot, V. and A. Pietrobelli (2005). 'Galien résussicité: *editio princeps* du texte grec du *De propriis placitis*'. *Revue des Études grecques* 118, 168–213.

Bravo García, A. (1982). 'Pedro Carnabacas y el fondo Hurtado de Mendoza de El Escorial: nuevas atribuciones y correcciones'. *La Ciudad de Dios* 195, 489–494.

Brock, A.J. (1929). *Galen: On the Natural Faculties*, Loeb Classical Library 71, Cambridge, MA.

Brock, S. (1991). 'The Syriac Background to Ḥunayn's Translation Technique'. *ARAM* 3, 139–162.

Brockmann, Ch. (2006). 'Philologische Annäherungen an Chirurgie und Anatomie. Beobachtungen an Galens Kommentar zu Hippokrates, De articulis'. In Carl W. Müller et al. (eds.), *Ärzte und ihre Interpreten*, Munich, 61–80.

Busse, A. (1891). *Ammonius in Porphyrii isagogen sive quinque voces*, Commentaria in Aristotelem Graeca 4.3, Berlin.

Busse, A. (1900). *Eliae in Porphyrii Isagogen et Aristotelis Categorias Commentaria*, Commentaria in Aristotelem Graeca 18.1, Berlin.

Busse, A. (1904). *Davidis Prolegomena et In Porphyrii Isagogen Commentarium*, Commentaria in Aristotelem Graeca 18.2, Berlin.

Caballero Sánchez, P. (2014). 'La *Geografía* de Tolomeo en un impreso anotado por Nicolás Múrmuris propiedad de Diego Hurtado de Mendoza'. *Estudios bizantinos* 2, 231–254.

Caius, John (1570). *De libris propriis / de libris suis*, London.

Calvus, M.F. (1525). *Hippocratis Coi ... octoginta volumina*, Rome.

Cantarero de Salazar, A. (2015), 'Reexamen crítico de la biografía del humanista Sebastián Fox Morcillo (*c.* 1526–*c.* 1560)'. *Studia Aurea* 9, 531–564.

Carpentieri, N., and T. Mimura (2017). 'Arabic Commentaries on the Hippocratic *Aphorisms*, vi.11: A Medieval Medical Debate on Phrenitis'. *Oriens* 45, 176–202.

Chartier, R. (1679). *Hippocratis ... et Claudii Galeni ... opera*, 13 vols., Paris.

Chinchilla, A. (1967). *Anales históricos de la medicina en general y biográfico-bibliográficos de la española en particular*, New York, 1967; facsimile of the originally edition published in 1841–1846.

Cohen-Skalli, A. (2007). 'Οἱ περὶ τὸν Ῥωμύλον: le motif du « fondateur » dans le fragment VII, 5 de la « Bibliothèque historique » de Diodore de Sicile'. *Revue de philologie, de littérature et d'histoire anciennes* 81, 229–242.

Congourdeau, M.-H. (1997). 'À propos d'un chapitre des *Éphodia*: l'avortement chez les médecins grecs'. *Revue des études byzantines* 55, 261–277.

Cornarius, J. (1538). *Hippocratis Coi medici ... libri omnes*, Basle.

Cornarius, J. (1546). *Hippocratis Coi medicorum omnium longe principis, Opera ... per Ianum Cornarium medicum physicum Latina lingua conscripta*, Basle.

Cottrell, É. (2009). 'An Arabic Manuscript of the Hippocratic Letters'. http://www.24grammata.com/wp-content/uploads/2013/08/Cottrell-24grammata.com_.pdf [accessed 13 July 2021].

Cottrell, É. (2016), 'سيرة أبقراط في المصادر العربية: حياته، رسائله، والقسم المشهور (Hippocrates' *Vita* in Arabic Sources: His Life, His Epistles, and the Famous Oath)'. In Pauline Koetschet,

Peter E. Pormann (eds.), *Naš'at al-Ṭibb al-ʿArabī fī l-qurūn al-wusṭā* (*La construction de la médecine arabe médiévale*), Publications de l'Institut Français de Damas, 131–142.

Coughlin, S. (2018). 'Athenaeus of Attalia on the Psychological Causes of Bodily Health'. In Chiara Thumiger and Peter Singer (eds.), *Mental Illness in Ancient Medicine: From Celsus to Paul of Aegina*, Studies in Ancient Medicine 50, Leiden, 109–142.

Coughlin, S. (forthcoming), *Athenaeus of Attalia: Fragments and Commentary.*

Coughlin, S. and O. Lewis (2020). 'Pneuma and the Pneumatist School of Medicine'. In S. Coughlin, D. Leith and O. Lewis (eds.), *The Concept of Pneuma After Aristotle*, Berlin Studies of the Ancient World 61, Berlin, 203–236.

Craik, E. (1998). *Hippocrates. Places in Man*, Oxford.

Craik, E. (2012). 'The Reception of the Hippocratic Treatise *On Glands*'. In Horstmanshoff, King, and Zittel (eds.), 65–82.

Craik, E. (2015). *The 'Hippocratic Corpus': Content and Context*, London.

Craik, E. (2017). 'Teleology in Hippocratic Texts: Clues to the Future?'. In Julius Rocca (ed.), *Teleology in the Ancient World: Philosophical and Medical Approaches*, Cambridge, 201–202.

Crespo Solana, A. and M. Herrero Sánchez, eds. (2002), *España y las 17 provincias de los Países Bajos. Una revisión historiográfica* (XVI–XVIII), 2 vols, Córdoba.

Cruser, H. (1531). *De morbis popularibus liber primus una cum tribus commentariis Galeni, Hermanno Cruserio Campesi interprete*, Paris.

Curtis, T. (2015). 'Author, Argument and Exegesis: a Rhetorical Analysis of Galen's *In Hippocratis de natura hominis commentaria tria*'. In Dean-Jones and Rosen, 399–420.

Dalen, E. van (2017a). 'The Rhetorical Strategies in the Arabic Commentaries on the Hippocratic *Aphorisms*: An Exploration of Metadiscourse in Medieval Medical Arabic', PhD thesis, University of Manchester.

Dalen, E. van (2017b), 'Subjectivity in Translation: Ḥunayn Ibn Isḥāq's Ninth-Century Interpretation of Galen's "Ego" in His Commentary on the Hippocratic *Aphorisms*'. *Oriens* 45, 53–79

Das, A., P. Koetschet, R.J. Hankinson, and M. Schiefsky (forthcoming). *Galen: Works on Human Nature II, translated with introduction and notes*. Cambridge Galen Translations. Cambridge.

De Boer, W. (1937). *Galeni de propriorum animi cuiuslibet affectuum dignotione et curatione / de animi cuiuslibet peccatorum dignotione et curatione / de atra bile*, Corpus Medicorum Graecorum 4.1.1, Leipzig.

De Lacy, P.H. (1978–1984). *Galen: On the Doctrines of Hippocrates and Plato*, Corpus Medicorum Graecorum 5.4.1.2, 3 vols, Berlin.

De Lacy, P.H. (1996). *Galen: On the Elements according to Hippocrates*, Corpus Medicorum Graecorum 5.1.2, Berlin.

Dean-Jones, L. and R.M. Rosen, eds. (2015). *Ancient Concepts of the Hippocratic: Papers Presented at the XIIIth International Hippocrates Colloquium*, Leiden.

Degen, R. (1978). 'Zur syrischen Übersetzung der Aphorismen des Hippokrates'. *Oriens Christianus* 62, 36–52.

Degen, R. (1981), 'Galen im Syrischen: Eine Übersicht über die syrische Überlieferung der Werke Galens'. In Vivian Nutton (ed.), *Galen: Problems and Prospects*, London, 131–166.

Deichgräber, K. (1930). *Die griechische Empirikerschule. Sammlung der Fragmente und Darstellung der Lehre*, Berlin.

Deichgräber, K. (1965). *Die griechische Empirikerschule*. 2nd ed., Berlin-Zurich.

Déroche, F. (1987–1989). 'Les manuscrits arabes datés du IIIe/IXe siècle'. *Revue des études islamiques* 55–57, 343–379.

Déroche, F. (1992). *The Abbasid Tradition. Qur'āns of the 8th to the 10th Centuries*, The Nasser D. Khalili Collection of Islamic Art 1, London.

Deusing, A. (1655). *De motu cordis et sanguinis itemque de lacte*. Groningen.

Diels, H. (1918). 'Hippokratische Forschungen V. Eine neue Fassung des XIX Hippokratesbriefes'. *Hermes* 53, 57–87.

Dietz, F.R. (1834). *Apollonii Citiensis, Stephani, Palladi, Theophili, Meletii, Damascii, Ioannis, aliorum Scholia in Hippocratem et Galenum*, 2 vol., Königsberg.

Diller, H. (1999). *Hippocratis De Aere Aquis Locis*, 2nd ed., *Corpus Medicorum Graecorum* 1.1.2, Berlin.

Dodge, B. (1970). *The Fihrist of al-Nadīm: A Tenth-Century Survey of Muslim Culture*, 2 vols. New York.

Dozy, R. (1881). *Supplément aux dictionnaires arabes*, Leiden.

Dunlop, D.M., ed. (1979). *The Muntakhab Ṣiwān al-ḥikmah of Abū Sulaimān as-Sijistānī*, The Hague, New York.

Duffy, J.M. (1983). *Stephani Philosophi In Hippocratis Prognosticum*, Corpus Medicorum Graecorum 11.1.2, Berlin.

Duffy, J.M. (1984). 'Byzantine Medicine in the Sixth and Seventh Centuries: Aspects of Teaching and Practice'. *Dumbarton Oaks Papers* 38, 21–27.

Duffy, J.M. et al. (1997). *John of Alexandria: Commentary on Hippocrates' Epidemics VI. Fragments, Commentary of an Anonymous Author on Hippocrates' Epidemics VI. Fragments, John of Alexandria: Commentary on Hippocrates' On the Nature of the Child*, Corpus medicorum Graecorum 11.1.4, Berlin.

Ecca, G. (2016). *Die hippokratische Schrift Praecepta. Kritische Edition, Übersetzung und Kommentar*, Serta Graeca 32, Wiesbaden.

Ecca, G. (2018), 'Note sul Vat. Urb. gr. 68 e sullo scolio a *Praecepta* 1'. *Seminari Romani di cultura greca* n.s. 7, 195–211.

Eijk, P.J. van der, ed. (1999). *Ancient Histories of Medicine: Essays in Medical Doxography and Historiography in Classical Antiquity*, Studies in Ancient Medicine 20, Leiden.

Eijk, P.J. van der, ed. (2005). *Hippocrates in Context. Papers read at the XIth International Hippocrates Colloquium. University of Newcastle upon Tyne. 27–31 August 2002*, Studies in Ancient Medicine 31, Leiden.

Eijk, P.J. van der (2012). 'Exegesis, Explanation, Epistemology in Galen's Commentaries on *Epidemics*, Books One and Two'. In Pormann (ed.), 25–47.

Eijk, P.J. van der (2015). 'On "Hippocratic" and "Non-Hippocratic" Medical Writings'. in Dean-Jones and Rosen (eds.), 17–47.

Edelstein, L. (1967). 'The Genuine Works of Hippocrates'. In Owsei T. and C. Lilian Temkin (eds.), *Ancient Medicine: Selected Papers of Ludwig Edelstein*, Baltimore, 133–144.

Ermerins, F.Z. (1859–1864). *Hippocratis et aliorum medicorum veterum reliquiae*, 3 vols., Utrecht.

Esteve, P.J. (1551). *Hippocratis Coi medicorum omnium principis Epidemiωn liber secundus, a Petro Iacobo Steve medico Latinitate donatus, et fussissimis commentariis illustratus, adiecta et singulis sententiis Graeca veritate, quo facilius diligens lector quanta sit servata fides intelligere possit*, Valencia.

Esteve, P.J. (1552). *Nicandri Colophoni poetae et medici antiquissimi clarissimique Theriaca, Petro Iacobo Steve medico valentino interprete et enarratore*, Valencia.

Expósito, L.M. (2004). 'El señorío laico de Burjassot (1568–1600). Primera parte: Bernat Simó, señor del lugar'. *El Nucli Antic*, Desembre, 41–43, available at https://www.centred-estudislocalsdeburjassot.es/app/download/4967581/JOSEP-ALEXANDRE-SIM-2.pdf; [accessed 26 March 2021].

Fernández Álvarez, M. (1966). *Política mundial de Carlos V y Felipe II*, Madrid.

Festugière, A.-J. (1948). *Hippocrate. L'ancienne médecine: introduction, traduction et commentaire*, Paris.

Flashar, H. (1962). 'Beiträge zur spätantiken Hippokratesdeutung'. *Hermes* 90, 402–418.

Flashar, H. (1964). 'Zum Proömium der Ps.-Aristotelischen Problemata Inedita'. *Hermes* 92, 249–251.

Flemming, R. (2008). 'Commentary'. In Hankinson (ed.) (2008b), 323–354.

Flemming, R. (2012). 'Antiochus and Asclepiades: Medical and Philosophical Sectarianism at the End of the Hellenistic Era'. In David Sedley (ed.), *The Philosophy of Antiochus*, Cambridge, 55–79.

Foesius, A. (1588). *Oeconomia Hippocratis*, Frankfurt.

Foesius, A. (1595). *Magni Hippocratis ... opera omnia*, Geneva.

Fortuna, S. (1997a). *Galeni De constitutione artis medicae ad Patrophilum*, Corpus Medicorum Graecorum 5.1.3, Berlin.

Fortuna, S. (1997b). *Galeno: A Patrofilo sulla costituzione della medicina. Testo e traduzione*, Corpus Medicorum Graecorum 5.1.3, Berlin.

Fortuna, S. (2012). 'René Chartier e le edizioni latine di Galeno'. In Véronique Boudon-Millot, Guy Cobolet, and Jacques Jouanna (eds.), *René Chartier (1572–1654) éditeur et traducteur d'Hippocrate et Galien*, Paris, 303–324.

Fortuna, S. (2018). 'Hippocrates' *Law* in the Middle Ages with the Edition of the Latin Translation and the Revision'. *Early Science and Medicine* 23, 299–329.

Fortuna, S., I. Garofalo, A. Lami, A. Roselli, eds. (2012), *Sulla tradizione indiretta dei testi medici greci: i commenti. Atti del IV seminario internazionale di Siena, Certosa di Pontignano, 3–4 giugno 2011*, Pisa, Rome.

Fuchs, L. (1532). *Hippocratis Epidemiarum liber sextus jam recens Latinitate donatus, Leonardo Fuchsio interprete. Addita est luculenta universi ejus libri expositio, eodem Leonardo Fuchsio authore. Adjecta insuper sunt ad calcem Graeca, ut diligens lector haec ipsa cum Latinis conferre possit*, Haguenau.

Fuchs, L. (1537). *Hippocratis medicorum omnium principis Epidemiων liber sextus, a Leonardo Fuchsio medico latinitate donatus, et luculentissima enarratione illustratus, jam recens non aestimandis vigilis ab autore recognitus, multisque in locis auctus, ac in lucem editus. Adjecta insuper sunt ad calcem Graeca, ut diligens lector haec ipsa cum Latinis conferre possit*, Basle.

Gaisford, T. (1848). *Etymologicum Magnum*, Oxford.

Ganz, J.C. (2018). *Intracranial Epidural Bleeding: History, Management, and Pathophysiology*, London.

Garofalo, I. (1994). 'Note filologiche sull'anatomia di Galeno'. *Aufstieg und Niedergang der römischen Welt* 37.2, 1790–1833.

Garofalo, I. (2010), 'Postilla a I commenti a *Epidemie I* e *II*'. *Galenos* 4, 255–256.

Garofalo, I., A. Lami, D. Manetti, and A. Roselli, eds. (1999). *Aspetti della terapia nel Corpus Hippocraticum. Atti del IXe Colloque International Hippocratique, Pisa 25–29 settembre 1996*, Florence.

Garzya, A. (1992). 'Appunti sull' ἐρωταποκρίσεις'. *Vetera Christianorum* 29, 305–314.

Garzya, A., R. Masullo (2004). *I problemi di Cassio Iatrosophista. Testo critico, introduzione, apparato critico, traduzione e note*, Naples.

Gibson R.K., Chr. Shuttleworth Kraus, eds. (2002). *The Classical Commentary: Histories, Practices, Theory*, Leiden.

Gil Fernández, L. (1997). *Panorama social del humanismo español (1500–1800)*, Madrid.

Gill, C., T. Whitmarsh, and J. Wilkins, eds. (2009). *Galen and the World of Knowledge*, Cambridge.

Giorgianni, F. (2006). *Hippokrates, Über die Natur des Kindes (De genitura und De natura pueri)*, Wiesbaden.

Golder, W. (2001). *Hippokrates und das Corpus Hippocraticum*, Würzburg.

Gorman, R.J. (2001). 'Oἱ περί τινα in Strabo'. *Zeitschrift für Papyrologie und Epigraphik*, 136, 201–213.

Gorris, J. de (1545), *Περὶ γονῆς, De genitura. Περὶ φύσιος παιδίου, De natura pueri … interprete Jo. Gorraeo … accesserunt ejusdem interpretis annotationes in eosdem libellos …*, Paris.

Gossen, H. (1920). 'Sabinus [25]'. *Realencyclopädie der classischen Altertumswissenschaft*, n. s. 1, col. 1600.

Gourevitch, D. (1992). 'Les lectures hippocratiques de Soranos d'Ephèse dans son traité des Maladies des femmes'. In J.A. Lopez-Ferez (ed.), *Tradados hipocraticos*, Madrid, 597–607.

Gourevitch, D. (2009). 'La bibliographie scientifique de Galien: l'exemple de Soranos'. In F. Le Blay (ed.), *Transmettre les savoirs dans les mondes hellénistique et romain*, Rennes, 245–258.

Gourevitch, D., P. Burguière, and Y. Malinas (1988–2000). *Soranus. Maladies des femmes*, 4 vols., Paris.

Gourmelon, É. (1572). *Hippocratis libellus de alimento a Steph. Gourmeleno … e graeco in latinum conversus et commentariis illustratus*, Paris.

Granjel, L.S. (1980). *La medicina española renacentista*, Salamanca.

Graux, Ch. (1880). *Essai sur les origines du fond grec de l'Escurial*, Paris.

Grimaudo, S. (2008). *Difendere la salute: igiene e disciplina del soggetto nel* De sanitate tuenda *di Galeno*, Naples.

Grmek, M. and F. Robert, eds. (1980). *Hippocratica—Actes du Colloque hippocratique de Paris, 4–9 septembre 1978*, Colloques internationaux du CNRS 583, Paris.

Grmek, M. and D. Gourevitch (1994). 'Aux sources de la doctrine médicale de Galien: l'enseignement de Marinus, Quintus et Numisianus'. *Aufstieg und Niedergang der römischen Welt* 37.2, 1501–1510.

Guardasole, A. (1997). *Eraclide di Taranto. Frammenti*, Naples.

Gurd, S.A. (2011). 'Galen on ἔκδοσις'. In Thomas Schmidt and Pascale Fleury (eds.), *Perceptions of the Second Sophistic and its Times. Regards sur la seconde sophistique et son époque*, Toronto, 169–184.

Gutas, D. (1998). *Greek Thought, Arabic Culture*, London.

Gutas, D. (2010). *Theophrastus on First Principles* (Known as his *Metaphysics*), Leiden.

Gutas, D. and L. Tarán (2012). *Aristotle's Poetics*, Leiden.

Ḥāfiẓ, M.M. al- (1989). *Ḥarīq al-ǧāmiʿ al-umawī wa-banāʾuhū (1311–1320 h.). Nuṣūṣ wa-waṯāʾiq*, Kuwait.

Hallum, B. et al. (2012), 'A New Manuscript: Istanbul, Süleymaniye Kütüphanesi, MS Ayasofya 3592'. In Pormann (ed.) (2012), 15–22.

Hankinson, R.J. (1992). 'Doing Without Hypotheses: the Nature of *Ancient Medicine*'. In López Férez (ed.), 55–67.

Hankinson, R.J. (2008a). 'Philosophy of Nature'. In Hankinson (2008b), 210–241.

Hankinson, R.J., ed. (2008b). *Cambridge Companion to Galen*, Cambridge.

Hankinson, R.J. (2009). 'Galen on the Limitations of Knowledge'. In Gill et al. (eds.), 206–242.

Hankinson, R.J. (2015). 'Galen on Hippocratic Physics'. in Dean-Jones and Rosen (eds.), 421–443.

Hankinson, R.J. (2017). 'Substance, Element, Quality, Mixture: Galen's Physics and His

Hippocratic Inheritance'. *Aitia* 7.2; https://doi.org/10.4000/aitia.1863 [accessed 26 March 2021].

Hankinson, R.J. (forthcoming) *Galen: The Nature of the Human Being*, translated with introduction and notes, in Das et al.

Hanson, A.E. (1998). 'Galen: Author and Critic'. In Glenn W. Most (ed.), *Editing Texts/Texte Edieren*, Göttingen, 22–53.

Hanson, M. (1999). *Hippocrates, On Head Wounds*, Corpus Medicorum Graecorum 1.4.1, Berlin.

Harvey, W. (1628). *De motu cordis et circulatione sanguinis*, Frankfurt.

Hasse, D.N. (2016). *Success and Suppression: Arabic Sciences and Philosophy in the Renaissance*, Cambridge, MA.

Hayduck, M. (1888). *Asclepii in Aristotelis Metaphysicorum libros Commentaria*, Commentaria in Aristotelem Graeca 6.2, Berlin.

Hayduck, M. (1891). *Alexandri Aphrodisiensis In Aristotelis Metaphysica Commentaria*, Commentaria in Aristotelem Graeca 1, Berlin.

Heeg, J. (1915). *In Hippocratis Prognosticum commentaria III*, Corpus Medicorum Graecorum 5.9.2, Leipzig et Berlin, 197–378.

Helmreich, C.G. (1893). *Claudii Galeni Pergameni Scripta Minora*, vol. 3, Leipzig.

Helmreich, C.G. (1904). *Galeni de Temperamentis*, Leipzig.

Hernández Morejón, A. (1967). *Historia bibliográfica de la medicina española*, 7 vols., New York, London; facsimile of the originally edition published in 1842–1852.

Hill, D.R. (1992). 'Mūsā (Banū)', *Encyclopédie de l'Islam*, 2nd ed., Leiden, vol. 7, pp. 639–640.

Hippocrates (1526). *Omnia Opera Hippocratis*, Venice.

Hippocrates (1538). *Hippocratis libri omnes, ad vetustos codices summo studio collati et restaurati*, Basle.

Hobson, A. (1999). *Renaissance Book Collecting: Jean Grolier and Diego Hurtado de Mendoza, Their Books and Bindings*, Cambridge.

Hobson, A. (2001). 'The Library of Diego Hurtado de Mendoza'. In *Actas del XVIII Congreso de la Association Internationale de Bibliophilie (Madrid 1993)*, Madrid, 39–51.

Houllier, J. (1576). *Coaca praesagia cum interpretatione et commentariis Jacobi Hollerii … nunc primum … Desiderii Jacotii Vandoperani opera in lucem editis*, Leiden.

Horstmanshoff, H.F.J., ed. (2010). *Hippocrates and Medical Education: Selected Papers Read at the XIIth International Hippocrates Colloquium, Universiteit Leiden, 24–26 August 2005*, Studies in Ancient Medicine 35, Leiden.

Horstmanshoff, H.F.J., H. King and C. Zittel, eds. (2012). *Blood, Sweat and Tears: The Changing Concepts of Physiology from Antiquity into Early Modern Europe*, Leiden.

Hutchinson, D.S. (1988). 'Doctrines of the Mean and the Debate Concerning Skills in Fourth-Century Medicine, Rhetoric and Ethics'. *Apeiron* 21.2, 17–52.

Ideler, J.L., ed. (1841). *Physici et medici graeci minores*, vol. 1, Berlin.

Ieraci Bio, A.M. (1995). 'L'ἐρωταπόκρισις nella letteratura medica'. In Claudio Moreschini (ed.), *Esegesi, parafrasi e compilazione in età Tardoantica. Atti del terzo Convegno dell' Associazione di Studi Tardoantichi*, Naples, 186–207.

Ieraci Bio, A.M. (2006). 'Un inedito commento anonimo ad Ippocrate (Aph. I 1)'. In Véronique Boudon-Millot et al. (eds.), *Ecdotica e ricezione dei testi medici greci. Atti del v convegno internazionale*, Naples, 253–272.

Ihm, S. (2002). *Clavis commentariorum der antiken medizinischen Texte*, Leiden.

Ilberg, J. (1889). 'Über die Schriftstellerei des Klaudios Galenos'. *Rheinisches Museum für Philologie*, 44, 229–238.

Ilberg, J. (1927). *Sorani Gynaeciorum libri IV, De signis fracturarum, De fasciis, Vita Hippocratis secundum Soranum*, Corpus Medicorum Graecoru 4, Leipzig, Berlin.

Iskandar, A.Z. (1989). *Galen. On Examinations by Which the Best Physician Is Recognised*, Corpus Medicorum Graecorum Supplementum Orientale 4, Berlin.

Joly, R. (2003), ed., *Hippocratis De diaeta*, Corpus Medicorum Graecorum 1.2.4, Berlin.

Jones, W.H.S. (1931). *Hippocrates*, vol. 4, Loeb Classical Library, Cambridge, MA.

Joosse, N.P. (2013). 'A Newly-Discovered Commentary on the Hippocratic *Prognostic* by Barhebraeus: Its Contents and Its Place within the Arabic *Taqdimat al-maʿrifa* Tradition'. *Oriens* 41, 499–523.

Joosse, N.P., Pormann, P.E. (2010). 'Decline and Decadence in Iraq and Syria after the Age of Avicenna? ʿAbd al-Laṭiīf al-Baghdādī (1162–1231) between Myth and History'. *Bulletin of the History of Medicine* 84, 1–29.

Joosse, N.P., Pormann, P.E. (2012), "Abd al-Laṭīf al-Baġdādī's Commentary on Hippocrates' *Prognostic*: A Preliminary Exploration'. In Pormann (ed.), 251–283.

Jouanna, J. (1992). 'Remarques sur la tradition arabe du commentaire de Galien aux traités hippocratiques des Airs, eaux, lieux et du Serment'. In J.A. Lopez-Férez (ed.), *Galeno: Obra, pensamiento e influencia*, Madrid, 235–251.

Jouanna, J. (1996a). 'L'éthique hippocratique chez Galien'. In H. Flashar, J. Jouanna (eds.), *Médecine et morale dans l'Antiquité*, Entretiens de la Fondation Hardt 43, Vandœuvres, Geneva, 221–253.

Jouanna, J. (1996b). 'Un témoin méconnu de la tradition hippocratique: l'Ambrosianus gr. 134 (B 113 sup.), fol. 1–2 (avec une nouvelle édition du Serment et de la Loi)'. In A. Garzya (ed.), *Storia e ecdotica dei testi medici greci*, Naples, 253–272.

Jouanna, J., (1996c). *Hippocrate. Airs, eaux, lieux*, Paris.

Jouanna, J. (1999). *Hippocrates*, Baltimore.

Jouanna, J. (2000). 'La lecture du traité Hippocratique de la *Nature de l'homme* par Galien. Les fondements de l'hippocratisme de Galien'. In Marie-Odile Goulet-Cazé (ed.), *Le Commentaire entre tradition et innovation*, Paris, 273–292.

Jouanna, J. (2002). *Hippocrate: La Nature de l'Homme*, Corpus Medicorum Graecorum 1.1.3, Berlin.

Jouanna, J. (2003a). *Hippocrate: Airs-Eaux-Lieux*, Paris.

Jouanna, J. (2003b). *Hippocrate. L'ancienne médecine*, Paris.

Jouanna, J. (2003c). 'La notion de nature chez Galien'. In Barnes and Jouanna (eds.), 229–268; translated in Jouanna (2012), 287–311.

Jouanna, J. (2012). *Greek Medicine from Hippocrates to Galen. Selected Papers by J. Jouanna*, translated by N. Allies, edited with a Preface by Ph. van der Eijk, Studies in Ancient Medicine 40, Leiden.

Jouanna, J. (2013). *Hippocrate. Prognostique*, Paris.

Jouanna, J. (2015). 'Les commentaires de Galien à Hippocrate, Épidémies I et Épidémies III: essai de comparaison sur les fiches de malades'. *Galenos* 9, 217–228.

Jouanna, J., ed. (2016). *Hippocrate. Épidémies I et III*, Paris.

Jouanna, J. (2018a). *Hippocrate. Le Serment, Les Serments chrétiens, La loi*, Paris.

Jouanna, J. (2018b). 'Textual History'. In Pormann (ed.), 38–62.

Jouanna, J. and M. Zink, eds. (2014). *Hippocrate et les hippocratismes: médecine, religion, société*, Paris.

Kamen, H. (1997). *Philip of Spain*, New Haven.

Kapetanaki, S., and R.W. Sharples (2006). *Pseudo-Aristoteles (Pseudo-Alexander)*, Supplementa Problematorum, Peripatoi 20, Berlin.

Karimullah, K.I. (2017). 'Transformation of Galen's Textual Legacy from Classical to Post-Classical Islamic Medicine: Commentaries on the Hippocratic *Aphorisms*'. *Intellectual History of the Islamicate World* 5, 311–358.

Karimullah, K.I. (2018). 'Translating Greek into Arabic and Syriac: Remarks on a New Contribution to the Field'. *Intellectual History of the Islamicate World* 6, 389–405.

Käs, F. (2010). 'Eine neue Handschrift von Ḥunain ibn Isḥāqs Galenbibliographie'. *Zeitschrift für Geschichte der arabisch-islamischen Wissenschaften* 19, 135–193.

Kessel, G. (2012). 'The *Syriac Epidemics* and the Problem of Its Identification'. In Pormann (ed.), 93 123.

Kessel, G. (2016). 'Appendix 4: Inventory of Galen's Extant Works in Syriac'. In Lamoreaux, 168–192.

Keyser, P.T. (2013). 'The Name and Nature of Science: Authorship in Social and Evolutionary Context'. In Markus Asper (ed.), *Writing Science: Medical and Mathematical Authorship in Ancient Greece*, Berlin, 17–62.

King, H. (1998). *Hippocrates' Woman*, London.

King, H. (2019). *Hippocrates Now*, London.

Klamroth, M. (1888). 'Über die Auszüge aus griechischen Schriftstellern bei al-Ja'qūbī'. *Zeitschrift der Deutschen Morgenländischen Gesellschaft* 42, 204–233.

Koch, K., ed. (1923). *De sanitate tuenda. (Matters of Health)*, Corpus Medicorum Graecorum 5.4.2, Berlin.

Kollesch, J. (1973). *Untersuchungen zu den pseudogalenischen Definitiones medicae*, Berlin.

Kollesch, J. and F. Kudlien (1965). *Apollonii Citiensis. In Hippocratis de articulis commentarius*, Corpus Medicorum Graecorum 11.1.1, Berlin.

Kollesch, J. and D. Nickel, eds. (1993), *Galen und das hellenistische Erbe. Verhandlungen des IV, internationalen Galen-Symposiums veranstaltet vom Institut für Geschichte der Medizin am Bereich Medizin (Charité) der Humboldt-Universität zu Berlin*, Stuttgart.

Kotter, B. (1968). *Die Schriften des Johannes von Damaskos I. Institutio elementaris, Capita philosophica (Dialectica)*, Berlin.

Kudlien, F. (1960). *Die handschriftliche Überlieferung des Galenkommentars zu Hippokrates 'De articulis'*. Deutsche Akademie der Wissenschaften zu Berlin. Schriften der Sektion für Altertumswissenschaften 27, Berlin.

Kudlien, F. (1972). 'Sabinus'. In Konrat Ziegler (ed.), *Der Kleine Pauly*, vol. 4, col. 1485.

Kudlien, F. (1981). 'Galen's Religious Belief'. In V. Nutton (ed.), *Galen, Problems and Prospects*, London, 117–130.

Kühlewein, H., ed. (1902), *Hippocratis opera quae feruntur omnia*, 2 vols., Leipzig.

Kühn, J.-H., U. Fleischer et al. (1986–1989). *Index Hippocraticus*, Göttingen.

Kühn, Karl Gottlob, ed. (1819–1833), *Galeni Opera Omnia*, 22 vols., Leipzig; repr. (1965), Hildesheim.

Kupreeva, I. (2014). 'Galen's Theory of Elements'. In Adamson, Hansberger and Wilberding (eds.), 153–196.

L'Alemant, A. (1557). *De flatibus liber ab Adriana Alemano … commentariis illustratus*, Paris.

Lamoreaux, J. C (2016). *Ḥunayn ibn Isḥāq on his Galen Translations: a Parallel English-Arabic Text*, Provo.

Langholf, V. (1977). *Syntaktische Untersuchungen zu Hippokrates-Texten. Brachylogische Syntagmen in den individuellen Krankheits-Fallbeschreibungen der hippokratischen Schriftensammlung*, Mainz.

Langholf, V. (1990). *Medical Theories in Hippocrates. Early Texts and the 'Epidemics'*, Untersuchungen zur antiken Literatur und Geschichte 34, Berlin.

Larusso, V. (2010). 'Tracce di esegisi alessandrina al *De methodo medendi* di Galeno in codici medievali'. In V. Boudon-Millot, A. Garzya (eds.), *Storia della tradizione e edizione dei medici greci*, Naples.

Lasserre, F., and P. Mudry, eds. (1983). *Formes de pensée dans la Collection hippocratique. Actes du IVe Colloque international hippocratique, Lausanne 21–26 septembre 1981*, Geneva.

Ledesma, M.J. (1547). *Prima primi Canonis Auicennae sectio, Michaele Hieronymo Ledesma Valentino Medico et interprete et enarratore*, Valencia.

Leigh, R. (2016). *On Theriac to Piso, attributed to Galen*, Leiden.

Leith, D. (2009a). 'The Qualitative Status of the *Onkoi* in Asclepiades' Theory of Matter'. *Oxford Studies in Ancient Philosophy* 36, 283–320.

Leith, D. (2009b). 'P.Oxy. LXXIV 4970'. *The Oxyrhynchus Papyri* 74, 52–55.

Leith, D. (2012). 'Pores and Void in Asclepiades' Physical Theory'. *Phronesis* 57, 164–191.

Leith, D. (2014). 'Galen's Refutation of Atomism'. In Adamson, Hansberger and Wilberding (eds.), 213–234.

Leith, D. (2015). 'Elements and Uniform Parts in Early Alexandrian Medicine'. *Phronesis* 60, 462–491

Lewis, O. (2017). *Praxagoras of Cos on Arteries, Pulse and Pneuma*, Studies in Ancient Medicine 48, Leiden.

Linden, J.A. van der (1645). *Aselli, Harvey, Spigelius, Walaeus. Opera quae extant omnia*, Amsterdam.

Linden, J.A. van der (1653). *Medicina physiologica*, Amsterdam.

Linden, J.A. van der (1659). *Hippocratis de circuitu sanguinis exercitationes XXVII D.D.D. Lucas Walckier*, Leiden.

Linden, J.A. van der (1660, 2nd ed. 1668). *De hemicrania menstrua historia et consilium*, Leiden.

Linden, J.A. van der (1665). *Magni Hippocratis Coi opera omnia*, Leiden.

Littré, É., ed. (1839–1861). *Œuvres complètes d'Hippocrate*, 10 vols., Paris.

Lloyd, G.E.R., ed. (1978). *Hippocratic Writings*, trans. W. Mann, rev. J. Chadwick, London.

Lloyd, G.E.R. (1988). 'Scholarship, Authority and Argument in Galen's *Quod animi mores*'. In Paola Manuli and Mario Vegetti (eds.), *Le Opere Psicologiche Di Galeno. Atti del Terzo Colloquio Galenico Internazionale Pavia 10–12 Settembre 1986*, Naples, 11–42.

Lloyd, G.E.R. (1991). 'The Hippocratic Question'. In id., *Methods and Problems in Greek Science: Selected Papers*. Cambridge, 194–223; updated version of original publication in *Classical Quarterly* 25 (1975), 171–192.

Lloyd, G.E.R. (1993). 'Galen on Hellenistics and Hippocrateans: Contemporary Battles and Past Authorities'. In Kollesch and Nickel (eds.), 125–143.

Lonie, I.M. (1981). *The Hippocratic Treatises On Generation, On the Nature of the Child, Diseases IV*, Berlin, New York.

López Férez, J.A., ed. (1992). *Tratados Hipocráticos (estudios acerca de su contenido, forma e influencia): actas Del VIIe Colloque International Hippocratique (Madrid, 24–29 de septiembre de 1990)*, Madrid.

López Piñero, J.M. (1979). *Ciencia y técnica en la Sociedad española de los siglos XVI y XVII*, Barcelona.

López Piñero, J.M. et al. (1983), *Diccionario histórico de la ciencia moderna moderna en España*, 2 vols., Barcelona.

Lorusso, V. (2010). 'Tracce di esegesi alessandrina al *De methodo medendi* di Galeno in codici medievali'. In V. Boudon-Millot, A. Garzya, J. Jouanna, A. Roselli (eds.), *Storia della tradizione e edizione dei medici greci, Atti del VI Colloqui internazionale (Paris 12–14 aprile 2008)*, Naples, 109–127.

Lyons, M. (1963). *Galeni in Hippocratis De officina medici commentariorum versio Ara-*

bica et excerpta quae ʿAlī ibn Riḍwān ex eis sumpsit, Corpus Medicorum Graecorum Supplementum Orientale 1, Berlin.

Joly, R. (1970). *Hippocrate. De la génération. De la nature de l'enfant. Des maladies IV. De foetus de huit mois*, Paris.

Joly, R., ed. (1977). *Corpus Hippocraticum. Actes du Colloque Hippocratique de Mons (22–26 septembre 1975)*, Mons.

Leven, K.-H. (2018). 'Ethics and Deontology'. In Pormann (ed.), 152–179.

Maas, P. (1952). *Textual Criticism*, Oxford.

Magdelaine, C. (1994). 'Histoire du texte et édition critique, traduite et commentée, des *Aphorismes* d'Hippocrate'. 3 vol., Thèse pour le Doctorat Nouveau Régime, Université de Paris-Sorbonne IV.

Manetti, D. (1985). 'Tematica filosofica e scientifica nel papiro fiorentino 115: un probabile frammento di Galeno in *In Hippocratis de alimento*'. In Walter Cavini et al. (eds.), *Studi su papiri greci di logica e medicina*, Florence, 173–213.

Manetti, D. (1992). 'P. Berol. 11739A e i commenti tardoantichi a Galeno'. In Antonio Garzya (ed.), *Tradizione e ecdotica dei testi medici tardoantichi e bizantini. Atti del convegno Internazionale, Anacapri 29–31 ottobre 1990*, Naples, 211–235.

Manetti, D. (1996). '῾Ως δὲ αὐτὸς Ἱπποκράτης λέγει: teoria causale e ippocratismo nell' Anonimo Londinense'. In Wittern and Pellegrin (eds.), 295–310.

Manetti, D. (2003). 'Galeno, la lingua di Hippocrate, e il tempo'. In Barnes and Jouanna (eds.), 171–220.

Manetti, D. (1999). '"Aristotle" and the Role of Doxography in the Anonymus Londiniensis (PBrLibr Inv. 137)'. In van der Eijk (ed.), 95–141.

Manetti, D. (2008). 'POxy2547: Iusj. 1–4'. In *Corpus dei papiri filosofici greci e latini* 2.1, Florence, 167–174.

Manetti, D. (2009). 'Galen and Hippocratic Medicine: Language and Practice'. In Gill et al. (eds.), 157–174.

Manetti, D. (2011). *Anonymus Londinensis de Medicina*, Berlin.

Manetti, D., ed. (2012). *Studi sul de indolentia di Galeno*, Pisa.

Manetti, D., (2014). 'Alle origini dell'Ippocratismo: tra IV e III sec.'. in Jouanna and Zink (eds.), 231–251.

Manetti, D. (2015). 'Medicine and Exegesis'. In Franco Montanari, Stefanos Matthaios, and Antonios Rengakos (eds.), *Brill's Companion to Ancient Greek Scholarship*, Leiden, 1126–1215.

Manetti, D. and Roselli, A. (1982). *Ippocrate. Epidemie. Libro sesto. Introduzione, testo critico, commento e traduzione*, Florence.

Manetti, D. and Roselli, A. (1994). 'Galeno commentatore di Ippocrate'. In *Aufstieg und Niedergang der römischen Welt* 37.2, 1529–1635.

Manetti, D. and Roselli, A. (1996). 'Note per una nuova edizione dei commenti di Galeno ai trattati chirurgici'. In Vegetti and Gastaldi (eds.), 77–87.

Mani, Nikolaus (1968). 'Jean Riolan II (1580–1657) and Medical Research'. *Bulletin of the History of Medicine* 42, 121–144.

Mansfeld, J. (1994). *Prolegomena. Questions to be Settled before the Study of an Author, or a Text*, Leiden.

Manuli, P. (1984). 'Lo stile del commento: Galeno e la tradizione ippocratica'. In Gabriele Giannantoni and Mario Vegetti (eds.), *La scienza ellenistica: atti delle tre giornate di studio tenutesi a Pavia dal 14 al 16 april 1982*, Naples, 375–394.

Martín Ferreira, Ana Isabel (1995). *El humanismo médico en la Universidad de Alcalá (siglo XVI)*, Alcalá de Henares.

Martínez Prieto, R. (2017). 'La recepción del humanismo médico en el *Libro de Theriaca* (1575) del boticario toledano Lorenzo Pérez'. In María Teresa Santamaría Hernández (ed.), *Traducción y transmisión doctrinal de la medicina grecolatina desde la Antigüedad hasta el mundo moderno: nuevas aportaciones sobre autores y textos*, Cuenca, 133–154.

Mewaldt, J. (1909). 'Galenos über echte und unechte Hippocratica'. *Hermes* 44, 111–134.

Mewaldt, J., G. Helmreich, and J. Westenberger, eds. (1914). *Galeni In Hippocratis de Natura Hominis; In Hippocratis de Victu Acutorum; De Diaeta Hippocratis in Morbis Acutis*, Corpus Medicorum Graecorum 5.9.1, Berlin.

Micheau, F. (1997). 'Mécènes et médecins à Bagdad au IIIe/IXe siècle. Les commanditaires des traductions de Galien par Ḥunayn b. Isḥāq'. In D. Jacquart (ed.), *Les voies de la Science grecque. Études sur la transmission des textes de l'Antiquité au XIXe siècle*, Paris, Geneva, 147–179.

Michler, M. (1968). *Die alexandrinischen Chirurgen. Eine Sammlung und Auswertung ihrer Fragmente*, Wiesbaden.

Migne, J.P. (1856–1866), *Patrologia Graeca*, 161 vols., Paris.

Militello, Ch. (2010). *I commentari all'Isagoge di Porfirio tra V e VI secolo*, Acireale.

Mimura, T. (2017a). 'Comparing Interpretive Notes in the Syriac and Arabic Translations of the Hippocratic *Aphorisms*'. *Aramaic Studies* 15, 183–199.

Mimura, T. (2017b). 'A Reconsideration of the Authoship of the Syriac Hippocratic *Aphorisms*: The Creation of the Syro-Arabic Bilingual Manuscript of the *Aphorisms* in the Tradition of Ḥunayn ibn Isḥāq's Arabic Translation'. *Oriens* 45, 80–104.

Moffat, John (1788). *The Prognostics and Prorrhetics of Hippocrates*, London.

Montero Cartelle, E. (2001). 'El médico filósofo en el siglo XVI'. In Juan Luis García Hourcade and Juan Manuel Moreno Yuste (eds.), *Andrés Laguna: Humanismo, ciencia y política en la Europa renacentista*, Valladolid, 93–121.

Morata, N. (1934). 'Un catálogo de los fondos árabes primitivos de El Escorial'. *Al-Andalus* 2, 87–181.

Moraux, P. (1977). 'Unbekannte Galen-Scholien'. *Zeitschrift für Papyrologie und Epigraphik* 27, 1–63.

Morgan, M.H., ed. (1914). *Vitruvius. Ten Books on Architecture*, Cambridge.

Morison, B. (2008). 'Language'. In Hankinson (2008b), 116–156.

Mouton, J.-M., Magdelaine, C. (2016). 'La transmission des textes médicaux grecs en arabe: le Commentaire au Serment d'Hippocrate attribué à Galien dans un manuscrit inédit de la Grande Mosquée de Damas'. In J.-L. Fournet, J.-M. Mouton and J. Paviot (eds.), *Civilisations en transition (II): sociétés multilingues à travers l'histoire du Proche-Orient*, Byblos, 169–193.

Mouton, J.-M., Sourdel, D., Sourdel-Thomine, J. (2013). *Mariage et séparation à Damas au Moyen Âge*, Paris.

Mouton, J.-M., Sourdel, D., Sourdel-Thomine, J. (2015). *Gouvernance et libéralités de Saladin d'après les données inédites de six documents arabes*, Paris.

Mudry, Ph. (1982). *La Préface du* De medicina *de Celse*, Bibliotheca Helvetica Romana 19, Rome.

Müller, I. (1901). *Claudii Galeni Pergameni Scripta Minora*, vol. 2, Leipzig.

Nachmanson, E. (ed.) (1918). *Erotiani Vocum Hippocraticarum collectio cum fragmentis*, Gothenburg.

Nares, R. (1808–1812). *Catalogue of the Harleian Manuscripts in the British Museum*, 4 vols, London.

Nicolás A. (1783/1788). *Bibliotheca hispana nova*, 2 vols, Madrid; repr. Torino, 1963.

Noja, S. (1984). 'Un nuovo anello nella trasmissione della cultura classica attraverso l'Islam: il manoscritto arabo del commentario di Galeno ai libri περὶ τόπων καὶ ἀέρων καὶ ὑδάτων di Ippocrate'. *Schede Medievali* 6–7, 42–51.

Nutton, V. (1979). *De praenotione ad Epigenem* (*Prognosis*), Corpus Medicorum Graecorum 5.8.1, Berlin.

Nutton, V. (1990). 'The Patient's Choice. A New Treatise by Galen'. *Classical Quarterly* 40, 236–257.

Nutton, V. (1993). 'Beyond the Hippocratic Oath'. *Clio Medica* 24, 10–37.

Nutton, V. (2000). 'Medical Thoughts on Urban Pollution'. In Valerie Hope and Eireann Marshall (eds.), *Death and Disease in the Ancient City*, London, 65–73.

Nutton, V. (2012a). '*Physiologia* from Galen to Jacob Bording'. In Horstmanshoff, King, and Zittel (eds.), 27–40.

Nutton, V. (2012b). 'The Commentary on the Hippocratic Oath Ascribed to Galen'. In S. Fortuna, I. Garofalo, A. Lami, A. Roselli (eds.), *Sulla tradizione indiretta dei testi medici greci: i commenti*, Pisa, Rome, 91–100.

Nutton, V. (2016). 'Galen. *Avoiding Distress*'. In Peter Singer (ed.), *Galen. Psychological Writings*, Cambridge, 43–99.

Oates, W.J. and E. O'Neill, Jr. (1938). Euripides. *The Complete Greek Drama in two volumes: Vol. 1 Hecuba, translated by E.P. Coleridge*. New York.

Omont, H. (1886–1898). *Inventaire sommaire des manuscrits grecs de la Bibliothèque Nationale et des autres bibliothèques de Paris et des Départements*, 2 vols., Paris.

Overduin, F. (2014). *Nicander of Colophon's* Theriaca*: A Literary Commentary*, Leiden.

Overwien, O. (2009), 'Die Bedeutung der orientalischen Tradition für die antike Überlieferung des Hippokratischen Eides'. In I. Garofalo, A. Lami, A. Roselli (eds.), *Sulla tradizione indiretta dei testo medici greci*, Pisa, Rome, 79–103.

Overwien, O. (2012), 'The Art of the Translator, or: How did Hunayn Ibn Ishaq and his School Translate?'. In Pormann (ed.), 151–169.

Overwien, O. (2015), 'The Paradigmatic Translator and His Method: Ḥunayn ibn Isḥāq's Translation of the Hippocratic *Aphorisms* from Greek via Syriac into Arabic'. *Intellectual History of the Islamicate World* 2, 158–187.

Overwien, O. (2018). 'Der medizinische Unterricht der Iatrosophisten in der "Schule von Alexandria" (5.–7. Jh. n. Chr.): Überlegungen zu seiner Organisation, seinen Inhalten und seinen Ursprüngen', *Philologus* 162, 2–14 and 265–290.

Palabıyık, N.Ö. (2019). 'An Unsung Hero of Oriental Studies in Leiden: Anton Deusing (1612–1666) and his Persian and Turkish Dictionaries'. *Lias* 46, 157–200.

Parker, G. (1998). *The Grand Strategy of Philip II*, New Haven.

Parker, G. (2014), *Imprudent King: A New Life of Philip II*, New Haven.

Pecquet, J. (1651), *Experimenta nova anatomica … Dissertatione anatomica de circulatione sanguinis et chyli motu*, Paris.

Perilli, L. (2000). 'La fortuna di Galeno filosofo. Un nuovo testimone dei commentari neoplatonici (Scholia Yalensia) al De elementis'. In Aldo Brancacci (ed.), *La filosofia in età imperiale. Atti del Colloquio (Roma, 17–19 giugno 1999)*, Naples, 87–135.

Peset, M. and J.L. Peset (1975), *Gregorio Mayans y la reforma universitaria. Idea del nuevo método que se puede practicar en la enseñanza de las Universidades de España, 1 de abril de 1767*, Valencia.

Peterson, D. (1977). 'Observations on the Chronology of the Galenic Corpus'. *Bulletin of the History of Medicine* 51, 484–495.

Petit, C., ed. (2018). *Galen's Treatise* Περὶ Ἀλυπίας *(De indolentia) in Context: A Tale of Resilience*, Studies in Ancient Medicine 52, Leiden.

Pétrequin, J.É. (1877–1878). *Chirurgie d'Hippocrate*, Paris.

Pietrobelli, A. (2012). 'La traduction arabe du Régime aux maladies aiguës d'Hippocrate: mise au point et nouvelles perspectives'. In S. Fortuna, I. Garofalo, A. Lami, A. Roselli (eds.), *Sulla tradizione indiretta dei testi medici greci: i commenti*, Pisa-Rome, 101–122.

Pognon, H. (1903). *Une version syriaque des Aphorismes d'Hippocrate*, Leipzig.

Pormann, P.E. (2004a). *The Oriental Tradition of Paul of Aegina's 'Pragmateia'*, Studies in Ancient Medicine 29, Leiden.

Pormann, P.E. (2004b). 'La querelle des médecins arabistes et hellénistes et l'héritage oublié'. In Véronique Boudon-Millot et Guy Cobolet, *Lire les médecins grecs à la Renaissance: Aux origines de l'édition médicale, Actes du colloque international de Paris (19–20 septembre 2003)*, collection Médic@, Paris, 113–141.

Pormann, P.E. (2005), 'The Physician and the Other: Images of the Charlatan in Medieval Islam'. *Bulletin of the History of Medicine* 79, 189–227.

Pormann, P.E. (2008). 'Case Notes and Clinician: Galen's Commentary on the Hippocratic Epidemics in the Arabic Tradition'. *Arabic Sciences and Philosophy* 18, 247–284.

Pormann, P.E. (2009). 'David Colville'. *Oxford Dictionary of National Biography*, Oxford. DOI: 10.1093/ref:odnb/98330

Pormann, P.E. (2010a). 'Islamic Hospitals in the Time of al-Muqtadir'. In John Nawas (ed.), *Abbasid Studies II: Occasional Papers of the School of 'Abbasid Studies, Leuven, 28 June–1 July 2004*, Orientalia Lovaniensia Analecta 177, Leuven, 337–382; reprinted in Pormann (2011a), vol. 1, pp. 136–178.

Pormann, P.E. (2010b). 'Medical Education in Late Antiquity: from Alexandria to Montpellier'. In Horstmanshoff (ed.), 419–441.

Pormann, P.E., ed. (2011a). *Islamic Medical and Scientific Tradition*, Critical Concepts in Islamic Studies, 4 vols, London.

Pormann, P.E. (2011b). 'The Dispute between the Philarabic and Philhellenic Physicians and the Forgotten Heritage of Arabic Medicine'. In id. (2011a), vol. 2, pp. 283–316; revised and updated English translation of Pormann (2004b).

Pormann, P.E., ed. (2012a). *Epidemics in Context: Greek Commentaries on Hippocrates in the Arabic Tradition*, Scientia Graeco-Arabica 8, Berlin.

Pormann, P.E. (2012b). 'The Development of Translation Techniques from Greek into Syriac and Arabic: The Case of Galen's *On the Faculties and Powers of Simple Drugs*, Book Six'. In Rotraud Hansberger, M. Afifi-Akiti and Charles Burnett (eds.), *Medieval Arabic Thought: Essays in Honour of Fritz Zimmermann*, London/Turin, 143–162.

Pormann, P.E. (2015). 'Al-Fārābī: The Melancholic Thinker and Philosopher Poet'. *Journal of the American Oriental Society* 135, 209–224.

Pormann, P.E., ed. (2018a), *Cambridge Companion to Hippocrates*, Cambridge.

Pormann, P.E. (2018b), 'The Arabo-Islamic Tradition'. In Pormann (2018a), 340–361.

Pormann, P.E., S. Barry, N. Carpentieri, E. van Dalen, K.I. Karimullah, T. Mimura, and H. Obaid (2017). 'The Enigma of Arabic and Hebrew Palladius'. *Intellectual History of the Islamicate World* 5, 252–310.

Potter, P., G. Maloney, and J. Desautels, eds. (1990), *La maladie et les maladies dans la Collection Hippocratique, Actes du VIe Colloque international Hippocratique* (*Québec 28 septembre–3 octobre 1987*), Quebec.

Preiser, G. (1969). 'Zur Hippokratesauffassung des Johannes Antonides van der Linden'. *Medizinhistorisches Journal* 4, 305–315.

Pritchet, Ch.D. (1975). *Iohannis Alexandrini commentaria in sextum librum Hippocratis Epidemiarum*, Leiden.

Radici, L. (2012). *Nicandro di Colofone nei secoli XVI–XVIII: Edizioni, Traduzioni, Commenti*, Biblioteca di *Thechnai* 2, Pisa, Rome.

Radt, S. (1988). 'Οἱ (αἱ etc.) περὶ + acc. nominis proprii bei Strabon'. *Zeitschrift für Papyrologie und Epigraphik* 71, 35–40.

Raiola, T., ed. (2018). *Sabini medici eiusque discipulorum fragmenta*, Biblioteca di Galenos 6, Pisa.

Raiola, T. (forthcoming), 'Per l'edizione dei frammenti di Sabino Ippocrateo'. In Véronique Boudon-Millot, Anna M. Ieraci Bio, Jacques Jouanna and Amneris Roselli, *Atti del VII colloquio internazionale di Ecdotica dei testi medici greci*, Naples, 67–82.

Revilla, A. (1936). *Catálogo de los códices griegos de la Biblioteca de El Escorial. Tomo I*, Madrid.

Richter, G. (1964). *Die Dialektik des Johannes von Damaskos. Eine Untersuchung des Textes nach seinen Quellen und seiner Bedeutung*, Ettal.

Riolan, J. (1653). *Opuscula nova anatomica*, Paris.

Rodríguez Mediano, F. and M. García-Arenal (2002). 'Diego de Urrea y algún traductor más: en torno a las versiones de los "plomos"'. *Al-Qantara* 23, 499–516.

Rolfinck, W. (1653). *Methodus cognoscendi et curandi adfectus particulares capitis*, Jena.

Roselli, A. (1998). 'L'anonimo *De medicina* (II 244–245 Dietz): prolegomena to the lecture of medical texts?'. *Filologia Antica e Moderna* 15, 7–25.

Roselli, A. (2000). 'Un corpo che prende forma: l'ordine di successione dei trattati ippocratici dall'età ellenistica fino all'età bizantina'. In Giovanni Cerri (ed.), *La letteratura pseudepigrafa nella cultura greca e romana: atti di un incontro di studi, Napoli, 15–17 gennaio 1998*, Naples, 167–195.

Roselli, A. (2010). 'Libri e biblioteche a Roma al tempo di Galeno: la testimonianza del *de indolentia*'. *Galenos* 4, 127–148.

Roselli, A. (2015). 'Galeno sull' autenticità del Prorretico I'. In Brooke Holmes and Klaus-Dietrich Fischer (eds.), *The Frontiers of Ancient Science, Essays in Honor of Heinrich von Staden*, Beiträge zur Altertumskunde 338, Berlin, 533–560.

Rosenthal, F. (1956). 'An Ancient Commentary in the Hippocratic Oath'. *Bulletin of the History of Medicine* 30, 52–87.

Roueché, M. (1974). 'Byzantine Philosophical Texts of the Seventh Century'. *Jahrbuch der österreichischen Byzantinistik* 23, 61–76.

Roueché, M. (1980), 'A Middle Byzantine Handbook of Logic Terminology'. *Jahrbuch der österreichischen Byzantinistik* 29, 71–98.

Rubin Pinault, J. (1992). *Hippocratic Lives and Legends*, Leiden.

Rutgers, J.H. (1849). 'Specimen medicum inaugurale exhibens editionem libri Hippocratis *De capitis vulneribus*'. MD thesis, Groningen.

Salanitro, G. (1987). 'A proposito della locuzione οἱ περί τινα'. *Sileno* 13, 241.

Santamaría Hernández, M.T. (2002). 'Nicandro latino en el humanismo médico valenciano: Pedro Jaime Esteve, traductor de los *Theriaca*'. In José María Maestre Maestre, Joaquín Pascual Barea, and Luis Charlo Brea (eds.), *Humanismo y pervivencia del mundo clásico. Homenaje al profesor Antonio Fontán*, 5 vols., Alcañiz, vol. 5, pp. 2579–2591.

Santamaría Hernández, M.T. (2003). *El humanismo médico en la Universidad de Valencia (siglo XVI)*, Valencia.

Santamaría Hernández, M.T. (2004a). '*Nicander Latinus*: la difusión latina de Nicandro en el siglo XVI'. *Humanistica Lovaniensia* 53, 125–173.

Santamaría Hernández, M.T. (2004b). 'La recuperación de los escolios a Nicandro en la exégesis renacentista del poeta'. In Ignacio J. García Pinilla, Santiago Talavera Cuesta (eds.), *Charisterion Francisco Martín oblatum*, Cuenca, 363–384.

Santamaría Hernández, M.T. (2004c). 'El léxico de Celso en una traducción de Hipócrates del siglo XVI: el libro II de las *Epidemias* de Pedro Jaime Esteve'. In Sergio Sconocchia and Fabio Cavalli (eds.), *Testi medici latini antichi (le parole della medicina: lessico e storia). Atti del VII Convegno Internazionale*, Bolognia, 353–373.

Santamaría Hernández, M.T., ed. (2011). *Miguel Servet. Escritos médicos: Apología contra Leonhart Fuchs. Doctrina completa de los jarabes. Introducción, edición crítica, traducción y notas*, Colección Ediciones Críticas 10. Cuenca.

Santamaría Hernández, M.T. (2012a). 'Pedro Jaime Esteve', 'Luis Collado', 'Pedro Jimeno', 'Miguel Jerónimo Ledesma'. In Juan Francisco Domínguez Domínguez (ed.), *Diccionario biográfico y bibliográfico del humanismo español (siglos XV–XVII)*, Madrid, 287–290, 224–228, 450–452, 469–471.

Santamaría Hernández, M.T. (2012b). 'El comentario de Pedro Jaime Esteve a los *Theriaca* de Nicandro (Valencia, 1552): Conjetura y traducción, o transmisión latina de los escolios griegos'. In Fortuna et al. (eds.), 149–185.

Santamaría Hernández, M.T. (2018a). 'El latín de la Medicina humanística y la barbarie médica. Claves lingüísticas de un enfrentamiento parcial'. In Astrid Steiner-Weber and Franz Römer (eds.), *Acta Conventus Neo-Latini Vindobonensis. Proceedings of the Sixteenth International Congress of Neo-Latin Studies (Vienna 2015)*, Leiden, 581–590.

Santamaría Hernández, M.T. (2018b). *Pedro Jaime Esteve. Nicandri Theriaca: traducción latina en verso (1552). Introducción, edición crítica, traducción y notas*. Colección Ediciones Críticas 25, Cuenca.

Santander Rodríguez, T. (1971), *Hipócrates en España (siglo XVI)*, Madrid.

Savage-Smith, E. (1996). 'Medicine'. In R. Rashed (ed.), *Encyclopedia of the History of Arabic Sciences* 3, London, 903–962.

Savino, Ch. (2012), 'Per una nuova edizione del Commento agli Aforismi di Galeno: la tradizione greca'. In Fortuna et al. (eds.), 29–57.

Savino, Ch. (2013). 'I commenti di Galeno'. *Lettre d'informations. Médecine antique et médiévale* n.s. 11, 1–31.

Savino, Ch. (2020a), *Galeni In Hippocratis Aphorismos VI commentaria / Galeno, Commento agli Aforismi di Ippocrate Libro VI. Testo, traduzione e note di commento*, Corpus Medicorum Graecorum 5.12.6, Berlin.

Savino, Ch. (2020b). 'Manus, quae supplevit, inscripsit scholia Theophili Protospatharii: Galien, Théophile et le commentaire mélange aux Aphorismes d'Hippocrate', *Byzantinische Zeitschrift* 113, 1025–1040.

Savino, Ch. (2021). '*Commentariis in Hippocratis librum Epidemiarum II uti non licet*: G.B. Rasario and the False "Galenic" Commentary on Epidemics II'. In Caroline Petit, Simon Swain and Klaus-Dietrich Fischer (eds.), *Pseudo-Galenica: The Formation of the Galenic Corpus from Antiquity to the Renaissance*, Warburg Institue Colloquia 34, London.

Savio, M. (2017). '"Un frammento per due": ΞΕΝΟΚΡΑΤΗΣ ο ΚΡΑΤΗΣ?'. In Gabriella Ottone (ed.), *Historiai para doxan. Documenti greci in frammenti: nuove prospettive esegetiche. Atti dell'incontro internazionale di Studi* (*Genova, 10–11 marzo 2016*), Rome, 278–283.

Schiefsky, M.J. (2005). *Hippocrates. On Ancient Medicine, Translated with Introduction and Commentary*, Studies in Ancient Medicine 28, Leiden.

Schöne, H. (1896). *Apollonius Citiensis in Hippocratis de articulis Commentarii*, Leipzig.

Serveto, M. (1537). *Syruporum Vniuersa Ratio*, Paris.

Sezgin, F. (1970). *Geschichte des arabischen Schrifttums III: Medizin-Pharmazie, Zoologie-Tierheilkunde*, Leiden.

Sezgin, F., ed. (2001). *Galen's Commentary On the Hippocratic Treatise On Airs, Waters, Places* (*περὶ ἀέρων, ὑδάτων, τόπων*) *in Arabic Translation*, Publications of the Institute for the History of Arabic-Islamic Science. Facsimile Edition 65, Frankfurt am Main.

Shuttleworth Kraus, Chr. (2002). 'Introduction: Reading Commentaries/Commentaries as Reading'. In Gibson, Shuttleworth Kraus, 1–27.

Sideras, A. (1994). 'Rufus von Ephesos und sein Werk im Rahmen der antiken Medizin'. *Aufstieg und Niedergang der römischen Welt* 37.2, 1077–1253.

Singer, P.N. (1996). 'Notes on Galen's Hippocrates'. In Vegetti and Gastaldi (eds.), 66–76.

Singer, P.N. (1997). *Galen: Selected Works*, Oxford.

Singer, P.N., ed. (2013). *Galen: Psychological Writings*, Cambridge Galen Translations, Cambridge.

Singer, P.N. (2018a). 'Note on MS Vlatadon 14: a Summary of the Main Findings and Problems'. In Petit (ed.), 10–37.

Singer, P.N. (2018b). 'New Light and Old Texts: Galen on his Own Books'. In Petit (ed.), 91–132.

Singer, P.N. and P.J. van der Eijk (2018). *Galen: Works on Human Nature I: Mixtures* (*De Temperamentis*), Cambridge Galen Translations, Cambridge.

Sluiter, I. (1995). 'The Embarrassment of Imperfection: Galen's Assessment of Hippocrates' Linguistic Merits'. in Philip J. van der Eijk, H.F.J. Horstmanshoff, Petrus H. Schrijvers (eds.), *Ancient Medicine and its Socio-Cultural Context. Papers read at the Congress held at Leiden University* (*13–15 April 1992*), *Clio medica* 27–28, 2 vols, Amsterdam, vol. 2, pp. 519–535.

Smith, W.D. (1979). *The Hippocratic Tradition*, Ithaca, NY.

Smith, W.D. (1994). *Hippocrates vol. 7: Epidemics 2 & 4–7*, Loeb Classical Library 477, Cambridge, MA.

Sorabji, R. (2005). *The Philosophy of the Commentators. 200–600 AD. A Sourcebook*, 3 vols., Ithaca, NY.

Sourdel, D. and J. Sourdel-Thomine (2006). *Certificats de pèlerinage d'époque ayyoubide. Contribution à l'histoire de l'idéologie de l'Islam au temps des Croisades*, Paris.

Spencer, W.G. (1935). *Celsus. On Medicine Books I–IV*, Loeb Classical Library 292, Cambridge, MA.

Sprengel, C. (1830). 'Pseudo-Dioscorides. Περὶ δηλητηρίων φαρμάκων … Περὶ ἰοβόλων'. Carolus G. Kühn (ed.), *Medicorum Graecorum opera quae exstant* 26.2, Leipzig, 1–91.

Strohmaier, G. (1970). 'Asklepios und das Ei'. In R. Stiehl, H.E. Stier (eds.), *Beiträge zur Alten Geschichte und deren Nachleben. Festschrift für Franz Altheim*, Berlin, 143–153, 448–454.

Strohmaier, G. (1974). 'Ḥunayn ibn Isḥāq et le serment hippocratique'. *Arabica* 21, 318–323.

Strohmaier, G. (1993). *Hellenistische Wissenschaft im neugefundenen Galenkommentar zur hippokratischen Schrift 'Über die Umwelt'*. In Kollesch and Nickel (eds.), 157–164.

Strohmaier, G. (2004). 'Galen's Not Uncritical Commentary on Hippocrates' *Airs, Waters, Places*'. In Peter Adamson, Han Baltussen and Martin W.F. Stone (eds.), *Philosophy, Science and Exegesis in Greek, Arabic and Latin Commentaries*, Bulletin of the Institute of Classical Studies. Supplement 83, 2 vols, London, vol. 2, pp. 1–9.

Strohmaier, G. (2012). 'Galen the Pagan and Ḥunayn the Christian: Specific Transformations in the Commentaries on *Airs, Waters, Places* and the *Epidemics*'. In Pormann (ed.), 171–184.

Subiza Martín, E. (1954). 'Los médicos de Felipe II. Aportación a su estudio'. *Archivo Hispano Americano de Historia de la Medicina* 6, 377–390.

Tassinari, P. (1997). *Galeno. Gli elementi secondo la dottrina di Ippocrate; I temperamenti*, Rome.

Tellechea Idígoras, J.I. (1965). 'Los jesuitas y la real pragmática de Felipe II de 1559. Un percance inquisitorial desconocido (1561)'. *Archivum Historicum Societatis Iesu* 25, 79–85; reprinted in id. (1977). *Tiempos recios. Inquisición y heterodoxia*, Salamanca, 268–271.

Tellechea Idígoras, J.I. (2000). 'Españoles en Lovaina en 1557'. In Werner Thomas and Robert A. Verdonk (eds.), *Encuentros en Flandes*, Leuven, 132–155.

Temkin, O. (1932). 'Geschichte des Hippokratismus im ausgehenden Altertum'. *Kyklos* 4, 1–80.

Temkin, O. (1991). *Hippocrates in a World of Pagans and Christians*, Baltimore.

Thivel, A., and A. Zucker, eds. (2002). *Le normal et le pathologique dans la Collection hip-*

pocratique. Actes du xe Colloque international hippocratique, Nice, 6–8 octobre 1999, 2 vols., Nice.

Tittmann, J.A.H. (1808). *Iohannis Zonarae Lexicon ex Tribus Codicibus Manuscriptis*, 2 vols., Leipzig.

Triller, D.W. (1766–1772), *Opuscula medica ac medico philosophica*, Frankfurt.

Ullmann, M. (1970). *Die Medizin im Islam*, Leiden.

Ullmann, M. (1977). 'Galens Kommentar zu der Schrift "De aere aquis locis"'. In Joly (ed.), 353–365.

Ullmann, M. (2002). *Wörterbuch der griechisch-arabischen Übersetzungen des neunten Jahrhunders*, Wiesbaden

Ullmann, M. and E.A. Schmidt (2012). *Aristoteles in Fes: Zum Wert der arabischen Überlieferung der* Nikomachischen Ethik *für die Kritik des griechischen Textes*, Heidelberg.

Université des sciences humaines de Strasbourg. Centre de recherches sur la Grèce antique (1975). *La Collection hippocratique et son rôle dans l'histoire de la médecine: colloque de Strasbourg*, 23–27 octobre 1972, Leiden.

Usener, H. (1859). *Alexandri Aphrodisiensis quae feruntur problematorum liber III et IIII*, Berlin.

Vagelpohl, U. (2011). 'In the Translator's Workshop'. *Arabic Sciences and Philosophy* 21, 249–288.

Vagelpohl, U., ed. (2014), *Galen: Commentary on Hippocrates' Epidemics Book I, Parts I–III. Edition of the Arabic Version with English Translation and Notes*, Corpus Medicorum Graecorum Supplementum Orientale 5.1. Berlin.

Vagelpohl, U., ed. (2016). *Galen: Commentary on Hippocrates' Epidemics Book II, Parts I–VI. Edition of the Arabic Version with English Translation and Notes*, Corpus Medicorum Graecorum Supplementum Orientale 5.2, Berlin.

Vallance, J.T. (1990). *The Lost Theory of Asclepiades of Bithynia*, Oxford.

Vallance, J.T. (1993). 'The Medical System of Asclepiades of Bithynia'. *Aufstieg und Niedergang der römischen Welt* 37.1, 693–727.

Vallés, F. (1559). *Claudii Galeni Pergameni de Locis Patientibus Libri Sex, cum Scholiis Francisci Vallesii Couarruuiani, in Schola Complutensi professoris publici*, Lyon, 1559.

Vallés, F. (1561). *In Aphorismos, & libellum de Alimento Hippocratis, Commentaria. Cum privilegio regis ad decennium*, Alcalá de Henares.

Vallés, F. (1562). *Octo librorum Aristotelis de physica doctrina versio recens et commentaria. Ad Philippum Hispaniarum Regem. Cum privilegio ad decennium*, Alcalá de Henares.

Vallés, F. (1567a). *Commentaria in Prognosticum Hippocratis. Authore Francisco Vallesio Covarrubiano, doctore medico, primarioque: medicae facultatis in Complutensi academia professore*, Alcalá de Henares.

Vallés, F. (1567b). *Galeni Ars medicinalis, Commentariis Francisci Vallesii Cobarrubiani doctoris medici, et in Complutensi academia primarii medicae facultatis professoris illustrata, Commentariola in libellum Galeni de inaequali intemperie*, Alcalá de Henares.

Vallés, F. (1569a). *Commentaria in libros Hippocratis de Ratione victus in Morbis acutis. Authore Francisco Vallesio Covarrubiano, doctore medico, primarioque; medicae facultatis in Complutensi academia professore. Cum privilegio*, Alcalá de Henares.

Vallés, F. (1569b). *Commentaria in libros Galeni de differentia febrium. Authore Francisco Vallesio Covarrubiano, doctore medico, primarioque; medicae facultatis in Complutensi Academia professore. Cum privilegio*, Alcalá de Henares.

Vallés, F. (1577). *In libros Hippocratis de morbis popularibus, commentaria magnam utriusque medicinae, theoricae inquam et practicae, partem continentia. Ad Philippum secundum, Hispaniarum regem potentissimum. Cum privilegio*, Madrid.

Van Nuffelen, P. (2014). 'Galen, Divination and the Status of Medicine'. *Classical Quarterly* 64, 337–352.

Vassès, J. (1550). *Libri epidemiorum Hippocratis primus, tertius, et sextus cum Galeni in eos commentariis, Johanne Vassaeo interprete*, Lyon.

Vega-Loeches, J.L. (2009). 'Sobre la primera traducción al inglés de la *Descripción breve* de El Escorial de Francisco de los Santos. *Lately consumed by fire* (1671), del entorno del conde de Sandwich'. *Anales de Historia del Arte* 19, 181–194.

Vegetti, M. (1999). 'Tradition and Truth: Forms of Philosophical-Scientific Historiography in Galen's *De Placitis*'. In van der Eijk (ed.), 333–357.

Vegetti, M. and S. Gastaldi (eds.). *Studi di storia della medicina antica e medievale in memoria di Paola Manuli*, Pubblicazioni della Facoltà di lettere e filosofia dell' Università di Pavia, Dipartimento di scienze dell'antichità 79, Florence.

Von Staden, H. (1989). *Herophilus: The Art of Medicine in Early Alexandria. Edition, Translation and Essays*, Cambridge.

Von Staden, H. (2002). '"A woman does not become ambidextrous": Galen and the culture of the Scientific Commentary'. In Gibson and Shuttleworth Kraus, 109–139.

Von Staden, H. (2006). 'Interpreting "Hippokrates" in the 3rd and 2nd centuries BC'. In Carl W. Müller et al. (eds.), *Ärzte und ihre Interpreten*, Munich, 15–47.

Von Staden, H. (2007). '"The Oath", the Oaths, and the Hippocratic Corpus'. In V. Boudon-Millot, A. Guardasole, C. Magdelaine (eds.), *La science médicale antique. Nouveaux regards. Études réunies en l'honneur de Jacques Jouanna*, Paris, 424–466.

Von Staden, H. (2009). 'Staging the Past, Staging Oneself: Galen on Hellenistic Exegetical Traditions'. In Gill et al. (eds.), 132–156.

Walaeus, J. (1640). *Epistulae duae de motu chyli et sanguinis*, Leiden.

Wallies, M. (1905). *Ioannis Philoponi in Aristotelis analytica priora commentaria*, Commentaria in Aristotelem Graeca 13.2, Berlin.

Walzer, R. (1944). *Galen on Medical Experience: First Edition of the Arabic Version with English Translation and Notes*, Oxford.

Wasserstein, A. (1982). *Galen's Commentary on the Hippocratic Treatise 'Airs, Waters, Places' in the Hebrew Translation of Solomon ha-Me'ati*, Proceeding of the Israel Academy of Sciences and Humanities N3, Jerusalem.

Weisser, U. (1989), 'Das Corpus Hippocraticum in der arabischen Medizin'. In Baader and Winau (eds.), 377–408.

Wellmann, M. (1912). 'Zur Geschichte der Medicin im Altertum'. *Hermes*, 47, 1–17.

Wenkebach, E. (1936). *Galeni In Hippocratis Epidemiarum librum III commentaria III*, Corpus Medicorum Graecorum 5.10.2.1, Leipzig.

Wenkebach, E. (1951). *Galeni adversus Lycum et adversus Iulianum libelli*, Corpus Medirocum Graecorum 5.10.3, Berlin.

Wenkebach, E. (1956). *Galeni in Hippocratis Epidemiarum librum VI commentaria I–VIII*, Corpus Medirocum Graecorum 5.10.2.2, Berlin.

Wenkebach, E. and F. Pfaff (1934). *Galeni In Hippocratis Epidemiarum librum I commentaria III; In Hippocratis Epidemiarum librum II commentaria V*, Corpus Medicorum Graecorum 5.10.1, Berlin.

Westerink, L.G. (1956). *Olympiodorus: Commentary on the First Alcibiades of Plato*, Amsterdam.

Westerink, L.G. (1962). *Anonymous Prolegomena to Platonic Philosophy*, Amsterdam.

Westerink, L.G. (1964). 'Philosophy and Medicine in Late Antiquity'. *Janus* 51, 169–177.

Westerink, L.G. (1967). *Pseudo-Elias (Pseudo David), Lectures on Porphyry's Isagoge*, Amsterdam.

Westerink, L.G. (1970). *Olympiodori in Platonis Gorgiam commentaria*, Leipzig.

Westerink, L.G. (1985–1995). *Stephani Atheniensis in Hippocratis Aphorismos Commentaria*, Corpus Medicorum Graecorum 11.1.3.1–3, Berlin.

Wilkins, J. (2013). *Galien: Sur le Facultés des Aliments*, Paris.

Withington, E.T. (1928). *Hippocrates. On Wounds in the Head. In the Surgery. On Fractures. On Joints. Mochlicon*, Loeb Classical Library 149, Cambridge, MA.

Witt, M. (2012). 'Galen's zweifache Kommentierung zu chirurgischen Schriften des Corpus Hippocraticum: *Methodus medendi*, Bücher 3–6 und chirurgische Hippokrates-Kommentare'. *Les Études Classiques* 80, 73–126.

Witt, M. (2014). 'Die verlorenen Galen-Kommentare zu den hippokratischen Schriften De ulceribus und De vulneribus in capite—Fragmentsammlung und Erläuterungen'. *Rheinisches Museum für Philologie* 157, 37–74.

Witt, M. (2015). 'Der "Schlag des Schusters" (D. 19,2,13,4 u. D. 9,2,5,3) aus (rechts)medizinischer und philologischer Sicht—ein Beitrag zur Geschichte der Contrecoup-Fraktur'. *Zeitschrift der Savigny-Stiftung für Rechtsgeschichte* 132, 459–468.

Witt, M. (2018a). 'Surgery'. In Pormann (ed.), 217–245.

Witt, M. (2018b). 'Fabio Calvo—Übersetzer, Herausgeber und Fälscher hippokratischer Schriften'. *Sudhoffs Archiv* 102, 33–88.

Wittern, R., and P. Pellegrin, eds. (1996). *Hippokratische Medizin und antike Philosophie:*

Verhandlungen des VIII. Internationalen Hippokrates Kolloquiums in Kloster Banz / Staffelstein vom 23. bis 28. September 1993, Hildesheim.
Zervos, S. (1901). *Aetii sermo sextidecimus et ultimus*, Leipzig.
Zwinger, Th. (1579). *Hippocratis Coi ... viginti duo commentarii tabulis illustrati*, Basle.

Index Locorum

General Index

www.ingramcontent.com/pod-product-compliance
Lightning Source LLC
Chambersburg PA
CBHW071327230926
51849CB00002B/331
9789004470194